DISCOU

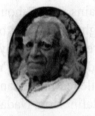

**"It is through your Body that you realize you are a Spark
of Divinity."**

—B.K.S. Iyengar

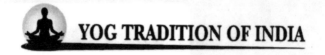

YOG TRADITION OF INDIA

Editorial Board:

Dr. S. F. Biria

Dr. Jitendra B. Shah

Mr. Prasant S. Iyengar

Yog is a pride possession of our great Indian tradition. It is a science, a faculty, a philosophy, a religion and a culture. The science of Yog contains entire thought of man. Yog knowledge can offer the highest goal and bliss of life. An anthology of the discourses were expounded by Prashant Iyengar for the students, scholars and sadhakas of Yog at different points of time. The readers, while learning Mantra Yog, Laya Yog, Hatha Yog, Raja Yog, Kundalini Yog, Nada Yog, Nama Yog as kinds of Jnana Yog, Karma Yog, Bhakti Yog and Dhyana Yog can get acquainted with many facets of Yog, They will learn that Yog is a way of Life. It is the sadhna of life. The engaging style of narration will appeal to the readers' brain and heart while they imbibe the knowledge of Yog, For easy comprehension, the words in the Sandhis are separated in the Sanskrit quotations. The books written by Prasant S. Iyengar selected to be published under the series are:

1. **Ashtanga Yoga of Patanjali:** *Philosophy, Religion, Culture, Ethos and Practices*
2. **Discourses on Yog**
3. **Manual on Humanics**
4. **Pranayama:** *A classical and traditional approach*

PRASHANT S. IYENGAR

DISCOURSES ON YOG

New Age Books

New Delhi (India)

DISCOURSES ON YOG

ISBN: 978-81-7822-481-7

First NAB Edition: Delhi, 2016

Published by
NEW AGE BOOKS
A-44 Naraina Industrial Area, Phase-I
New Delhi (India)-110 028
E-mail: nab@newagebooksindia.com
Website: www.newagebooksindia.com

NAB Cataloging-in-Publication Data
DISCOURSES ON YOG
ISBN 978-81-7822-481-7
(About the Series, Yog Foreword,
Contents, Glossary)

Printed and published by
RP Jain for NAB Printing Unit
A-44, Naraina Industrial Area
Phase-I, New Delhi-110 028. India

TRADITION OF YOG

There are many traditions in classical yog and there is great scope for research. But all classical yog find trace in what the Mahabharata mentions:

हिरण्यगर्भो योगस्त वक्ता नान्यः पुरातनः।

Mahabharata later clarifies that the Hiranyagarbha is Paramatma Sriman Narayana who is the Sarva-Antaryami and He is the first speaker of yog. Hiranyagarbha Yog has been maintained in bits and pieces in Pancharatra. Ahirbudhnya Samhita mentions that He gave discourses on chitta-vritti nirodha kind of yog which has Abhyasa-Vairagya and Ishvara-Pranidhana as means. The schemes of Ashtanga Yog too find a mention here. This is the basis of Patanjali's Yog. This main stream of yog received many contributions. Apart from the Pancharatra originated Vaishnava Agamas, the other major contributions were from Tantras, Shaiva agamas and Shakta Agamas. Many of the yogic concepts of Kriya, Mudra and Bandha were given by Shaiva-Shakta agamas and Tantras. The North Indian tradition of yog was greatly influenced by these. So much so that Lord Shiva became the source of yog for them. Hatha-yogic tradition has strong base in Shaiva cult of yog. The Natha-Sampradaya puts Adinath (Shiva) as origin of yog. We have great texts such as Hatha yog pradipika, Gheranda samhita, Shiva samhita and prolific works ascribed to Gorakhnath.

Dattatreya who advised yog to Sankruti must also be considered here. This piece of instruction is preserved for us in the Shandilya Upanishad. Gheranda rishi in his samhita has the yog where he puts Pratyahara before Pranayama while usually all traditions maintain the Pranayama to Prattyahara process. This is quite a significant revolution.

The Bhagwad Gita revived the Karma yog tradition which Bhagwan Himself says was instructed earlier (in Vaikuntha) to Vivasvan (Surya). The Gita mentions the main forms of yoga which are

- **Jnana Yog**

- **Dhyana Yog**

- **Karma Yog**

- **Bhakti Yog**

There is great significance when Vyasa calls Gita as Brahma vidya, Upanishad and Yog shastra in the colophone of each chapter. Each chapter is called as a kind of yog and thus eighteen chapters give us eighteen yogs.

The Yogopanishads posit that Ashtanga Yog is fount-hole of all various yogs. Then there are different yogs in different levels. The first level is Ashtanga Yog. The second level is Mantra Yog of sixteen limbs. The third yog is Laya yog of nine limbs and the fourth yog is Hatha Yog of six limbs. These are graduations and not cults or schools. Classical yog was maintained intact until about late 18th century. Then yog was slowly being compromised and was opened out to greater mass of people.

With the advent of 20th century, classical yog was greatly compromised and pop versions came up to appeal to a greater community and yog now remains to be a consumer product in our era.

Today, yog has only "feel-good" purpose for even those who claim to be students of yog. Another case to bow before time!

कालाय तस्मै नमः।

PRASHANT S. IYENGAR
Pune, July 2015

ॐ

योगेन चित्तस्य पदेन वाचाम्
मलं शरीरस्य च वैद्यकेन ।
योऽपाकरोत्तं प्रवरं मुनीनाम्
पतंजलिं प्रांजलिरानतोऽस्मि ।।

आबाहुपुरुषाकारं शंखचक्रासिधारिणम् ।
सहस्रशिरसं श्वेतं प्रणमामि पतंजलिम् ।।

सहस्रशीर्षाय विद्महे विष्णुतत्त्वाय धीमहि
तन्नो शेष: प्रचोदयात्

ॐ नमो ब्रह्मादिभ्यो
ब्रह्मविद्यासंप्रदायकर्तृभ्यो
वंशऋषिभ्यो नमो गुरुभ्य:

YOG FOREWORD

An anthology of the discourses given by Prashant Iyengar in Marathi in the Ramamani Iyengar Memorial Yog Institute, Pune for exploring some aspects of Yog was published in 2004. It gives us great pleasure to publish the First Volume of these discourses translated in English.

Yog is a science, a faculty, a philosophy, a religion and a culture. The discourses were given for the students, scholars and *sadhakas* of Yog. They are being published so that philomaths of Yog in and outside the Institute also should be benefitted.

Yog is a pride possession of our great Indian tradition. The project is designed to introduce it to the curious students. The science of Yog contains entire thought of man. The *sadhanaa* of Yog Vidya can offer the highest goal and bliss of life. The greatness of this science is expounded in the beginning of the book.

It is impossible to think about man without thinking about the natural phenomena around him as he is born out of it. This thought is extremely interesting, wonderful and engrossing. A human being does not exist only in visible physical body but has trinity of body-the triple body as gross, subtle, causal. This is spiritual knowledge. The discourses lucidly explain the three kinds of body, the five *koshas* and the six plexi.

Next comes Ashtanga yog in all its aspects. This Ashtanga Yog is the basis of all kinds of Yog such as Jnana Yog, Karma Yog, Bhakti Yog, Mantra Yog, Laya Yog, Hatha

Yog, Raja Yog, Kundalini Yog, Nada Yog, Nama Yog. This seminal thought is put forth with appropriate evidences. The basis of Yog sadhana is the trinity of yajna, dana or charity and tapa or penance. One chapter explains this path and culture of Yoga as it is not only relevant but very significant in the modern world.

The part of physiology is interesting, brain storming and important from the point of view of Yog sadhana. The science of Yog is brimful of psychology. Hence the discourses on Yog psychology have become unforgettable.

One amazing thought here is about the freedom of an individual. It is proved logically that this does not stand in opposition to self control but is in line with it. While describing Mantra Yog, Laya Yog, Hatha Yog, Raja Yog, Kundalini Yog, Nada Yog, Nama Yog as kinds of Jnana Yog, Karma Yog, Bhakti Yog and Dhyana Yog the readers can get acquainted with many facets of Yog. They will not fail to be aware that Yog is a way of life. It is the sadhana of life. The engaging sytle of narration will appeal to their brain and heart while they imbibe the knowledge of Yog.

The words in the Sandhis are separated in the Sanskrut quotations in order that all the readers should understand their meaning easily.

The Publishers 'Yog' are thankful to Dr. Adavi and Dr. Supriya Sahasrabuddhe who translated the discourses from Marathi into English and to Dr. Vijaya Deo for her help in proof reading.

We sincerely thank the students from England for sponsoring this publication.

To explain or summarize the profound sciences that deal with mysticism is the job of the sages. Any Tom or Dick can never be entitled to do that. And yet – Even though King Eagle cannot gauge the expanse of the sky, paltry insects also try to fly according to their mean capacity.

This effort is similar to that.

Prashant Iyengar

CONTENTS

Discourse 1

The Glory of Yog

योगात् परतरं पुण्यं योगात् परतरं शिवम् ।
योगात् परतरं सूक्ष्मं योगात् परतरं न हि ।।

The seer in the *Upanishad* is praising *Yog* here without any exaggeration or hyperbole. He is just stating a fact. The seer proclaims :

Nothing is greater than *Yog*;

Nothing is more sacred than *Yog*;

Nothing is finer than *Yog*;

The knowledge coming from *Yog* is absolutely limitless;

The knowledge coming from *Yog* is supreme;

Is not *Yog* truly magnificent ? Is not *Yog* truly magnanimous ?

Greatness of Yog

The *yogic* path shows the way for the upliftment of entire humanity, right from an ordinary individual to the godly and saintly men. So, all of them regard it with the highest reverence. Every step in the spiritual progress of man has importance of *yog*. The *Bhagavadgita* is taken to be a treasure trove of philosophy and a celestial song by Lord *Krishna* who is rightly called *Yogeshvara* and whose life story is an incarnation of *Yog* and philosophy. Every chapter of *Bhagavadgita* declares at the end that it is a part of *yog shastra*, universal philosophy of *yog*. Every chapter relates to a particular facet of *yog* which is clear from their ending lines. For example, the chapters have their titles, *Bhakti Yog, Karma Yog, Vibhuti Yog,* etc. Every piece of advice in the *Gita* is called a kind of *yog*. The spiritual aspirant can see the greatness of *yog* through the *Gita*, too.

The *Vedas* hold that the human body is the entire cosmos in micro or atomic form and it houses the Universal Spirit with all the divinities. The science of *yog* thinks of the world in the same way. It comprises of the different yogic paths-*yog* (union with reality), *viyog* (eradication of negative attributes), *prayog* (experimentation), *viniyog* (employment of positive inherent qualities) and *upayog* (utilization of supplementary virtues from outside). *Shama* (peace of mind), *dama* (self-restraint), *titiksha* (endurance), *uparati* (dispassion), *jnanavairagya* (knowledge and renunciation), and *shantisamadhana* (tranquillity and contentment) constitute the six aspects of spiritual wealth. The means and manner of attaining them and the fruits thereof are thoroughly spelt out in the science of *yog*. *Yog* is an experimental subject. So in *prayog* we have to experiment with the qualities like *brahmacharya, satya,* etc. In *Yog* practice also we have to do experiments in *asanas* with lab psychosis. Only then can we know and see the best or the most virtuous path.

Much of *yog* is based on *vi-yog* or expulsion or excising. We need to expel *tamasic* nature, *rajasic* nature, viciousness and ignorance. Strangely, *yog sadhana* is primarily *vi-yog sadhana*. Spiritual development is attained by following a certain prescribed course of action (*yog*). All these *Yogas* are attainable. On attaining these, man effects his own development towards the goal of fulfilment.

In like manner, the eradication of negative attributes (*viyog*) is also necessary. The ways of eliminating sorrows, lust and the necessity for their elimination are essential knowledge for human ripeness. We should get rid of genetic and allergic diseases (*Adhidaivika*), self-inflicted diseases (*Adhyatmika)* and diseases caused by the imbalance of elements in the body (*Adhibhoutika*).

2

We also have to overcome our endless desires, *shadripus* i.e. the six-fold enemies of lust (*kama*), anger (*krodha*), avarice (*lobha*), infatuation (*moha*), jealousy (*matsara*), and audacity (*mada*), and the five afflictions (*kleshas*) of ignorance (*avidya*), egotism (*asmita*), attachment (*raga*), hate (*dvesha*), clinging to existence (*abhinivesha*), arrogance and pride. The science of *yog* has analysed in a logical manner these various aspects, and has established sure means of eliminating the above negative attributes - thus proving to be of supreme value to the spiritual aspirants. In the same way, the word *prayog* is synonymous with the *kriyas* for the purification of the body (*kaya shuddhi*), mind (*manas shuddhi*), and intellect (*chitta shuddhi*). It has prescribed ways for the development of the physical body and the causal body, i.e. for the body, speech and mind. Similarly, *viniyog* is the process of employing the inherent qualities of virtue (*satva*), auspicious thoughts (*shubhavasana*), residue of the virtues of past birth (*purvasukruta*), and merit (*punya*) and divine attributes (*daiviguna* and *daivisampada*). How *upayog* comes into play is demonstrated by the manner in which we may utilize the rich spiritual heritage, the tradition of excellence of *Bharatavarsha,* and above all the good fortune of the association with saints, ascetics and *yogis -* all of which are obtainable in large measure and at all times. Thus the various *yog sadhanas* (of *yog, viyog, prayog, viniyog,* and *upayog*) are described in a logical and threadbare manner, in the science of *yog.*

The Human body

'शरीरम् आद्यम् खलु धर्मसाधनम्' – the body is the essential prerequisite for spiritual realization – is an established principle of *Dharma.* Even though the body is the source of various ailments and sorrows, it also is an instrument of acquiring merit, piety and

3

knowledge. The above saying of *Kalidas* gives the body a fundamental status and suggests a concept far beyond the idea of mere flesh and blood. The science of *yog* has classified different levels of the body into *sthula* (gross), *sukshma* (subtle), *karana* (causal), and *mahatkarana* (intelligence). Thus, viewed in this comprehensive sense, the corporeal body is the means of man's fulfilment. The science of *yog* is a study in entirety of all the aspects of human existence and it can show a path of fulfilment to every human being.

All the twenty-four principles (*tattvas*) of *Prakriti* (Nature) exist in this limited corporeal body. The entire Universe is manifested in it. Therefore, thought must be given to the relationship of the Universe and the individual soul. The Universe consists of the seven upper worlds (*Bhuhu, Bhuvaha, Svaha, Mahaha, Janaha, Tapaha* and *Satyam*). The seven subterranean regions are *Atala, Vitala, Sutala, Talatala, Mahatala, Rasatala* and *Patala*. The human body is composed of all the elements of the Cosmos. The nature and characteristics of the Universe and the human body in general requires careful attention. The individual is composed of the five gross elements of earth, water, fire, air and ether (space) and the subtle elements (*tanmatras*). One has to consider the nature and functions of all these aspects. The individual is composed of all these elements of *tattvas*. Thus, man is not merely an object of medical or anatomical sciences, but is to be considered as a part of the Cosmos. Anatomical science tells about the gross external body. Psychology tells about the external behaviour of man. Man is, however, not determined by only these characteristics since he possesses many more attributes, such as his subliminal impressions (*samskaras*) and the higher levels of the subtle sheaths of the body (*koshas*). Man has been existing

4

since the beginning of creation. These *samskaras* have been stored in the process of his metempsychosis. How much of it is dawned upon the modern science of psychology ? So some people are led to think that it is a pseudo-science.

Man's physical body has to be viewed in its entirety. It consists of the five elements of nature viz., earth, water, fire, air and ether; the five *tanmatras*; the seven constituent elements (*dhatus*) i.e., chyle, blood, flesh, fat, bone, marrow and semen. In addition there is the ego principle (*Ahamkara*), cosmic intelligence (*Mahat-tattva*) and finally the primordial Nature (*Mula-Prakriti*). All this is to be understood from the *Samkhya* philosophy of *Kapila* which is the very basis of the science of *yog*. Man has been existing since the beginning of creation. His corporeal body also contains all these elements (*tattvas*). In addition, man's body houses the soul. Thus the science of *yog* is a complete philosophical system (*Darshana*) which enables one to understand all the aspects of the nature of man. Other philosophies are inadequate, in that they indulge in mere hair-splitting arguments. However the science of *yog* embodies all the essential ingredients for a complete understanding of the human system. Medical science merely explains the causes of man's ill-health and the means of its eradication. Man's real nature is beyond the reach of medical science. Modern psychology is likewise inadequate for understanding the total man. It only tells us about his actions and behaviour, his sub-conscious and lower mind, etc.

The gross body consists of chyle, blood, flesh, fat, bone, marrow, and semen produced by the five gross elements, necessitating purificatory measures of the body, and elimination of sorrow and diseases. This gross body hovers between birth and death. It exists for one life-time only, but the *jiva* (individual soul) journeys through eighty-four lakh wombs along with the *sukshma sharira* (subtle body). This *sukshma sharira* is not subject to death even once. Its end comes only once at the time of final release on attaining *Mokhsa* or salvation. The *sukshma sharira*, like the gross body, also possesses the same characteristics of food, water, breath, movements and rest, and can be cast off like the gross body. Knowing this, an easy way is suggested for achieving this highest value in life. *Japa* or uttering of the Lord's name (*Nama-sadhana*), and meditation on his form are a powerful means, which aid in its attainment. The practice of *yog* in the development of the *sukshma sharira* enables it to prepare for a higher birth in this very life. The practice of *yog* can bring about transformation of the causal body within the gross body. The gross body possesses a subtle divinity.

The practice of *yog* can transform the external and internal behaviour of the individual by controlling the six mystical plexi of the body, *shatchakras,* the subtle energy channels of *nadis, panchpranas,* the three important nodes of *granthis-Vishnu, Shiva* and *Brahma granthis.* The science of *yog* shows the process of refining the seven constituent elements of the body (chyle, blood, etc.), the five elements (earth, water, etc), the five vital airs, the three *granthis,* the five sheaths of the body, the three humours of wind *(vata),* bile *(pitta)* and phelgm (*kapha*), the three *gunas* (*satva, rajas* and *tamas*), the five *upa-pranas* etc. Man's internal state has to change for this. Externally, man may have distinct characteristics, but internally there exist several disparate undercurrents. His apparent behaviour is mistaken for his character. Metaphysically, it is said "स्वभाव: अक्षर: उच्यते" – one's nature is unalterable. We assume man's apparent behaviour or temperament to be his true nature. Such and such a person is irritable, such and such a person is calm or is lazy, or active, or bold, or timid,

6

or pleasure-seeking, etc. All these are facets of apparent behaviour or temperament. However, there are times when, due to the ill-effects of the *shadripus*, there is a play of innumerable states of mental activity. We see different outward behavioural patterns e.g. of bold or timid, brutal or compassionate, happy-go-lucky, dallying or industrious and devout, irritable or tranquil. The irony of it is that quite often the irritable person gets angry with his own irritability, so also the man of a calm disposition is irritated with his tranquility. Man is a peculiar creature so that sometimes even a bold person is diffident of his own boldness, so also the timid person is even proud of his own cowardice! In short, quite often, man feels awkward regarding his own good points as also the wicked man feels proud of his wrong doings. If a person is determined to weep or grieve, he will do so in spite of his virtues or for the lack of them, and also possibly on account of his own wickedness. In short, any fanciful reason could be good enough for a person who is bent on weeping or grieving.

Human Mind

Mind is actually not bound by the mere physical limitations. Human body is formed of five sheaths. The *sukshma sharira* is beyond the gross body. Man's mind existed before his birth and will remain even after his death. Therefore, for a real understanding of man's nature there is no alternative to the science of *yog*. What is the essence of man's nature ? His corporeal body and the various organs have their origin in Nature (*Prakriti*). What is his cosmic or universal characteristic ? Man journeys through Nature's processes of creation and dissolution and a correct perception is necessary in this regard. It is not really correct to say that man comes into this world with birth and dies in death. He is actually constantly moving with the wheel of time and the cycle of creation. It would therefore be relevant to recognize the importance of Time. Time is both the cause and effect of everything in this world. Time consists of a succession of moments, as well as a collection of moments. Every moment is a constituent of the Reality of creation. Every happening is associated with time. "There is a time for everything" is practical everyday experience, which is both logical and scientific. Sequence of events is real. The different time periods ranging from the second to minute, hour, day, week, month, year, era, age, etc., all these are surprisingly only the products of imagination. Our idea of time is unreal, illusory and deceptive. While thinking about time, man has to say ultimately at one moment 'Kalaya tasmai namaha' and stop [O Time, we are nothing before you. We bow before you.]. Time is the product of Prakriti, which is erroneously supposed to be founded on reality - the absurdity of this idea sends the brain spinning. While studying the cosmos, it will be recognised that Ishvara is lodged in the minutest unit of time, creation, and soul. He is the Cause of the supreme attainment of the highest value of liberation or salvation or Moksha. Man can attain the highest on realising the Self, the highest bliss, which is not external but within himself, and in order to do this, he will have to obtain the knowledge of the Self. Yog is the surest means of attaining this Self-knowledge.

The point to be made here is that in order to transform a man's temperament and behaviour, knowledge of the six plexii is necessary. yogshastra demonstrates the technique for his transformation. For effecting the transformation, an investigation into the six-fold chakras is helpful. As a consequence of this effort, it is possible to evolve a fundamental transformation in man's panchaprana, panchatattva, vata, pitta, and kapha, or, tridosha.

If we say that the word manava or mankind is derived from the word *manas* or mind, the truth of the dominance and control of *manas* over mankind is easily understood. We are human beings, not merely on account of possessing our two hands, and our ability to stand on our two legs, but essentially because of our mind, which is far beyond logic, understanding and intellect. Mind, which is present in this corporeal body of six feet is profounder than the ocean, higher than Mount Everest and more expansive than the sky. This fact eludes our attention. The sun exhibits itself and at the same time illuminates the world, but on the other hand, the mind enlightens the entire Universe, but is hidden in the self. In order to discover this hidden mind and to secure direct Self-perception, there can be no alternative to *yogshastra*. Just as the sea is nothing but water, so also the mind is constituted of the subtle and the abstract. So also *yogshastra* is nothing but science of mind, consciousness and psyche. In all senses, *yog* is the science of mind, intellect and ego. Complete knowledge of the human mind is contained in *yogshastra*. The focal point of mind is "I". "I" also belongs to the first person in grammar. Thus, mind is firmly attached to this "I". To detach this "I" from the Self by tangible means is extremely difficult. *yogsadhana* does this task very easily. Just as we can remove a thorn from the foot, and minutely observe it, so also the spiritual aspirant can remove his "I", and observe and study it in the test-tube of the *yogic* laboratory. This can be called the science of 'witnessivity'.

Every moment, unfathomable, all the while bubbling with bizarre, strange, spasmodic and unpredictable activities - this is mind. Despite that, *yogshastra* encompasses this infinite mind. In reality, these mind *vrittis*, movements or thought waves are incapable of estimation. But *yogshastra* has analysed this problem logically, and it postulates that, even though the *vrittis* are infinite in number, they are either

9

afflicted or unafflicted, and can be classed into only five types. There can be no sixth type of *vritti.* Afflicted or defective *vrittis* cause man's downfall, and unafflicted or pure *vrittis* result in his upliftment. Thus, however complicated be the mind-activity, *vrittis* are strictly limited only to five types without a sixth one. It is emphasised that *yogshastra* has simplified the analysis in a marvellous manner, by classifying the *vrittis* into five groups only. *Yogshastra* has thus established a profound and clear principle by separating and classifying the different *vrittis*, by describing their cause and effect, and by defining their afflicted and unafflicted states. Mind, actually, is unfathomable. It is considered to be deeper than the ocean, high as the skies and infinitely expansive.

''असंशयं महाबाहो मन: दुर्निग्रहं चलम् ।'' This statement is made by Lord *Krishna* Himself. It is *shloka* 35 in Chapter 6 of the *Gita.* To win one's own mind is more difficult than winning a whole army of Napoleon or Alexander. The power to control the unrestrained mind is described in *yogshastra,* and it can be attained through *yogsadhana. Yogshastra* has evolved a discipline regarding the mind which cannot be found anywhere else. *Yogshastra* contains a scientific study of the total human body and the mind. Man is made up of several constituent elements, such as the organs of perception and of action and the mind; in addition, he has the physiological constituents, such as lungs, stomach, spleen, liver etc. There is, however, a subtle aspect regarding the above constituents of the human system which requires to be stressed and which is explained in *yogshastra.* All these constituents have five characteristic features according to this *shastra. Grahana,* the functional form of the sensation of organs; *svarupa,* the substantive form; *asmita,* the 'I'ness behind the senses and organs; *anvaya, sattva, raja, tama* constituents, *arthavatva*, purposiveness which has *bhogarthata* and *apavargarthata* are the five features. It may be observed that the eye is located in a hollow and does the job of seeing. It is able to see an object which is its function but that is not its true nature. The mere superficial action of a sweeper in doing the job of sweeping is definitely not his true nature. He has his own independent individual character. Thus each constituent of the human system has its unique functional aspect and though the differences in their functional aspects are cognizable, they are really directed by the man's "I" or ego. The organs and limbs are in reality the active constituents of the mind. They have their own "I" consciousness, which is the product of the three *gunas*. Finally, the experience of joy and sorrow and final emancipation is the aim and purpose, and this purposiveness is the basis of the above five forms - such is the extraordinary and established postulate of *yogshastra*. The *yog* practitioner has his own kind of experience and extraordinary predilection. For example, any organ such as the abdomen or liver acquires a different nature from its functional form, through the practice of *shavasana* and meditation. After the *vrittis* are restrained and one attains *samadhi*, all the senses and organs are absorbed in their pristine state.

Prana

Prana is inherent in the *vrittis* of attachment and detachment of a person. The source of man's existence and external manifestation is *prana*. It has the greatest contribution to man's character and individuality. It is the basis of all man's physical, mental, perceptive, emotional, and intellectual activities. The great significance of *prana* is borne out by the following shloka of the *Atharva Ved* :

"प्राणाय नमो यस्य सर्व इदं वशे ।

यो भूत: सर्वस्थ: ईश्वर: यस्मिन् सर्व प्रतिष्ठितम् ।"

'*Prana* is the Lord of the Universe. All is controlled by Him. All is contained in *prana* only."

The above *shloka* gives a fitting description of *prana*.

"प्राणो वा इदं सर्व प्राणो वा रुद्र:

प्राणो आदित्य: प्राणो वसव: प्राणो वै हरि: ।"

According to the above, *prana* is seen to be all-prevading. The *Prashnopanishad* declares that *prana* comprises of all that is included in the three worlds :

"प्राणस्य हि वशे सर्व त्रिदिवे यत् प्रतिष्ठितम् ।"

The following is a mantra from the *Yajurveda* which is worth noting :

"राजा मे प्राण: । प्राणो वै बलम् । प्राणो वै अमृतम् ।"

And in the *Chhandogya* and *Bruhadaranyaka Upanishads* we have :

"यो ह वै ज्येष्ठं श्रेष्ठं च वेद ज्येष्ठश्च श्रेष्ठश्च ह वै भवति ।

प्राणो वा ज्येष्ठश्च श्रेष्ठश्च ।"

Such is the glory and supremacy of *prana*. *Yogshastra* gives us the sacred knowledge of *prana*. All of man's internal and external activity takes palce through *panchaprana*, due to *panchaprana*, and for *panchaprana*. *Panchaprana* exists in man's physical, mental, intellectual and emotional states. *Yog* has the means of controlling this *panchaprana*. *Yogshastra* is the very science of *prana*. An ancient commentary on the *Samkhyakarika, contained in the Yuktidipika,* makes the following observations :

The internal action of *prana* is Breathing. Its external action is self-confident action.

The internal action of *apana* is Excretion and Reproduction. Its external action is successful retreat.

The internal action of *samana* is Digestion of food intake. Its external action is co-operation, co-ordination.

The internal action of *vyana* is Nerve conduction all over the body. Its external action is pride or arrogance such as brandishing a dagger, the threatening action of taking out a sword from its sheath.

The internal action of *udana* is Conducting arterial pulsation of the temporal and brain region. Its external action is living together, piety, generosity, samaritanism.

Prana plays an important role in the understanding of the corporeal body, the mind and the moulding of intellectual excellence. In the practice of *yog*, *prana* is not only the prime mover but it is all-in-all. Man's internal and external transformation takes place through *prana*, i.e. only through the pranic technique of *yogsadhana*. *Yog* has the capability of fully controlling the *panchapranas* and the *pancha upapranas*. It is by controlling *prana* that a *yogi* can control the three worlds. The entire process in *Ashtanga Yog* right from the first *yama* or ethical discipline of *ahimsa*, non-violence is controlled by *prana*. The *ashtamahasiddhis*, the eight major yogic powers of a *yogi* are generated through *prana*. *Yog shastra* thoroughly expounds the pranic principle with all its ramifications. The entire sacred knowledge of *prana* is contained in *yogshastra*.

'I' consciousness

Firstly, it is interesting to note that when we are immersed in thinking, all the organs including the abdomen, liver, etc., are in a

13

subtle state. When we experience sorrow, they, too, are listless. In *shavasana* and meditation the organs and senses remain in their pristine state. Secondly, just as we have "I-ness" and "mine-ness', the senses and organs too have their "I-ness" and "mine-ness". In accordance with the *samkhya* philosophy all the senses and organs come from the "I" consciousness. For this reason the senses and organs possess the nature of the ego or self-identity. There is a third feature possessed by these very organs. Every creature in the Universe is the product of the three *gunas* of *sattva, rajas* and *tamas*. The fourth feature is the relationship of the organs with the *gunas*. Further, according to teleology, there are only two purposes for the existence of the senses and organs. These senses and organs exist in order to experience joy, sorrow and infatuation i.e. *bhoga* and emancipation i.e. *apavarga* or *moksha*. Thus, the fifth and final characteristic feature of the organs and senses is that of experiencing joy and sorrow or final liberation. In this way, all the faculties and organs of the body will be found to consist of the five characteristic features of *grahana,* etc. and they are described in the *Patanjali's yogsutras* in a succinct, illuminating and meaningful manner.

In the so-called intellectually oriented modern society, individual freedom is given an exaggerated importance. In ordinary parlance individual freedom is intended to mean unfettered action. In this context the nature of "I" and "mine" have to be recognized clearly and without self-deception. What we ordinarily understand by "I" is faulty, and perhaps dangerous and fraught with misery. For achieving perfect freedom, selflessness and self-determination are necessary. *Yog* is the sure way for its achievement. This is a matter to be considered with seriousness by the sociologists, psychologists and humanitarians. The discernment of the "I" principle or "I"-ness has

14

been delineated in all its ramifications in *yogshastra*. The entire philosophy of *yog* centers round this "I"-principle. Everyone has the sense of 'I' which is totally deceptive and misconceived. The *yog sadhana* helps the practitioner to identify the 'I' in its pristine form. The intuitive perception of "I" results from the application of the "I"-consciousness. It is the *yogis*, the ascetics and the saints, who possess this perception, who can really tell us the nature of this "I". Only they can explain the real nature of individual freedom and its niceties. Today, however, the self-willed individuals profess to know everything about individual freedom. Not only is this very dangerous but also utterly regrettable and ruinous. The total point of view of "I" is explained in *yogshastra* and direct perception of the Self is attained through *yogsadhana*.

Yog Shastra

Man's miseries are boundless, and there are innumerable reasons for his sorrows. *Yogshastra* demonstrates to us a very profound and logical analysis of man's unhappy state. In addition it also shows the way and manner of attaining emancipation.

Sorrows are of three kinds. *Adhibhautika* are externally radiated. e.g. dog bite, snake bite, bacterial infection. Their causes may lie in climatic conditions. These are inclemencies caused by factors outside us. *Adhidaivika* are celestially radiated sorrows such as caused by fate, malefic planetary conditions as appear in horoscopes. For *Adhyatmika* freedom the individual will have to be free from the six enemies. It is pertinent to recall, here, the definition of *yog* given in the *Bhagavadgita* :

"तं विद्यात् दुःखसंयोगवियोगं योगसंज्ञितम् ।" This definition in *shloka* 23 of the *Gita* is given in the sixth *adhyaya*. The prime reason for this misery in life is a mistaken sense of duty and determination

15

of action, error of judgement, carelessness or wrong conduct. Understanding of both *Dharma* and *karma* is genuinely necessary for counteracting human misery. Ignorance of *Dharma* and *karma*, is responsible in large measure for man's miseries. *Yogshastra* deals with the study of *Dharma* and *karma* in detail. *Yogshastra provides the panacea, which is achieved through the practice of yog and yogic* discipline.

Yogshastra has made a study of *Dharma* and *karma*, and also of the mind. Practice of *Dharma* is of central importance and is the *sine qua non* of spirituality. *Yog* shows the proper path of *Dharma* and *karma*, and transports man to the highest upliftment and effortlessly takes him to his spiritual fulfilment. The two most important factors in *yog*, which lead man to his development are knowledge of *Dharma* and *karma*. These two factors enable the spiritual aspirant to acquire the desirable, and to discard the undesirable. Eventually, *Yog* takes man even beyond these two opposites. Such is the glory of the art and science of *yog*. This *yogdharma* enables man to achieve the highest excellence in life, both temporal and spiritual.

'आचारप्रभव: धर्म:',

यत: अभ्युदयनि:श्रेय: संसिद्धि: स: धर्म: ।

'धर्मस्य प्रभु: अच्युत:'

यत्र योगेश्वर: कृष्ण: यत्र पार्थ: धनुर्धर: ।

तत्र श्री: विजयो भूति: ध्रुवा नीति: मति: मम ॥

'यत: धर्म: तत: जय:'

'धर्म: रक्षति रक्षित: ।

The above *shlokas* regarding *Dharma* are noteworthy in the above context.

16

Yogshastra comprises a thorough study of man's temporal and spiritual life. The nature of the corporeal body, the mind, *praana,* intellect, *Dharma* and *karma*, spiritual culture, *sadhana*, worship or *upasana*, have been discussed in it. How the average man should lead his life, and how those who have realized the supreme value of life should shed their mortal coil in death so that they may not be bound to die again, is effectively conveyed by this *shastra*. We will consider further, the various aspects of *yog, jnana, shastra, Dharma, Kala*, and *samskriti*.

We will also consider the highest *Dharma, abhyudaya*, the road to success, the supremely pure, subtle, and auspicious facets of *yogshastra* as far as possible and to the best of our knowledge through this garland of *yog.* The art, science, philosophy and religion of *yog* teach commoners how to live a fruitful life. Right from the moment of awareness of life, man has been facing the string of *yaksha prashna*-What is the purpose of life? Where is the beginning and where is the end? What is my destined role in this drama of life? The questions are endless. The sign of question mark [?] has a full stop in itself. We can certainly turn to *yogshastra* to try to get the answers. It has the unique power to make us turn inwardly for these efforts. In this sense it is a complete science. We will be now dealing with this divulgence of *yogshastra* to the best of our abilities. This is the first flower of the garland.......

Shri Krishnaarpanam astu

✢ ✢ ✢

Discourse 2

Knowledge of the Universe and Nature

Man and Universe

Man is a part of the Universe. Man lives in nature and the universal principle exists in man. Naturally, in order to make a thorough and complete enquiry in the nature of mortal man one has to analyze the character of the Universe, along with that of the origin and material causes of Nature. Man is a constituent part of Nature, but modern science is so preoccupied with the material and apparent aspects of nature, in order to make happy his material life, that it has ignored this fact. Unless the origin of man's existence is known, it will not be possible to know man's original nature. Man is born through the process of creation of the Universe. The universe is born out of the manifest and the unmanifest, the gross and the subtle, the temporal and the spiritual. *Prakriti,* which is the cause of the universe, is also a responsible factor of the creation of man. Thus the time and manner of creation of the universe should be a matter for exploration.

One way of realizing man is to try to know the twenty-four *tattvas* of *Prakriti.* To begin with, Man is created through the cosmic process of *Prakriti,* hence it is necessary to have knowledge of the process. We know that cosmology today is the science of the origin and structure of the Universe, especially as studied in astronomy. Ontology is a subject of study in philosophy concerned with the nature of existence. Teleology studies the purpose of the phenomenon of existence. *Yogshastra* has all these sciences in its ken. Its cosmology divides the universe into three tiers—Terrestrial world, Extra-terrestrial or celestial world and Infernal world. The principles of these worlds are of three kinds, Matter, Infra-matter and supra-matter. The metaphysists of *yog, Patanjali* and the *samkhya* philosophers, hold

18

that the universe has only two fundamental principles, abstract *Purusha* and concrete *Prakriti*. This is the starting point of *yog* ontology. *Yog* teleology strongly believes that the cosmos is not chaos and it does have a purpose. The dual purpose is *bhoga* and *apavarga*. This is just an introduction of the vast studies of *yogshastra*.

It is essential to think of man as a part of the Universe and Nature for a comprehensive study of him. Thus, without consideration of the Universe, Nature and the world in which he lives, it is not possible to understand Man. Man is formed through the creative process of the cosmos. Man is shaped by the same process as the Universe, which is constituted of the manifest and the unmanifest, the sentient and the insentient, the gross and the subtle, the temporal and the spiritual elements. The how and why of the creation of man as well as that of the Universe are interlinked. It is only logical that it is so. The *samkhya* philosophy has postulated twenty-four *tattvas.* It is pertinent to consider these *tattvas* or evolutes. The reality of man's nature is to be understood through the study of metaphysics. The knowledge of cosmology, ontology and teleology concerning man can be acquired by a study of *yog* philosophy.

The nature of *Prakriti* is made up of the three *gunas.* Firstly it affects the physical inanimate objects of the Universe and secondly it influences the animate senses and the organs of living organisms. *Samkhya* and *yog* contain the knowledge of these influences. The soul which consists of the eternal, infinite and *non-Prakritic* consciousness pervades the sphere of *Prakriti.* The soul is *non-Prakritic* and contrary to *Prakriti* and undisturbed by it; therefore, man cannot be considered as a mere mass of flesh. In this context a metaphysical approach to the concept of soul becomes necessary and is as much indispensable as it is invaluable. The structure of the Universe is due to the twenty-four *tattvas* of *Prakriti.* All these *tattvas* and the entire infinite Universe are contained in the human body of finite size; this is indeed an amazing and awesome phenomenon! It is therefore logical to consider this universal aspect of the individual-his *gross-sukshma sharira*.

According to the *puranas*, there are seven regions of the upper world viz., *Bhu, Bhuva, Sva, Maha, Jana, Tapa* and *Satya* and the seven regions of the nether world are *Atala, Vitala, Sutala, Talaatala, Mahatala, Rasatala* and *Patala*. All these fourteen regions are ensconced in the human body. So the knowledge of man has to comprise also of the knowledge of the existence of the three worlds-the lower world, the earth and the upper world. A complete knowledge of man is not merely that of the parts of his body like his skin, skeleton, bone, fat, marrow and even of his mind. *Prakriti* consists of five primary elements of earth, water, fire, air and ether. These elements are the constituents of the physical body. Their nature, function and purpose have to be considered while studying the human system. Their atomic nature is represented by the *tanmatras*. These primary and subtle elements are the evolutes of *ahamkara* or the cosmic principle of ego. This ego is not merely the mind ego. The ego principle or *tattva* is the source of the *tanmatras*. The *ahamkara tattva* is evolved from the *Mahattattva* which is the great principle-the intelligence, as distinct from *manas*. *Yogshastra* has investigated the fundamental nature of these subtle principles with regard to the individual human being. Indian *rishis* felt the significance of such a study. The individual soul inevitably traverses between creation and dissolution. It is a matter of obvious knowledge that man has to move along with the cycle of time, the nature of which has to be understood. Birth and death, days, nights and weeks, centuries and ages, creation and dissolution, cycles of nature are the inevitable consequence of Time. Time is the sum total of moments. Moments are realistic in every sense of the term but the constituted time spans of seconds, minutes, hours, days, months, centuries etc are not realistic. This fact is mind boggling. A moment which is a measure of time is a product of Nature, and according to metaphysics, the time-cycles of hours, weeks, months, years, centuries, ages, even the *manvantaras* and the *mahakalpas* are all metapsychological illusions. How far is the concept of time real or unreal? This is truly a challenge to the brain. It is something more than blind faith or idealistic postulate. *Ishvara* is the Inner Controller within the individual. He is both the means as well as the end. He is the sole means of Supreme Peace. Thus *yogshastra* opens the way for achieving the Supreme Goal. The more the intellectual pursuit is deliberated the more confounding it is. It can only split the brain while affinity to *Ishvara* who is the internal ruler and *Antaryami* pacifies the mind.

The three Gunas

Yogshastra tells us that Nature is the product of three *gunas*, and the evolutes viz. the senses and the organs. The Eternal Soul is ever-present in the vast expanse of Nature. We have to recognize this metaphysical principle. In this infinity of the expanse of Nature it is imperative to realize that this Soul is unaffected by *Prakriti* and exists within the consciousness of the Universe but, surprisingly, is untouched by it.

In our tradition of *samkhya* and metaphysics, *Prakriti* is constituted of the three *gunas* of *sattva, rajas* and *tamas.* We should understand the *sattvic, rajasic* and *tamasic* nature of man. It will then be possible to obtain a proper management of the *gunas.* The *satva* content has to be increased and the *rajasic* and *tamasic* content considerably reduced. The association with the saintly and the virtuous can bring about the aforesaid *satvic* management of these *gunas.* These *gunas*

21

are present in the corporeal body, mind and intellect. Knowledge of this fact is important for the spiritual aspirant. The manifestation of these three *gunas* can be better understood with the help of a table of the three *gunas*.

Sattvaguna	Rajoguna	Tamoguna
equity, equanimity	activity	obstructing
luminosity	actionism	obscuring
lightness	workaholism	heaviness
purity		lethargy
piety, sublimity	motivation	languor
nobility	multifaceted personality	timidity
faith in god	versatility	ignorance
reverence for parents, elders and noble ones	turbulence	sloth
belief in life after death	kinetic	inactivity
virtuosity, wisdom	hardworking	pessimistic
gratitude, courtesy, memory	persistent	giving sorrows
tolerance, forbearance	self-respect	taking sorrows
thirst, constancy	pronounced	vice
for knowledge	self-esteem	wickedness
all noble qualities	incompassionate	atheism
among human beings	ostentatious	brutality
	envious	
	jealous	
	aspirations	
	valour	
	strength	
	prowess	
	sensuality	
	impulsive in delights and sorrows	

22

The *sattva guna* which is the first column of the table is clear and lucid. This *guna* is extremely subtle i.e. it is totally opposite to the gross. A *sattvic* man pays attention to the purification of his mind and is averse to impiety. He is devout and respectful to his elders. He has faith in God and *Dharma*. He can discriminate between good and evil, he believes in transmigration, *Karma* and its *phala* or fruit. He finds happiness in the path of virtue. He possesses gratitude, has thirst for knowledge and is honest, forbearing and sincere by nature. He has radiant *medha, buddhi* and a sense of equanimity. His memory harbours only the auspicious and not the evil thoughts. He has filtration of memories. The thoughts about other people's sins or malice, injustice imposed by others, thoughts of revenge, etc. are things to be forgotten. These go into oblivion without much delay. On the other hand, goodness in other people, our duty towards them, etc. are to be remembered and retained in the mind. Retentivity, intelligence, and balance are obvious signs of his *vrittis*. The *rajoguna,* is the originator of action. It is multifaceted. About *rajas* the *Gita* says: 'रजस:तु फलं दु:खम् ।' A *rajoguni* person experiences multitude of sorrows. Such a person displays vigour, is self-opinionated and easily gets ruffled. He can be heartless, hypocritical and covetous, but he also possesses brave nature. He is avaricious and greedy and has the habit of inordinately magnifying his joys and sorrows.

Tamoguna produces darkness, heaviness, sluggishness, fear, ignorance, excessive sleep, laziness, inaction, grief, intoxication, sorrow, unrighteousness, atheistic nature, inhuman cruelty - all these attributes are motivated by *tamas,*

Vrittis in the mind of man are a result of these three *gunas.* The *gunas* are the subtlest evolutes of *Prakriti,* the gross and the subtle, the sentient and the non-sentient- all these elements of the Universe

23

are affected by the activity of the three *gunas*. *So* also, the seven upper regions of the higher world, and the seven subterranean regions of the lower world are made up of the three *gunas*. There is predominance of *rajoguna* on this earth. *Satyaloka* or the upper world is predominantly comprised of *sattva* and in the nether world the main element is *tamas*. These *gunas* are present in relative proportions in all the manifestations of the Universe. Among the plants, the basil *(tulasi)* plant is pre-eminently *sattvic*. Saints, kind-hearted people and animals like the cow obviously possess a greater proportion of *satva*. The wealthy, the powerful, the warring class are endowed with more of *rajas*. The tea and coffee plants which yield stimulating drinks have *rajoguna*. Feral beasts, cobras, pythons, kites, bats, etc., opium, tobacco, licentious and pleasure seeking people - all these are manifestations of intensity of *tamoguna,*

Modern science tells us that the Universe is comprised of three types of sub-atomic particles. Nuclear physics states that at the nucleus of the atom is the neutron, and the protons and electrons revolve round the nucleus. This is the limit of the knowledge of physical science. The ancient science of creation goes beyond this limitation. The mind, intellect and ego are subtler than the subatomic particles. *Sattva, rajas* and *tamas* are *prakritic gunas* i.e. born out of nature, and are more subtle than the protons, electrons and neutrons. The united action of the varying proportions of these *gunas* is the cause of this amazing diversity in the Universe. Even the different elements of the lower world are a product of the relative levels of the three *gunas.*

According to the *samkhya* philosophy, substances become different according to different proportions of *sattva, raja and tama*. For example, water has different names and forms depending on the context of its contents of the *gunas* and of its use. e.g. *Ganga* water is *satvic,* whereas drainage water possesses excess of *tamoguna.* The *sattvic* quality of water depends on our spirit of consecration. If the ordinary water of a municipal tap undergoes treatment of divine spell, it could be *tirtha* or sacred. Its inherent quality can be transformed by one's mental approach, the nature of its use and the purpose for which it is used. Water can be sprinkled on an individual either for bestowing a boon or for giving curses. Objectively, however, water is the compound H_2O, according to the science of chemistry. However a subjective attitude towards this compound of hydrogen and oxygen imparts to it a quality of subtle difference. The quality changes, depending upon this subjective attitude. *Samkhyashastra,* therefore, gives us a supramaterial concept of water which is beyond the ambit of physical science. The *satva* and *rajas* content in the five physical elements depend upon the degree of consecration, distinctiveness and purpose. For example, the sacrificial fire burns in the *yajna,* and fire also burns in the cremation ground. Objectively, both the fires are identical but in accordance with the order of the *gunas* these two fires become different in nature. This concept of difference does not fit within the logic of physical science. The science which can transcend the physical, alone, can give an explanation for this. The physical science has its own limitations. The supraphysical science or the divine knowledge offers an invaluable elucidation. It offers explanation for the subtle difference between the fires in the above two examples. The aim, observance, solemnity and performance of rituals with the fire of the same intensity, all these create differences in the content of the *gunas* of the fire. These concepts are the gifts of the profound wisdom of our seers.

The effect of the *gunas* can also be seen on money. The worth of a hundred rupee note is the same in any field of business, yet every hundred-rupee note differs in its outcome. The inherent *guna* of the note depends upon whether it is obtained by stealing, by killing someone, by fraudulent means or whether it is hard-earned money. In practical life we say "the money has not proved to be beneficial", which means that we are deprived of its real value to us. However, money which is honestly earned grants us hundred-fold benefits. Its personal value or subjective value is qualitatively different from its business or objective value. This substantial difference in value is based on the effect of the *gunas* and is entirely dependent on their qualitative content.

The Universe is composed of the three *gunas* by God's *Maya* or will. Though the nature of the Universe seems to be physical, there is a divine quality present in each of the *pancha mahabhutas*. The divinity of the *prithvi tattva* or earth is *prithvi devata*. *Ap(water)* and *téj* (fire) have *Varuna* and *Agni* respectively as their deities. The deity of *Vayu* is *Vayudevata* and *Akash* or ether has the eight regents of the cardinal points of the Universe, *Digdévatas*. The entire Universe is divine in nature. It is the abode of the Divine. There is a consciousness even in inanimate objects like mud, stone, gold, silver as well as in birds and animals, insects and ants, and human beings. This consciousness is none other than Divinity. For this reason it has been said दैवी हि एषा etc. The prayer to *Devi* in the *Saptashati* says :

या देवी सर्व भूतेषु शक्तिरूपेण संस्थिता ।
नमस्तस्यै नमस्तस्यै नमस्तस्यै नमो नमः ॥

The *Bhagavadgita* gives several examples with regard to these *gunas* of *sattva*, *rajas* and *tamas*. Food, sport, thoughts, sacrificial rites, energy, austerity, enjoyment, invocation, charities, knowledge, activity, endurance, devoutness, ego, capabilities, bravery, vivacity, etc. are imbued with the three *gunas.* This principle is analyzed in the seventeenth and eighteenth chapters of the *Gita,* and is of invaluable importance in spiritual *sadhana.* Our seers have always seen gross matter, outward activity and external manifestation in the context of their *gunas.* Such an approach taught to us by their wisdom and sagacity is unique to our culture. In chemistry, the chemical elements are denoted by symbols like H, O etc. The chemical formula for water is H_2O i.e. two atoms of hydrogen combine with one atom of oxygen to form water. This fact is known to a student of modern science. In our *samkhya* philosophy, amusingly, H and O are also provided with S R T content i.e. *sattva, rajas* and *tamas.* Water used for worship and religious ceremonies, according to the above S R T principle will be constituted of H_2O + S=800, R=5 and T=l. If it is drainage water, then to H and O must be added S =10, R = 5 and T = 100, i.e. the *tamasic* content is increased hundred-fold. The *satva* content of *Ganga* water is the highest. If we compare the contents of this water with those of the river Thames in England, we conclude that the Thames is *tamasic. Tamasa* or Thames is *tamasi.* Laboratory tests have confirmed that bacteria when released in the *Ganga* are destroyed, while in the Thames bacteria increase when released in it. Then again, there is a sea of difference in the diamond of the ear-ring of the wife of a wine-shop owner and the diamond of the alligator-shaped ear-ring of *Vitthala* of *Pandharpur.* The materialist scientist will not be able to discriminate between the two. The spiritual intuition of the *rishis* alone can see and reveal this difference. This concept of difference is at the basis in the science of *yog.* While explaining the principles of the *samkhya* system, sage *Patanjali* declares that the living beings in the Universe are predominantly *rajasic* and *sattvic,* whereas the insentient objects that are incapable of feeling are predominantly *rajasic* and *tamasic*. This enables us to understand the metaphysics of the three worlds. The Universe consisting of the three worlds is a three-fold manifestation of the material of gunas. It is celestially constituted and has a spiritual substrate. The celestial world has preponderance of *sattva*, while the terrestrial has *rajas* and the infernal has *tamas*. According to the *Vedantic* precept, the Universe is illusory. Thus the *Gita* says; दैवी हि एषा गुणमयी मम माया दुरत्यया I (7 : 14)

Shakti – Universal consciousness

The Universe is a manifestation of *Shakti* or the Universal consciousness. Each and every substance has a divine consciousness. The *Shakti* of one substance is unlike that of the others. The mind well-versed in *vedic* lore easily understands the purport behind the above-quoted hymn. The *vaidic* person achieves life's fulfilment by experiencing the divine grace of *Shakti* with a spirit of humility. The *Rudra,* a holy text, has two sections known as *chamaka* and *namaka*. Of these two sections, *chamaka* manifests the profound sense of gratitude of the *vaidic.* We should listen to it attentively and contemplate upon it seriously. The universal consciousness is also inherent in food, water, flowers, fruits, etc. All these objects are utilized by the *vaidic* in a spirit of humility for a *sattvic* purpose. He knows that the divine influence is present in the senses and organs. According to the *vaidic* person, God's creation and Nature are meticulously planned by Him to cater to all the human needs and we have to be grateful for this. For example, the expecting mother prepares in advance woolen apparel for the baby. Saint *Tukaram* has lucidly described in his abhang that Nature makes provision of milk in the mother for the baby in advance. In modern times, we come across the term "eco-system". This notion is already deeply embedded in our ancient system. It is inherently eco-friendly. The contents of the *chamak* section of the *Rudra* are ennobling in this regard. The *vaidic* says:

Rudra hymn

वाजश्च मे । प्रसवश्च मे प्रयतिश्च मे प्रसितिश्च मे धीतिश्च मे क्रतुश्च मे स्वरश्च मे श्लोकश्च मे श्रावश्च मे श्रुतिश्च मे ज्योतिश्च मे सुवश्च मे प्राणश्च मेऽपानश्च मे व्यानश्च मेऽसुश्च मे चित्तं च मे आधीतं च मे वाक् च मे मनश्च मे चक्षुश्च मे श्रोत्रं च मे दक्षश्च मे बलं च मे ओजश्च मे सहश्च मे आयुश्च मे जरा च मे आत्मा च मे तनूश्च मे शर्म च मे वर्म च मे अङ्गानि च मे अस्थानि च मे परूषि च मे शरीराणि च मे ।

ज्यैष्ठ्यं च मे आधिपत्यं च मे मन्युश्च मे भामश्च मे अमश्च मे अंभश्च मे जेमा च मे महिमा च मे वरिमा च मे प्रथिमा च मे वर्ष्मा च मे द्राघुया च मे वृद्धं च मे वृद्धिश्च मे सत्यं च मे श्रद्धा च मे जगच्च मे धनं च मे वशश्च मे त्विषिश्च मे क्रीडा च मे मोदश्च मे जातं च मे जनिष्यमाणं च मे सूक्तं च मे सुकृतं च मे वित्तं च मे वेद्यं च मे भूतं च मे भविष्यश्च मे सुगं च मे सुपथं च मे ऋद्धं च मे ऋद्धिश्च मे क्लृप्तं च मे क्लृप्तिश्च मे मतिश्च मे सुमतिश्च मे ।

शं च मे मयश्च मे प्रियं च मे अनुकामश्च मे कामश्च मे सौमनसश्च मे भद्रं च मे श्रेयश्च मे वस्यश्च मे यशश्च मे भगश्च मे द्रविणं च मे यन्ता च मे धर्ता च मे क्षेमश्च मे धृतिश्च मे विश्वं च मे महश्च मे संविच्च मे ज्ञात्रं च मे सूश्च मे प्रसूश्च मे सीरं च मे लयश्च मे ऋतं च मे अमृतं च मे यक्ष्मं च मे अनामयत् च मे जीवातुश्च मे दीर्घायुत्वं च मे अनमित्रं च मे अभयं च मे सुगं च मे शयनं च मे सूषा च मे सुदिनं च मे ।

ऊर्क् च मे मे सूनृता च मे पयश्च मे रसश्च मे घृतं च मे मधु च मे सग्धिश्च मे सपीतिश्च मे कृषिश्च मे वृष्टिश्च मे जैत्रं च मे औद्भिद्यं च मे रयिश्च मे रायश्च मे पुष्टं च मे पुष्टिश्च मे विभु च मे प्रभु च मे बहु च मे भूयश्च मे पूर्ण: च मे पूर्णतरं च मे अक्षितिश्च मे कूयवाश्च मे अन्नं च मे अक्षुच्च मे व्रीहयश्च मे यवाश्च मे माषाश्च मे तिलाश्च मे मुद्गाश्च मे खल्वाश्च मे गोधूमाश्च मे मसुराश्च मे प्रियंगवश्च मे अणवश्च मे श्यामकाश्च मे नीवाराश्च मे ।

अश्मा च मे मृत्तिका च मे गिरयश्च मे पर्वताश्च मे सिकताश्च मे वनस्पतयश्च मे हिरण्यं च मे अयश्च मे सीसं च मे त्रपुश्च मे श्यामं च मे लोहं च मे अग्निश्च मे आपश्च मे वीरूधश्च मे ओषधयश्च मे कृष्टपच्यं च मे अकृष्टपच्यं च मे ग्रामाश्च मे पशव: अरण्याश्च मे यज्ञेन कल्पन्ताम् वित्तं च मे वित्तिश्च मे भूतं च मे भूतिश्च मे वसु च मे वसतिश्च मे कर्म च मे शक्तिश्च मे अर्थश्च मे एमश्च मे इतिश्च मे गतिश्च मे ।

अग्निश्च मे इन्द्रश्च मे सोमश्च मे सविता च मे सरस्वती च मे पूषा च मे बृहस्पतिश्च मे मित्रश्च मे वरुणश्च मे त्वष्टा च मे धाता च मे विष्णुश्च मे अश्विनौ च मे मरुतश्च मे विश्वे च मे देवा पृथिवी च मे अंतरिक्षं च मे द्यौश्च मे दिशश्च मे मूर्धा च मे प्रजापतिश्च मे ।

अंशुश्च मे रश्मिश्च मे अदाभ्यश्च मे अधिपतिश्च मे उपांशुश्च मे अन्तर्यामश्च मे ऐन्द्रवायवश्च मे मैत्रावरुणश्च मे आश्विनश्च मे प्रतिप्रस्थानश्च मे शुक्रश्च मे मन्थी च मे आग्रयणश्च मे वैश्वदेवश्च मे ध्रुवश्च मे वैश्वानरश्च मे ऋतुग्रहाश्च मे अतिग्राह्याश्च मे ऐन्द्राग्रश्च मे मरुत्वतीयाश्च मे माहेन्द्रश्च मे आदित्यश्च म पौष्णश्च मे हारियाजनश्च मे।

इध्मश्च मे बर्हिश्च मे वेदिश्च मे धिष्णियाश्च मे चमसाश्च मे ग्रावाणश्च मे स्वरवश्च मे उपरवाश्च मे अधिषवणे च मे द्रोणकलशश्च मे वाय्व्यानि च मे

पूतभृच्च मे आधवनीयश्च मे आग्रीधं च मे हविर्धानं च मे गृहाश्च मे सदश्च मे पुरोडाशाश्च मे पचताश्च मे अवथुथरच मे स्वगाकारश्च मे ।

अग्निश्च मे धर्मश्च मे अर्कश्च मे सूर्यश्च मे प्राणश्च मे अश्वमेधश्च मे पृथिवी च मे अदितिश्च मे दितिश्च मे द्यौश्च मे शक्करीरंगुलयो दिशश्च मे यज्ञेन कल्पन्ताम् सामश्च मे वत्साश्च मे त्रिवत्साश्च मे आत्मा च मे प्राणो यज्ञेन कल्पताम् व्यानो यज्ञेन कल्पताम् ऋक् च मे मनो यज्ञेन कल्पताम् यज्ञेन कल्पताम् समानो यज्ञेन कल्पताम् यज्ञो यज्ञेन कल्पताम् ।

The *vaidic* recites the above hymns in praise of Nature. *Cha mé, cha mé- all this is for me-* so says the *vaidic* with all *humility-* thus qualifying himself for absorption of the *sattva* from Nature. In the *shlokas* of the *Taittiriya Samhita*, (4-7-1 to 4-7-10), it is said that all the *tattvas,* all the birds and animals and everything here is the manifestation of the Self. This lofty ecological principle has been asserted with utmost gratitude. The notion that the divine consciousness exists in the entire Universe is again obvious here. The entire Universe is the Lord's *Maaya.* The *vaidic* devotee firmly believes that the cognitive senses of sound, touch, sight, taste and smell enable him to absorb the divinity in Nature. Among the *vaidics* there is a sect of *Shaktas* who exalt Goddess *Shakti* who represents female personification of the Divine Consciousness. They believe that *Shakti* is the essence of knowledge, intelligence, faith, memory and all the cognitive senses. In the *Saptashati* it has been stated :

या देवी सर्वभूतेषु ज्ञानरूपेण संस्थिता ।

नमस्तस्यै नमस्तस्यै नमस्तस्यै नमो नमः ।।

In the same way, the *Saptashati* also states that *Shakti* is the support of all the other faculties :

या देवी सर्वभूतेषु विद्यारूपेण संस्थिता

या देवी सर्वभूतेषु बुद्धिरूपेण संस्थिता

या देवी सर्वभूतेषु धृतिरूपेण संस्थिता

या देवी सर्वभूतेषु चेतना इति अभिधीयते

या देवी सर्वभूतेषु स्मृतिरूपेण संस्थिता

या देवी सर्वभूतेषु निद्रारूपेण संस्थिता

The five *tanmatras* are infra-atomic structure of elements, meaning particles of elements. The above manifestations, *vidya, buddhi, dhruti, chétana, smruti, nidra* are divine in nature as declared in the *Saptashati*. It is amusing to note that in Sanskrit language all our virtuous qualities such as faith, compassion, affection, tenderness, fortitude are feminine in gender whereas, all evil qualities such as pride, foolishness, cruelty are masculine in gender! Even so, in the practice of the *vaidic Dharma*, there is an overflowing sense of gratitude and sublimity for the divine manifestations in the senses and organs, too. This gives rise to a flood of *Bhakti* or devotion in the *vaidic* devotee. In the *Taittiriya samhita* it is said आकाशात् वायु:, वायो: अग्नि:, अग्ने: आप्, आपभ्यां पृथ्वी, that is to say, the sky or ether is the source of the foregoing elements. The metaphysics of *samkhya* tells us that the *akashatattva* comes from the subtle primary element of sound or *nada*. It is *akasha* which makes this possible. The *vaidic* humbly asserts - "All this is created from sound and word." All manifestations in the Universe are sound-based. The following *shloka* asserts the same thing -

नादरूपो स्मृतो ब्रह्मा नादरूपो जनार्दन: ।

नादरूपा परा शक्ति: तस्मात् नादात्मकं जगत् ॥

The primordial sound is "*Omkar*". All creation is generated from *Omkar* which is pure and sacred. The Universe is God's *Maya* or will. Lord *Krishna* says in the *Gita*:

दैवी हि एषा गुणमयी मम माया दुरत्यया । (7 : 14)

Or

मया अध्यक्षेण प्रकृति: सूयते सचराचरम् । (9 : 10)

That is to say, the living Universe is created by God's will. He further says :

मम योनिर्महत् ब्रह्म तस्मिन् गर्भं ददामि अहम् ।। (14 : 3)

The *Shakti* principle is the Mother of the Universe, according to the *Gita*. According to the *Vaishnava* philosophy, this creation is the energy of *Vishnu*. It is stated in the *Upanishad*:

ईशावास्यम् इदं सर्वम् यत्किंच जगत्याम् जगत् ।

The whole Universe is pervaded by God. So the Universe is founded on a metaphysical principle. This is the conviction of the *vaidic*. The Universe is created according to the plan of the Divine. In its atoms and sub-atoms breathes the Divine Principle. In the *Brahadaranyaka Upanishad* there is a section *Antaryami Brahmana*. Therein is described the underlying spiritual base of the Divine arrangement. This section of the *Upanishad*, *Shruti*, is highly philosophical, poetic and enthralling. It is the very basis of the *vaidic* belief. *Ishvara* is not imagined to be an emperor sitting on a majestic throne. In the third *shruti* of the third chapter we find the following description:

33

यः पृथिव्यां तिष्ठन् पृथिव्या अन्तर:, यं पृथिवी न वेद
यस्य पृथिवी शरीरम् यः पृथिवीमन्तरो यमयति एष त आत्मा अन्तर्यामी
अमृत: ।।

योऽप्सु तिष्ठन् अद्भ्योऽन्तर: यमापो न विदु: यस्या: आप:
शरीरम् योऽपोऽन्तरो यमयति एष त आत्मा अन्तर्यामी अमृत: ।।

यः अग्नौ तिष्ठन् अग्ने: अन्तर: यम् अग्निर्न वेद यस्याग्नि:
शरीरम् योऽग्निमन्तरो यमयति एष त आत्मा अन्तर्यामी अमृत: ।।

योऽन्तरिक्षे तिष्ठन् अन्तरिक्षादन्तर: यमन्तरिक्षं न वेद
यस्यान्तरिक्षं शरीरम् योऽन्तरिक्षमन्तरो यमयति
एष त आत्मा अन्तर्यामी अमृत: ।।

यो दिवि तिष्ठन् दिव: अन्तर: यं द्यौर्न वेद यस्य
द्यौ: शरीरम् यो दिवमन्तरो यमयति एष त
आत्मा अन्तर्यामी अमृत: ।।

यो दिवि तिष्ठन् दिवोऽन्तर: यं द्यौर्न वेद यस्य द्यौ:
शरीरम् यो दिवमन्तरो यमयति एष त आत्मा अन्तर्यामी अमृत: ।।

य आदित्ये तिष्ठन् आदित्यादन्तर: यमादित्यो न वेद यस्यादित्य:
शरीरम् य आदित्यमन्तरो यमयति एष त आत्मा अन्तार्यामी अमृत: ।।

यश्चन्द्रतारके तिष्ठन् चन्द्रतारकादन्तरो यं चन्द्रतारकं न वेद यस्य
चन्द्रतारकं शरीरं
यं चंद्रतारकमन्तरो यमयति
एष त आत्मा अन्तर्यामी अमृत: ।।

य आकाशे तिष्ठन् आकाशादन्तरो यम् आकाशो न वेद यस्याकाश:
शरीरं य आकाशमन्तरो यमयति एष त
आत्मा अन्तर्यामी अमृत: ।।

यस्तमसि तिष्ठन् तमसोऽन्तर: यं तमो न वेद यस्य तम:

शरीरम् यस्तमोऽन्तरो यमयति एष त आत्मा अन्तर्यामी अमृत: ।।

यस्तेजसि तिष्ठन् तेजसोऽन्तर: यं तेजो न वेद यस्य तेज:

शरीरम् यस्तेजोऽन्तरो यमयति एष त आत्मा

अन्तर्यामी अमृत: । इत्यधिदैवतम् अथाधिभूतम् ।।

य: सर्वेषु भूतेषु तिष्ठन् सर्वेभ्यो भूतेभ्योऽन्तर: यं

सर्वाणि भूतानि न विदु: यस्य सर्वाणि भूतानि शरीरम्

य: सर्वाणि भूतान्यन्तरो यमयति एष त आत्मा

अन्तर्यामी अमृत: इत्यधिभूतम् अथाध्यात्मम् ।।

य: प्राणे: तिष्ठन् प्राणादन्तर: यं प्राणो न वेद

यस्य प्राण: शरीरम् य: प्राणमन्तरो यमयति, एष त आत्मा अन्तर्यामी

अमृत: ।।

यो वाचि तिष्ठन् वाचोऽन्तर: यं वाक् न वेद यस्य वाक्

शरीरम् यो वाचमन्तरो यमयति एष त आत्मा

अन्तर्यामी अमृत: ।।

यश्चक्षुषि तिष्ठन् चक्षुषोऽन्तर: यं चक्षुर्न वेद यस्य

चक्षु: शरीरम् यश्चक्षुरन्तरो यमयति एष त आत्मा अन्तर्यामी अमृत:।।

य: श्रोत्रे तिष्ठन् श्रोत्रादन्तर: यं श्रोत्रं न वेद

यस्य श्रोत्रं शरीरम् य: श्रोत्रमन्तरो यमयति

एष त आत्मा अन्तर्यामी अमृत: ।।

यो मनसि तिष्ठन् मनस: अन्तर: यं मनो न वेद यस्य मन: शरीरम् यो

मन: अन्तरो यमयति एष त आत्मा अन्तर्यामी अमृत: ।।

यस्त्वचि तिष्ठन् त्वचोऽन्तर: यं त्वड्. न वेद यस्य

त्वक् शरीरम् यस्त्वचमन्तरो यमयति एष त आत्मा

अन्तर्यामी अमृत: ।।

यो विज्ञाने तिष्ठन् विज्ञानादन्तर: यं विज्ञानं न वेद यस्य

विज्ञानं शरीरम् यो विज्ञानमन्तरो यमयति एष त आत्मा

अन्तर्यामी अमृत: ।।

यो रेतसि तिष्ठन् रेतसोऽन्तर: यं रेतो न वेद यस्य रेत:

शरीरं यो रेतोऽन्तरो यमयति एष त आत्मा अन्तर्यामी

अमृत: ।। अदृष्टो द्रष्टा, अश्रुत: श्रोता अमन्तो मन्ता अविज्ञातो

विज्ञाता न अन्योऽतोऽस्ति द्रष्टा न अन्य: अत:

अस्ति श्रोता न अन्य: अत: अस्ति मन्ता न अन्य: अत:

अस्ति विज्ञाता एष त आत्मा अन्तर्यामी अमृत: ।।

अत: अन्यत् आर्तम्; ततो होद्दालक आरुणिरुपरराम ।।

Meaning of the hymn

That Which, standing on the Earth is other than the Earth, Whom the Earth goddess knows not, Whose body the Earth is, That Which internally governs the Earth ; That is thy soul, the Inner Controller, immortal and devoid of all worldly attachment. That verily, is the Soul of the Universe.

That Which resides in water but is other than Water, Whom the god of waters knows not Whose body the Water is That Which resides in and controls the Water. That verily is thy Immortal soul and Inner Controller.

That Which has the abode in Fire but is other than Fire, Whom the god of Fire knows not That very Fire which is Its body That Which internally restrains the god of Fire That verily is thy Immortal soul and Inner Controller.

That Which lives in Space, but is other than Space and Who is not known to the god of Space, Whose body is this very Space That Which controls the god of Space from inside, That is thy Immortal soul and Inner Controller.

That Which pervades the Wind but is other than the Wind-god, Whom the god of the winds knows not, Whose body is this Wind. That Which internally directs the god of the winds, That is thy Immortal soul and Inner Controller.

That Which is in the Heavens, but is other than the Heavens, Whom the Deity of the Heavens knows not, Whose body the Heavens are, That Which resides internally and controls them. That is thy Immortal soul and Inner Controller.

That Which dwells in the Sun, but is other than the Sun-god, Whom the Sun-god does not know, Whose body the Sun-god is. That Which resides in and controls the Sun. That is thy Immortal soul and Inner Controller.

That Which resides in the Quarters but is other than these, Whom the god of the Quarters knows not, Whose body these Quarters are, Who controls the Deity of the Quarters from inside, That is thy Immortal soul and Inner Governor.

That Which dwells in the moon and the stars but is other than these, Whom the god of the moon and stars knows not, Whose body these are, Who controls them from inside, That is thy Immortal soul and Inner Controller.

In the same manner, the *shlokas* which follow refer to the Sky, Darkness, Light, All Beings, *Prana,* Speech, Sight, Hearing, Mind, Skin, Intelligence, the Seed/semen/egg.

The last *shloka* reads as follows :

That Which is not seen but is the Seer, is unheard of but is the Listener, is not perceived but is the Perceiver, is unknown but is the Knower, there is no other seer, no other listener, no other conceiver than Him. There is no other Knower. This is thy Immortal Soul and Inner Controller. Except Him, all else is perishable. *Uddalaka* became silent after listening to this.

Shri Krishnaarpanam astu

✤ ✤ ✤

Discourse 3

The Esoteric Anatomy (गूढशरीर)

य:पृथिव्यां तिष्ठन् पृथिव्या अंतर: यं पृथिवी न वेद, यस्य पृथिवी
शरीरम् य: पृथिवीमन्तरो यमयति एष त आत्मा अंतर्यामी अमृत: ।।

... अदृष्टो द्रष्टा अश्रुत: श्रोता अमतो मन्ता
अविज्ञातो विज्ञाता न अन्य: अत: अस्ति द्रष्टा न अन्य:
अत: अस्ति श्रोता न अन्य: अत: अस्ति मन्ता न अन्य:
अत: अस्ति विज्ञाता, एष त आत्मा अंतर्यामी अमृत: ।।

The above quote from the *Antaryami Brahmana* in the *Brahadaranyaka Upanishad* is demonstrative of the spiritual substrate of the Universe. This Inner Controller referred to in the above quote is the Immortal *Purusha*. He, the *Antaryami*, is the supreme pervading spirit of the Universe. The above-mentioned *Brahmana* describes that *Purusha* as the support of the Universe which is constituted of the physical elements, the celestial elements and the spiritual elements. He is the support of *Shakti, Narayana, Shiva, Bhagavanta*, the Internal Controller of everything in the Universe and the source of supreme holiness and bliss. This principle has been expounded in the *Védanta*. It is emphatically stated that the Supreme Spirit is present in every atom and sub-atom of the Universe, which is also the substrate of the entire Universe. The *Taittiriya Aranyaka* states, 'अंतर्निविष्ट: शास्ता जनानां सर्वात्मा'. *Purusha or Paramatma* is the Internal Controller.

God and Temples

The *védic* postulate also says that *Paramatma* exists not only in the temples or in the heavens, but He pervades the entire Universe.

39

The modern intellectual diehards, while deriding the firm faith of the *vaidic* in God, say, "God is not found in the temples nor is He present in the idol, nor is He found in places of pilgrimage; since He is all-pervading, it is not necessary to go to temples." A religious man, however, believes that even though God is all-pervading, He has also to be visualized in the idol as an object of adoration. This truth can be discerned in *Ramanuja's* philosophy of *Vaishnavism.* Though it is true that God is all-pervading, He is imminent in the idol. The temples and pilgrimage centers are sanctified by saints. Again, majority of people find it difficult to concentrate on God without an idol. Lord *Krishna* says in the *Gita*,

क्लेश: अधिकतर : तेषां अव्यक्तासक्तचेतसाम् (12.5)

It is very hard to concentrate on the Principle which is not visible to the external eyes. So, temples do help the common man to worship God. It is too much to expect from them that they worship God without an idol.

The *Bhagavadgita* in its tenth chapter, has explained how and where to seek the places of divine influence.

Human body

According to the *védic* metaphysics the *adhidaivika* substrate and the spiritual postulation are involved in the Universal manifestation. This *védic* tenet is fundamental to all our knowledge and experience, *Dharma, Karma, Shastra, Upasana, Samskriti and Sadhana.* Man is the micro-model of the vast infinite Universe; man's corporeal body houses the entire Universe. It is clear, therefore, that a thorough investigation of man's physical body has been made in *yogshastra* from three different perspectives. The first is the gross material body. It is formed of the seven essential ingredients (*dhatus*), such as chyle, blood, flesh, fat, bone, marrow and semen. They are formed into different masses of flesh and bone. The corporeal body or *pinda deha* is formed from these masses. This body consists of mental faculties and skeletal-muscular, nervous, circulatory, respiratory, digestive, excretory, reproductive and psycho-mental systems. There is a mutual alliance, proximity, co-ordination, balance amongst these systems which gives us physical and mental health. Even if one of these constituents loses its balance, the result will be all round disorder in health and consequent misery. In spite of the progress made by modern medical science and of the modern knowledge of human anatomy, there is a lack of a holistic approach towards the corporeal body. That is because the knowledge of its subtler aspects is beyond this advancement of knowledge. Modern medical science will have to take support of *yogshastra* for a complete understanding of human existence; otherwise there could be no great improvement in the present state of knowledge. The knowledge of the *sukshma sharira* or esoteric anatomy has not even risen on the horizon despite the astonishing progress claimed by the modern sciences. Even the study of the systemic body is incomplete because of this deficiency.

The subtle or Esoteric body

Yogshastra has investigated the *sukshma sharira* in addition to the gross body. Along with the seven *dhatus* of the body, it has also considered esoteric physiology. Esoteric physiology is a study of six plexii and their governance of the body, the *panchapraanas* and their role and also their application in human evolution in spiritual pursuit. Effective use of the knowledge of the energy released by the *panchapranas* and their operation is disclosed by *yogshastra* for the upliftment of man. This body is made up of five *koshas*, *Annamaya-* food profuse, *Pranamaya - prana* profuse, *Manomaya -* mind profuse,

Vijnanamaya - soul profuse, and *Anandamaya* - bliss or divinity profuse. We marvel at the insights attained by radiologists in understanding internal aspects of body but *yogshastra* is already way ahead in its penetrations and has discovered plexii, *koshas* and the eternal *sukshma sharira.*

It is necessary to peep into our ancient knowledge of *Ayurved* to know the entire system of this corporeal body, consisting of the seven *dhatus.* *Yogshastra* admits of the existence of the three cardinal *tridoshas* or humours which are mentioned in *Ayurved.* The lustre and upkeep of the body depend on these *tridoshas.* Both these sciences acknowledge the influence of these three humours on the seven *dhatus.* The vitiation of these humours causes diseases within the body. For example, the imbalance of *vata* results in pain. The muscles become weak, resulting in discomfort, fatigue, and rheumatism. The body becomes dull and frigid, and there is loss of weight. The mind becomes unsteady and confused, and loses firmness. There is loss of strength. The body with preeminence of *pitta* or bile is fair and lustrous. Also the body of athletes, gymnasts and sportsmen is endowed with *pitta* but it is also prone to acidity and arthritic conditions. The imbalance of *pitta* in the body results in paleness. In such a condition, the body can undergo physical strain, but it is prone to hyperacidity. Alcoholics generally have a bilious nature. Such persons are irritable, they lack endurance and are bad-tempered and hotheaded. Persons having imbalance of *kapha* or phlegm lack emotion, are lazy and susceptible to colds.

Physical and mental ailments have bearings on the *tridoshas* and *trigunas.* Therefore, *Ayurved* has a concept of *dinacharya* and *rutucharya*, it emphasizes on adaptation to habits and life styles appropriate to changing seasons. In short, an imbalance in the

42

proportions of the three humours results in various psychosomatic disorders. *Ayurvedic* literature contains this knowledge. The body is influenced by these three *doshas* and the three *gunas, sattva, rajas, tamas.* The medical science of *Ayurved* propounded by the ancient *rishis* should be studied by those who are interested.

Yogshastra emphasizes more on the esoteric than on the exoteric body. The *shastra* describes the six *chakras, nadis* and *granthis* such as *Brahma granthi, Rudra granthi* and *Vishnu granthi*, which are not physical, but are esoteric in nature. *Yogshastra* describes these *granthis.* It is possible to manage physical well-being and to eliminate suffering with the knowledge of the influence of these *nadis, granthis* and *panchpranas.* This knowledge and application leads one to the attainment of esoteric consciousness. The art of controlling the *nadis* and the six plexii leads to proper management of the *sukshma sharira. Yogshastra* also holds the unique concept of the *panchapranas* and advises practices with reference to six plexii and *nadis* but it is different from that mentioned in *Ayurved.*

The plexii

The corporeal body contains five sheaths. The physical body is *Annamaya.* It is created and sustained by food. It finally merges into food itself. The six-fold plexii work on and control the *pranamaya sharira.* This endows man with mental, intellectual and intuitional faculties that distinguish him from other creatures. All this is related to the six plexii. Man's inclinations, emotions, desires and other mental faculties depend on the *chakra* management. The differences of mentality, intellectuality and emotionality among individuals are because of their *chakras. Yogshastra* gives ways, practices and techniques which can completely transform the individual consciousness. It demonstrates the *chakra* technology. There is a relationship between the six plexii and the five *pranas* which governs the body and mind.

We shall now describe the plexii and their relationship with the body, mind and the five *pranas*. The first *chakra* is known as the *Muladhara chakra*. It is situated at the root of the spine. The second *Svadhishtthana chakra* is situated in the genital region. The third *Manipuraka chakra* is situated within the naval region. The fourth *Anahata chakra* is in the heart. The fifth *Vishuddhi chakra* is situated in the throat. The sixth *Aajna chakra* is located between the eyebrows. These *chakras* can be activated by *yog sadhana*. The seventh *Sahasrara chakra* which transcends the other six is situated at the crown of the head and its activation by the Divine Grace results in *moksha* or salvation.

Muladhara chakra

Man is engrossed in the biological instincts for hunger, sleep, fear and copulation. All these instincts of living creatures have their origin in the *Muladhara chakra*. Man's biological tendencies and natural propensities are dictated by this *chakra*. This *chakra* supports the primary element of earth in the body and is controlled by the *Apana*. Intimately connected with this *chakra* are many *bandhas*, *mudras* and *kriyas* in *yog sadhana*. If consciousness rises above the *Muladhara chakra*, then only will spiritual evolution takes place and the lower nature of the individual is elevated. This is related with *Brahmacharya*.

Svadhishtthana chakra

The *genital chakra* or *Svadhistthana chakra*, is the substrate of an individual's personality. Living beings are susceptible to fear. Fear can be beneficial as well as destructive. It has its roots in this *chakra*. Beneficial or positive fear is responsible for survival of living beings and it also promotes their good fortune and well-being. The negative

44

aspect of fear causes breakdown in the individual's emotional, intellectual and mental faculties. Management of this *chakra* corrects diseases arising out of *jaladosha* and *vatadosha*. The *Apana Vayu* influences this *chakra* and the primary element of water in the body. It corrects "I"-ness problems, and problems on account of superiority and inferiority complexes. The positive and constructive aspect of the trio of fear, courage and the complexes is a necessity for spiritual uplift. *Mahamudra*, and *Uddiyana bandha* are foundational and basic for the *Svadhishtthana*. Diseases associated with the primary element of water can be corrected with practice of these *bandhas* and *mudras*.

Manipuraka chakra

Manipuraka or *Udara chakra* works on *Agnidosha* and digestive disorders which are due to imbalance in the bile. The *Chhandogya Upanishad* states in this regard, अन्नमयो हि सौम्यमना: I". Thus, according to the ancient wisdom, mind is sustained with food. Digestion of food and mental faculties are interrelated. The subtlest form of the food that is eaten becomes the mind. The food eaten is processed in three divisions--gross, middle and subtle. The gross becomes faecal matter, middle forms the flesh, muscles and bones, and the subtle becomes the mind. Digestion nourishes the body cells. The mind is shaped by the manner of absorption and assimilation. The *Manipuraka chakra* is instrumental in strengthening the mind-cells also. *Satvic* food along with *yog sadhana* and regiment of *ahara, vihara, achar* and *vichara* augment the process of evolution of mind. *Brahmacharya, Dhyana yog* and *Mantra yog* accelerate this process. The *Manipuraka chakra* is an important *chakra*, and works against depression, fear and timidity resulting in the proper development of the mind cells. This *chakra* is governed by the *Samana*. It is the focal point of the *vaishvanara* in the body.

45

Anahata chakra

The fourth, *Anahata chakra*, is situated in the region of the heart. It is the source of feelings of affection, emotional attachment, compassion, tenderness, generosity, friendship, fondness etc. It is the source of devotion and spiritual knowledge. The Lord has said in the *Gita*:

सर्वस्य च अहं हृदि संनिविष्टो ।
मत्त: स्मृति: ज्ञानं अपोहनं च ।। (15 : 15)

or

ईश्वर: सर्वभूतानां हृद्देशे अर्जुन तिष्ठति ।
भ्रामयन् सर्वभूतानि यंत्रारूढानि मायया ।। (18 : 61)

The physical heart is the same in all beings, yet the *Hrudaya chakra* is more dominant in woman than in man. The *Anahata kriya* is useful in cases of emotional upsurges, confusion and mental weakness. It is also instrumental in unravelling the mysteries of spiritualism. Lungs are air profuse and proximate to this *chakra*, so it is the locus of element of air. This *chakra* is *pranic* in nature and *prana* governs this *chakra*.

Vishuddhi chakra

The fifth *chakra* is the *Vishuddhi chakra* or *Kantha chakra*. Man differs from animals because he possesses ability to think. He thinks with the mind and determines with the intellect. This *chakra* works on disorders of mind and can change it positively. A *yogi* can control his hunger and thirst with the help of *kriya* on this *chakra*. The physical element of *Akasha* or space has the locus in this *chakra*. The ethereal vibrations of this *chakra* transmute man's thoughts and make him a *yogi*. It is called the *Vishuddhi chakra* because it cleanses the thought processes. *Patanjali's sutra* in this regard is as follows:

कंठकूपे क्षुत्पिपासानिवृत्ति: ।

This *chakra* is controlled by the *Udana*. *Yogasana, pranayama* and *jalandhara kriya* operate on this *chakra* which works on disorders of throat, thyroid and voice. The prescribed remedy for uncontrolled thoughts is the *jalandhara kanthakriya*.

Ajna chakra

The sixth *chakra* is the *Ajna chakra* or the *Bhrukuti chakra*. Man's will-power is attributed to this *chakra*. The power necessary for executing his will is derived from this *chakra*. The *Ajna chakra* is of vital importance for achieving firm and balanced will. Defective or weak will causes pain and misery. The *chakra* works on pride, arrogance and depression. Deficiency of will-power is the cause of lust and evil desires, further resulting in immense grief. The *Yajurved* contains a propitious aphorism in this respect. Firm, supportive and constructive will-power is attainable through special *yogsadhana*.

Sahasrara chakra

The seventh *chakra* is the *Sahasrara chakra*. This *chakra* is responsible for salvation of the individual. At the time of his death the *prana* of a *yogi* breaks through this *chakra* and is released. In case of others, the *prana* passes through any other of the nine openings in the body, generally through the anus.

Plexii and personality

For a comprehensive evaluation of the above *chakras* again in relation to the esoteric physiology and the psychomental faculties we will consider the following:

The first, *muladhara chakra* is governed by the *apana* and *prithvi* elements. The *muladhara* is connected with diseases of the anus and generative organs. Sexual diseases due to lust are associated with this *chakra*.

Imbalance in the *svadhishtthana chakra* gives rise to disorders on account of *jaladosha* and *vatadosha*. Malfunctioning of this *chakra* creates psychological problems of inferiority complex, fear complex, "I"-ness and superiority complex and also those related to liver and bile. Such tendencies and propensities result in discomfort caused by inflammation of joints etc and imbalance of *vata*.

The *manipuraka chakra* is associated with disorders of *vata* in the abdomen and those arising out of *Agnidosha*, resulting in anger and resentment, and diseases of the bile.

The *anahata chakra* is connected with diseases of lungs and chest. Emotional and mental afflictions, those related to phlegm and respiratory disorders are related with this *chakra*.

The *vishuddhi chakra* works on throat disorders, disorders of the thyroid gland and on thoughtless behaviour due to *shadripus* like *kama*, *krodha*, etc. that produce many afflictions.

The *ajna chakra* works on the brain, intellect and vision. It cures the mindset of arrogance and over-confidence. Thus the six plexii, *panchapranas*, and *panchabhutas* are all linked with man's happiness and misery, his sense of pleasure and pain, and psychological, mental, emotional and intellectual aspects.

Yogic techniques ensure a balance in the functions of these evolutes of *Prakriti*. The techniques include *yogasanas, pranayama, bandhas* and *mudras*. It is essential for the *sadhaka* to practise these *kriyas*. These *kriyas* need not be practised by an advanced *yogi*. An accomplished *yogi* establishes the methodology of coordinating the principles of *hathayog, layayog* and *rajayog* from the point of view of their bearing on the *plexi* for evolving a *yogic* mind.

Panchaprana

Apart from the body of flesh and bones, there is much more to man, which is made up of mindset and engendered by the *pranic* body. This is set up by the six *plexii*. These decide the physical and mental constitution of an individual. The *panchapranas* are housed in the *pranamaya kosha*. As far as the physical body is concerned, X-ray photographs of normal individuals will be the same. However, an insight into the minds of these individuals will reveal that they can never be alike. This is because the influence of the *pranamaya kosha* or esoteric body differs from individual to individual.

What is *panchaprana*? While regarding *panchaprana* we have to consider two aspects. The first is the *panchamahaprana- prana, apana, vyana, samana* and *udana*. The movement of these *pranas* in the body makes it lustrous, vigorous and active. Secondly, there are the five *upapranas- naga, kurma, krukara, devadatta* and *dhananjaya*. The science of *Aayurved* takes into account the influence of the *pranas* in the well-being of the body. *Yogshastra*, however, considers them with more profound insight. The *Ayurvedic* knowledge of *panchaprana* is related to the corporeal frame, the gross body, the position of the humours, ill-health and medicament. Due to the difference in the two systems, there has to be a difference in the remedial approach. One should not view the idea of *praana* of *yogshastra* from the view-point of *Ayurved*. *Ayurvedic* experts lack knowledge regarding *praana* as it is considered in *yogshastra*. *Yogshastra* transcends the limits of mere physical well-being and elucidates how the spiritual aim of final accomplishment can be attained.

The body houses the *panchapranas* and the five *upapranas*. There is a continuous movement of the *upapranas* through the countless *naadis* or energy channels housed in the body. These *nadis* come together at the junction of the navel or *nabhi chakra* and the heart or *hrudaya chakra*. The navel is the source of seventy two lac and seventy-two thousand *nadis*. These channels further have branches and sub-branches. From the heart arise hundred and one *nadis*. A hundred of them have branches. Each one of these branches has seven million two hundred seventy-two thousand branches. Amongst all these *pranic* channels, only ten are important. The three most important of these are the *Ida*, *Pingala* and *Sushumna*. Though the entire *prana* pervades the entire corporeal frame, it is divided into *panchapranas* because of their different locations as well as their different functions. Just as the sea is one vast expanse, at different locations it is named differently, such as Pacific, Mediterranean, Atlantic, Arabian, Caspian, etc. In the same way, the *prana* is referred to by different names. In the *Jabala Darshanopanishad* it is said, "Where from comes *prana*?" The main *prana* which enters the nose enters the hollow of the abdomen as *samana*; as *udana* in the hollow of the throat. The very *prana* pervades in the hollow below the navel as *vyana* and *apana*. The *pranic* actions vary according to the respective locations of the *pranas*. The action of the *prana* in one part of the body such as nose is completely different from its action in another functional area such as head or abdomen.

In the *Samkhyakarika* there is an ancient commentary known as *Yuktidipika*. It has a stimulating assertion saying that each *prana* has two unique functions - the external and the internal. The main internal action of the prana consists in breathing through the two nostrils. Its external action is manifested in the outward demeanour. When a soldier or a policeman brandishes a smart salute, there is an element of ego in the action. It may be noted here that the salute of a soldier is an ego cult despite being a salute, while the salute usually has to be out of reverence and respect with humility.

The *apana* internal activity relates to the functions of excretion and reproduction. Its external action results in the exercise of caution. At times it is preferable to effect a safe retreat like taking two steps backward before proceeding one step forward. Such a mental attitude is created by the *apana*.

The internal function of *samana* is in creating internal balance within the nutrients taken in the body. That is why the food eaten through the mouth nourishes the entire body with the food energy converted into blood for the whole body. The internal action of this *prana* is to provide energy from the tip of the toe to the crown of the head. The external action of *samana* is manifested in the mindset for coordinating, collaborating and integrating for practising the equity principle in social life.

The internal action of *udana* is to execute blood circulation above the heart region. It may be noted here that heart needs to pump blood to the areas above. It conveys blood from the throat to the region of the mouth and from the heart to the brain. Blood flows downwards of its own accord by law of gravity; hence no force is required to make blood flow downwards. The external manifestation of *udana* is that of "I"-ness. The aggressiveness in wielding the sword out of its sheath is an example of its external manifestation.

By the internal action *vyana* permeates and activates the whole body through the nervous system. The mindset of adoration and affection which binds individuals together and of affinity and friendship and their outward gestures are the external manifestations of the *vyana*.

This account of the *panchapranas* in *Yuktidipika* is relevant in the study of *yogshastra*.

According to the *Brahmavidya Upanishad*, the organs of action and speech, the locomotive organs, the excretory organ and the generative organ are influenced by the five *pranas*. *Upapranas* regulate the sense organs of touch, sight, hearing, taste and smell. *Upapranas* can bring a positive influence on these five sense organs through the practice of *pranayama* and meditation. Although the fourth limb of *yog* is called *pranayama* which has positive effects on the intellectual refinement of the practitioner, surprisingly, it is *upa-pranayama* in nature. Only for convenience is it called *pranayama*. The *Mahapranas* i.e. *prana, apana, samana, vyana, udana* are concerned with the organs of action. These *pranas* flow through the *nadis*. The network of these countless *nadis* is present not only in the physical body, but also in the mental, intellectual and emotional aspects. The *yogic kriyas*, especially *pranayama*, and the function of these *nadis* bring yogic culture in *chitta*. In addition, the body consisting of the *saptadhatus*, the ten organs and senses, and the internal consciousness also gets refined by the *yogic* process.

Nadis

The important point to be stressed here is that the concept of the nadis in *yogshastra* differs from that in the *Ayurved*, and also that in astrology. The concept of *nadi* in *Ayurved* relates to the physical plane viz. the *tridoshas* of *vata, pitta* and *kapha*, the *saptadhatus* and physical diseases. The astrological concept is concerned with the effect on the psyche, of the disposition of the planets, their conjunction, etc. In *yog*, transformation and spiritual elevation take place on account of *pranayama, dharana and dhyana* and of proper functioning of the *nadis*. It is closely connected with functioning of the *panchapranas* and the *panchamahabhutas* in the body. Some of the prominent *nadis* help the *yogi* to acquire the *ashta siddhis*. They are *anima, laghima, garima, mahima, prapti, prakami, ishitva,* and *vashitva.* The *nadis* control his senses and organs, and reform hunger, thirst, consciousness, movements, conduct and powers. This cannot happen in case of an ordinary individual. In case this is imposed, it will develop debilitating condition or inside revolt in him. An ordinary individual becomes weak due to fasting, whereas the *yogi* acquires spiritual strength and a glow after fasting. The function of the *nadis* effects yogic transformation in the body, mind and *indriyas.* The body of the ordinary individual remains healthy only as long as the flow of blood through the arteries and veins is normal. These *nadis* do not work efficiently in old age and the result is decay and, diseases. In contrast, the *yogi's* body remains remarkably fit and his thoughts and actions are endowed with an exemplary prowess. In modern parlance, his body is traffic-worthy for *prana!* Proper trafficking of *prana* effects the *yogic* nature in the seeker and also in the accomplished. For attaining this, he assiduously practises *yogasanas, mudras, kriyas, bandhas* and *pranayama.*

Shri Krishnaarpanam astu

✜ ✜ ✜

Sukshma Sharira

Sukshma Sharira or sublte body

Sukshma sharira – It is a proven principle of *yogshastra* that the evolution of the *sukshma sharira* is effected mainly by *japa* i.e. recitation of *mantras* and God's name and His *dhyana* or meditation. Mere physical nutrients can not nourish the *sukshma sharira*. It also does not get relaxation through mere sleep. The physical exercises, evacuation of the bowels, etc. does not affect the *sukshma sharira*. We will consider the relevance of *japa* in a separate topic and consider the technique, procedure and practice of *japa*.

Man experiences pleasures and pain through the *sukshma sharira*. The *sukshma sharira* is affected by *vasanas* or cravings. Worldly sorrows are the result of the interplay of desires and actions in the individual. Hindu *Dharma* has prescribed a remedy. The remedy consists in faithful chanting of *mantras* and *nama*, practice of austerity, *yog sadhana* and inclination towards spiritualism. The *sukshma sharira* is subject to hunger, thirst and it needs all that the gross body requires such as water, air, cleanliness. These needs are fulfilled if one practises *japa*. The *sukshma sharira* is affected by *karma*, consisting of both positive as well as negative actions, as mentioned in the *Dharmashastra* or the religious code. Pursuit of the spiritual path for the invisible but phenomenal can give the remedy for the maladies of the *sukshma sharira*, in fact, it is a panacea for all the sufferings of the *sukshma sharira*.

It is often believed that there is no antidote to man's *karma* or destiny, but this is not true. Man's *karma* can however be influenced by *sadhana* of the *sukshma sharira*, *sukshma deha*, *linga deha* or *vasana deha*. The *samkhyashastra*, which is the foundation to *yog* shastra, describes in detail the constitution of the sukshma sharira. The ninth sutra of the third chapter on this point states, 'समदशैकं लिंगं'. The aforementioned seventeen (saptadasha) elements exist at the time of creation and all of them dissolve at the time of deluge. While commenting on the 40th karika of Ishvara Krishna in Samkhyatattvakaumudi, Vachaspati Mishra says :

महत्अहंकारदशेंद्रियपंचतन्मात्रपर्यंतम्
एतेषां समुदाय: सूक्ष्मं शरीरम् ।।

The above definition of the sukshma sharira is quite clear. Man's corporeal or visible body, is formed of the six physical sheaths (shatkaushika) of back, belly, thighs, limbs, chest and head. These six sheaths are formed of flesh and bone. They are different from the panchakoshas of our being. For example, the thirty-ninth karika of Vachaspati Mishra further explains that this psycho-physical emotional sheath possesses maternal and paternal aspects. This thought is very interesting and is beyond the thinking of modern science. He states that skin, blood and flesh have maternal characteristics and those of the muscles, bones and marrow are paternal in nature. Thus the somatic body has six sheaths and our total existence is described in terms of the five koshas, the Annamaya, Pranamaya, Vijnanamaya, Manomaya and Anandamaya. Another variation of the samkhya system has prescribed sixteen evolutes of Prakriti. These are the ten indriyas,- senses and organs,- the five tanmatras, and the antahakarana or consciousness. The ten indriyas referred to here are not the gross physical organs of sense and action. They are subtle in nature. They are not ten senses as they appear in a body but they are tendencies behind the ten senses. So even a blind man would have tendencies for sight and a deaf man would have tendencies for audition and so forth. The evolution or devolution of the human mind is affected by the *sukshma sharira*. Human sorrows have their source in this *sukshma sharira*. The modern remedial sciences, including psychiatry, on the maladies of human body and mind, have not even sighted the roots of human sorrows. The Freudian division of consciousness offers very little help here and today we see that his sex-oriented theories are being substantially challenged.

Importance of Japa

The ups and downs in a man's life are due to the movements within the *sukshma sharira*. The emotion of sorrow has its source in the *sukshma sharira* which is the indestructible origin of the gross or visible body. Western medicine, including psychiatry, has no ultimate remedy for this state of mind. The success rate among psychic cases does not go beyond seven per cent. The sure remedy is prescribed by *yogshastra*, in the form of *japa, namasankirtana, dhyana* and worship. It is the ancient Hindus who have discovered an antidote for complex human sorrows. This has been possible because of deep insight into human existence and psyche. Relief from disease of the gross physical body can be secured by formal medical treatment. This body is subject to hunger and thirst. Its needs are cleanliness, exercise and excretion. In the same manner, the *sukshma sharira* has subtle needs which cannot be appeased by material substances like foodstuffs, air, water, physical rest and exercise. The fulfillment of these needs is obtained through subtle channels. In this respect, it is to be noted that *japa* is food, *japa* is air and water, *japa* is the tonic. Japa is medicine, *japa* is rest, exercise and excretion and purification. Japa is bath. Japa is everything for the *sukshma sharira*. It is the breath of the *sukshma sharira*. This great asset of *japa* is mentioned in *mantrayog*. The *Bhagavadgita* significantly states :

56

'यज्ञानां जपयज्ञोऽस्मि ।' (10.25) Having thus discussed the *Adhidaivika* and *Adhibhautika* aspects of the *sukshma sharira*, now we will try to understand the *Adhyatmika* aspects of the *sukshma sharira*.

Pinda and Brahmaanda

We have seen that the material manifestation of the Universe has a celestial structure and a spiritual substrata. The universe in its apparent form seems to be material. However, the wisdom scan points out that it is *Adhidaivika* constitution. The celestial forces seem to be like particles of matter and the *Adhyatmika* aspect is at the substratum. Marvellously the six foot human body has a miniature universe in itself. Thus the expression — as is the macrocosm so is the microcosm,- as the *Brahmanda* is, so the *pinda* is. For, this everchanging body and the journey of the body from birth to decay and death has a substrate — which is eternal, changeless, indestructible, formless and dimensionless in nature. The body, like every other substance in the Universe, has a spiritual substratum. This soul is devoid of form, is imperceptible for the senses, mind and consciousness. It is minuter than the atomic and larger than the most colossal. This is the principle of *Atma*, a metaphysical entity. This *Atma* is the unborn, eternal, primeval, mystical and transcendental principle. It is not just merely a hairsplitting philosophy. It is the focal point of the *Shrutis* and the *Smritis*. The Hindu philosophy is neither a polemic warfare nor an airy thought speculation or hairsplitting intellectual gymnastics as is the case with other philosophies but it postulates, divulges and reveals this spiritual principle – the *Atma*. The *Brahadaranyaka Upanishad* describes it – 'य: प्राणे तिष्ठति स आत्मा सर्वांतर:' The Indweller (*Paramatman*) resides at the centre of our being i.e. in the heart. He is the Inner Controller. In chapter 10, *shloka* 20, of the *Bhagavadgita*, the Lord

57

says : 'अहम् आत्मा गुडाकेश सर्वभूताशयस्थित: ।' O *Gudhakesha*, I am the central principle of all the living beings. In the *Shvetashvatara Upanishad* it is stated : 'एको देव: सर्वभूतेषु गूढ: निवेशित: सर्वव्यापी सर्वभूतांतरात्मा कर्माध्यक्ष: सर्वभूताधिवास: साक्षीचेता केवलो निर्गुण: च ।'. There is only one divine principle in all the beings and this divinity is all pervasive, the indwelling soul and presiding force behind all activities of beings and yet it stays merely as a witness and absolutely in isolation from all universal phenomenalism and also transcends the basic *gunas* i.e. *sattva, raja, tama* which constitute the universe. The *Brahadaranyaka Upanishad* states in the *Antaryami Brahmana* :

'य: आत्मनि तिष्ठान् यम् आत्मा न वेद यस्य आत्मा शरीरम् य आत्मा अंतरो यमयति एष त आत्मा अंतर्यामी अमृत: ।'. The *Gitaa* states in the 18th chapter : 'ईश्वर: सर्व भूतानां हृद्देशे अर्जुन तिष्ठति' भ्रामयन् सर्वभूतानि यंत्रारूढानि मायया ।। (18 : 61) *Krishna* says, O *Arjuna*, *Ishvara* resides in the heart of all living beings. He moves them as if they are mounted on a roulette machine, the *Maya*. All these expressions point to the spiritual substrate of the corporeal body.

As mentioned earlier, *Yogshastra* gives us an insight into the nature of the gross body as well as that of the *sukshma sharira*. Man is born in the Universe and *Ishvara*, the Creator of this Universe, is the Indweller of the heart. The human being is constituted of all the elements of the Universe. Man might be taken as an object among countless objects in the universe right from minute bacteria to the gigantic stars in the skies, but it is not so. The awe-inspiring fact is that man is a miniature universe by himself. Man has a different mould as compared to the inanimate objects like stones, stars, minute sand particles, atoms, and even animals like elephants, horses. Man

58

is the microscopic manifestation of the entire Universe. The Universe and the individual are inextricably intertwined – this is the fundamental metaphysical principle.

Creation of the Universe

It is important to understand the manner of the creation of the Universe in order to understand the inherent characteristics of man. The whole Universe at the time of Creation is in an extremely numinous and unmanifested state. There is an interesting dialogue between the spiritual master *Aruni Uddalaka* and his disciple *Shvetaketu*, regarding the Universe. In the *Chhandogya Upanishad, Shvetaketu* asks : "*Guruji*, how has the banyan tree come to be here?" *Guruji* replies : "My Child, pluck a fruit and bring it to me." *Shvetaketu* brings the fruit. *Guruji* asks him to peel it and observe what was inside. *Shvetaketu* replies : "There is a seed inside." *Guruji* asks him to break the seed and tell him what he saw inside. "Also break what you see inside", *Guruji* instructs him. "*Acharya*, I see nothing in it", he replies. *Guruji* then says, "This tree is formed from nothing, but how can something be produced from nothing? Hence, whatever you see inside the seed which is broken, seems as though there is nothing. It is unmanifest".

It is thus seen that the tree evolves from the unmanifest state into the seed, from the seed to the bud and from the bud to the plant which finally develops into the full-fledged tree. Then from the *Mahattattva*, the cosmic principle or the Universal consciousness, is evolved the *ahamkara* and the other subsequent evolutes. One branch of the evolutes consists of the *panchamahabhutas* and the five *tanmatras* forming the gross Universe, and the other branch consists of the mind and the ten *indriyas*,- the senses and organs. The Universe is thus manifested by means of these evolutes.

59

All these Universal principles exist in man. Man's fundamental nature has its roots in the three *gunas*. *Mahat*, the cosmic intelligence, the five *tanmatras*,- subtle primary elements, *buddhi*,- intelligence, *indriyas*,- senses and organs, the *saptadhatus* or the seven physical ingredients of the body, the five subtle elements and the five physical elements are all influenced by the collective action of the *gunas*. *Atma* is non-*Prakritic*. All else comes from *Prakriti*, and the evolutes of *Prakriti*, and these evolutes are influenced by the collective action of the three *gunas*. In the *samkhya* system, the *Purusha* is *Atma*. पुरे शेते इति पुरुष – the One who lives in the *pura* or body is *Purusha*. *Purusha* is thus defined. There are nine outlets in the physical body and the *Purusha* or *Atma* is dormant in it. It is devoid of gender, form, *guna*, *avastha*, caste or creed. *Atma* is the divine principle. The Lord says in the *Gita* : "मम एव अंश: जीवलोके जीवभूत: सनातन: I" (15 : 7) The eternal soul of living beings in the universe is only one of my aspects. It is the Inner Controller of all the atoms and sub-atoms in the Universe. Man cannot be studied in toto by any science of physiology, biology or for that matter, psychology. The nature of man transcends the limitations of the physical and mental sciences. He is basically and inherently spiritual - a point which should be noted by the *yogsadhaka*.

Yogshastra regards the complete man not only objectively but also in a subjective way. In the process, it understands that man is not only beyond the body but also beyond the mind. Empirically man is summed up in body and mind but man is far beyond these aspects. This inducts him to the core aspect which is metaphysical and spiritual. So also it makes him understand that man is made up of the five *koshas*, the three bodies and *Adhibhautika*, *Adhidaivika* and *Adhyatmika* aspects. Thus man cannot be summed up in his existence to 'I'-ness and 'mine'-ness. Objectivistic studies enable man to understand what man is and what he is made up of, while subjectivistic studies give him knowledge of why he is made up like that. These studies will also help man attain the supreme good, here and hereafter. In philosophy this is called *iha* and *paramarthika*, supreme good or also *abhyudaya* and *nihshreyasa*. *Yogshastra* helps man to attain virtuosity. Virtuosity is the supreme merit in this world and leads to ultimate and eternal accomplishment which is *moksha*. Therefore this is a complete science, escorting man from a rudimentary beginning in spiritualism to the ultimate destination of liberation. This science is one's friend, guide and philosopher, thus in itself a *guru* and rightly hailed as a supreme *vidyaa*. This is testified in the *Bhagvadgita*. Every chapter of it has been named as a form of *yogvidya*. It is designated with the name of the part of *yogvidya* with which it is concerned. It is known as *yogshastra*. The ending of each chapter would reveal this fact. The first chapter is called the "*Arjuna Vishada Yog*". This is followed by *karma yog, karmasanyasa yog, bhakti yog, akshara brahma yog, Purushottama yog, vibhuti yog, daivasurasampadvibhaga yog,* etc. The *Gita* is complete with *yogvidya*. *Yog* has many forms such as *jnana yog, hatha yog, raja yog, mantra yog, laya yog, nama yog, kundalini yog, nada yog*. The variety is truly astonishing. The *sadhaka* finds it difficult when it comes to choosing the kind of *yog* appropriate for him. *Gurus* there are many, but to identify '**The Guru**', and nobody else, is possible only with the blessing of God. We will consider the question of securing the proper *Guru* who can teach the *yog* of the aspirants' aptitude in the next topic.

Shri Krishnaarpanam astu

✤ ✤ ✤

Discourse 5

Introduction to Spirituality

Ashtanga Yog – the Foundational Yog

The peak of a mountain may be scaled from various directions. It could be from the north, south, east or west, and even though the effort, experience, modus operandi and the landmarks from various directions would be different, ultimately, the same peak is scaled. Similarly, *yog* is the peak, and it can be accessed in various ways.

Traditionally, it is believed that there are four major forms of *yog* and then there are multiple sub-forms. These four forms of *yog* are *jnana yog, karma yog, dhyana yog* and *bhakti yog.* Further, each of these four specialized spiritual disciplines has sub-divisions. The goal of these four is one and the same, i.e. *Parama Abhyudaya-* Supreme Accomplishment. *Ashtanga yog* of *Patanjali* is the basic and foundational course for all the various forms of *yog.* The seed of the various forms of *yog* are planted in the field of *ashtanga yog*, and the trees of the different *yogas* grow in the field of *ashtanga yog.*

Just as in a kitchen garden, we grow different types of vegetables and fruits of various tastes as well as flowers with different fragrances from the same ground and soil, similarly *ashtanga yog* can be a ground for all forms of *yog.*

We can take the example of the field of education. Here we have the choice of studying different branches. It is possible to obtain graduate, postgraduate or doctoral degrees in the chosen branch. However, at the start there will be a foundational common course for all the various disciplines. The basic ABC of education is necessary for advanced study. *Ashtanga yog,* like the ABC of education, is a foundational ground for all the various forms of *yog* and occupies a pivotal position in *yogshastra*. Only afterwards is it possible to take up any of the specializations like *nada yog, dhyana yog, tantra yog, kundalini yog*. One cannot suddenly get up and say that he would practise *jnana yog* or awaken his *kundalini shakti!* This would amount to sheer folly. It would be incorrect to presume that one could become a *yogic* aspirant without proficiency in *ashtanga yog*. It is imperative not to overlook this aspect.

Branches of Yog

As mentioned before, there are four main branches of *yog*, i.e. *jnana yog, bhakti yog, karma yog* and *dhyana yog*, and these have several sub-branches. *Jnana yog* can be *raja yog* or *tarka yog*. *Karma yog* can be sub-divided into the *karma yog* which is based on *jnana*, and *karma yog* based on *bhakti*. *Bhakti yog* can be sub-divided into *nama yog, japa yog* and *nada yog*. By means of any of these, the goal of *bhakti* is reached.

There are several forms of *dhyana yog* like *mantra yog, laya yog, hatha yog, raja yog, japa yog, nada yog, kundalini yog, nama yog, tarka yog* and *tantra yog*. Meditation can evolve from the different techniques in all these various modes and various forms which are all *yogic* forms. However, the mother of all *yogas* is *ashtanga yog*. The alphabets of all forms of *yog* are fashioned in *ashtanga yog*.

Even if it is stated that *yogvidya* begins with *ashtanga yog*, in fact, it was possible to do so in the *vedic* period. The texts of *yog* were written in the classical times. The culture during that period was different from that of today. We are now divorced from the *vedic* faith as well as the religious tradition of yore, and so we are unable to undertake the practice of *yogvidya* even from those first primary steps of *ashtanga yog*. The sages had devised *yogshastra* at a time when the society was founded on the *vedic* faith.

The formal education of the child in the past, started at the age of five. Today the child's pre-primary stage of education commences two years earlier. During these two years, the lower K.G. and the higher K.G. have come into force. In some other cases there is also a pre-nursery course. Fortunately for us, no education can be forced on the child before its birth and the child is allowed to play on the mother's lap for one or two years at least!

At present, just as a child has to undergo a pre-primary course at the beginning of education, so also there are certain preliminaries to be followed before becoming qualified for the practice of *ashtanga yog*. The social system in the times of *Patanjali, Yogeshvara Krishna, Jnaneshvara,* and *Yajnyavalkya*, was based on three core principles of *yajna* (sacrifice), *dana* (munificience) and *tapas* (austerity). In the first two limbs or stages of *ashtanga yog* i.e. *yama* (ethical disciplines) and *niyama* (ethical observances) are included *ahimsa* (non-violence), *satya* (truthfulness), *asteya* (non-stealing), etc. Our present society is blind to these principles. These great and perpetual values are taken to be outdated and useless in practical life. In fact, it is necessary to inculcate these core principles into our modern social system for developing fitness for *ashtanga yog*. Our culture today has become pleasure-centred and self-centred. Selfishness is at its zenith. Consumerism and pleasure-seeking are today's models of conduct. We have become slaves to the TV culture. We run after things useful for our material comforts like cars or bungalows. Social contacts are cherished on purely materialistic considerations. In *vedic* times the social fabric was untainted. If *Patanjali* were to incarnate in the present age, he would perforce prescribe a preparatory course for *ashtanga yog*.

As discussed before, there are three core principles in our *dharma* and *samskriti*. Without these principles of *yajna, dana* and *tapas*, the practice of *vedic Dharma* and *vedic* rituals would lose all merit. It is mandatory for the spiritual aspirant to have faith in these principles. Such preliminary conditioning of the aspirant is obligatory before he undertakes the path of *ashtanga yog*. After attaining proficiency at this stage, the beginner becomes qualified for the second stage i.e. *kriya yog. samprajnata* or *dhyana yog* is practised after this. *Patanjali* has described this Supreme *Yog* of self-realization in the first chapter (*samadhi pada*) of his *yogsutras*. *Kriya yog* is explained in the beginning of the second chapter *sadhana pada*, and in the middle of the chapter *Patanjali* has explained *ashtanga yog*. In the *sadhana pada, kriya yog* is meant for the aspirant, and in the *samadhi pada*, there is the Supreme *yog* of Self-realization for the advanced aspirant. The three stages of *sadhaka* can be described as *adhamadhikari-* neophyte, *madhyamadhikari-* proficient and *uttamadhikari-* accomplished. Several lives are consumed for reaching the stage of accomplishment. *Ashtanga yog* is the foundational *yog* in the *sadhana pada*.

In the contemporary educational system, there are the secondary and higher secondary courses of ten and twelve years respectively. Normally a total period of not more than fifteen years is required for getting a degree. This itself is quite a long duration. But in the field of *yog,* even a period of fifty or sixty years may not be enough to reach the preliminary stage. In the sixth chapter of the *Gita*, the Lord has said, '**अनेकजन्मसंसिद्धौ ततो याति परां गतिम् ।**'. (7 : 45) It means that after the efforts of numerous births, the aspirant can hope to reach the Ultimate Goal. This fact is likely to amaze the so-called modern educated individual. Today people find it difficult to spend even ten or fifteen years for learning a fine art. But the *yogic* journey takes several births and yet the true aspirant does not get disheartened.

Ashta-angas

Ashtanga yog, kriya yog and the *paramoccha* or Supreme *yog* are the stages of development in *yog*. *Yama, niyama, asana, pranayama, pratyahara, dhyana, dharana* and *samadhi* are the eight limbs of *ashtanga yog*. There are five *yamas- ahimsa, satya, asteya, brahmacharya,* and *aparigraha*. The *niyamas* consist of *shaucha, santosha, tapa, svadhyaya* and *Ishvarapranidhana*. *Asanas* are of four types. The first type consists of psychosomatic *asanas*. These relate to the physical body stage. They consist of twisting, stretching, etc. of the body and they are beneficial for physical and mental conditions. The second type is iconographic in nature, that means the visual images are associated with a movement. This type is associated with the *panchapranas* and consists of *asanas* of a higher level. The third type consists of *asanas* of the neutrality type i.e. they remove the influence of dualities. The *asanas* of the fourth and still higher stage are archetypal, that means they underlie all the theories and methodologies of *yogasanas*. They range from the body-mind state to the abstract *dhyana* state. For example, *shirshasana* is first performed at the body-mind level. The second stage is associated with the *panchapranas*. Then it proceeds to the stage without the two opposites which is a neutrality state, and finally merges with the *dhyana* state, giving the perfected *shirshasana*.

Pranayama, too, has similar stages of evolvement. The first stage consists of inhalation, exhalation and holding the breath. Next comes the realization of the five vital *pranas* or *panchapranas* and their involvement in the *pranayamic* process. The stages of *pranayama* consist of *pranasomatic, pranamanasic, pranapsychosomatic, udanayama, pranachaitik* and then *pranavatmaka, mantranvita, japanvita, dhyananvita.* The *pranayama* of a *yogi* is associated with *dhyana.*

Pratyahara is withdrawal of the senses into the mind and it has two aspects. The first type is practical; the mind can be unruffled even if it is affected by worldly afflictions. The second one is preparatory to *dhyana* in *ashtanga yog* and is the *yogic pratyahara.* It is created out of *pranayama.*

Dharanaa, dhyana and *samadhi* are confinement, meditation and absorption. They are the subsequent limbs of *ashtanga yog* and are initially in the mental state. The *sadhaka* is in the meditative mode of the mind. Then onwards he rises to the *pranic* and *chaittic* levels which lead to the pure *samskarika* level, and ultimately to the highest, *paramoccha yogic* level. Generally, neophytes like us struggle for concentration on the psychological plane.

Kriya Yog

The second stage in *ashtanga yog* is that of *kriya yog.* It consists of three limbs out of the eight. This *yog* is triangular, the three sides being *tapa, svadhyaya* and *Ishvarapranidhana.* This *yog* develops in conjunction with these three features. The noteworthy point is that fivefold afflictions or *panchakleshas* of *avidya, asmita* (I-consciousness), *raga,*(attachment), *dvesha,* and *abhinivesha (*fear of death*)* are weakened by this process. *Jnana yog* is the antidote to *avidya. Karma yog* is the antidote to *asmita, dhyana yog* for *raga* and *dvesha,* and *bhakti yog* for *abhinivesha.* These four *yogas* are instrumental in eradicating the *panchakleshas. Ashtanga yog incorporates the basics of these four yogas.* A *yogi* can be strongly influenced by any one of the aforesaid four branches. Then the *yogi* becomes a qualified *yogi* and proceeds towards *Kaivalya.* He is released from worldly life, and then onwards he proceeds towards *samadhi,* the supreme *yog.*

Just as a coin has two sides, *samadhi sadhana* has the two sides of *abhyasa* and *vairagya. Abhyasa* and *vairagya* constitute *yog sadhana. Abhyasa* means effort to steady the mind and is lack of thirst for objects of the senses. That is why *Patanjali* says, 'अभ्यासवैराग्याभ्याम् तन्निरोध: ।' This *sadhana* is striving for restraining *vrittis* of the *chitta* which comprises mind, intellect, ego and consciousness. This restraint is a way of concentration. The calibre of this *sadhana* can be mild, middle or intense. *Chittavrittinirodhaha* is the foundation of all the *yogas,* from the lowest to the highest. *Yog* culminates in *samadhis* of two kinds,- *samprajnata* or cognitive trance and *asamprajnata* or ultra- cognitive trance. These practices evolve in phases. They are in the following order. 1] purification of *chitta* 2] meditation on personal deities or noble symbols and sound forms 3] *Pranika japa* 4] *pranayamika japa* 5] meditation on *Om* 6] trance on *Om* 7] *Adhyatma Prasad* i.e. bestowal of spiritual bounty and grace 8] *Rutambhara prajna* or truth bearing wisdom faculty 9] *Samskarashuddhi* or purification of subliminal impressions 10] Restraint of the above tendencies 11] *Dharma megha samadhi* i.e. torrential downpour of supreme virtue which washes out all defects and sins in the consciousness 12] *Kleshanasha* or destruction of all afflictions 13] Spiritual accomplishment 14] Reversal of the three *gunas* 15] Isolation from *gunas* i. e. Liberation. This is the pathway of *yogasadhana.*

Shri Krishnaarpanam astu

✤ ✤ ✤

Discourse - 6

Patanjala Sadhana-1

Patanjali has laid down a three-stage *Sadhana* in his *yogasutras;* for the initiate, the intermediate and the evolved *(uttamaadhikaris)* aspirants. The first stage of the *sadhana* generally extends for a long period. This is but natural. a neophyte has to bear in mind that this stage may even take more than one or two decades. We have repeatedly asserted what the *Gitaa* says:

अनेकजन्मसंसिद्धौ ततो याति परां गतिम् । (7 : 45)

The *yogi* achieves the supreme stage only after *sadhana* of many births.

The foundational stage of the *sadhana* is *ashtanga yog*. Different types of *yog* blossom on the soil of *ashtanga yog*. As mentioned earlier, it is possible to grow various plants and fruit trees in the same common field. The same soil can offer hot chillies and sweet mangoes, colourful roses and white jasmine and so on. So also, any type of *yog* can be nurtured with appropriate *sadhana* on the same foundation of *ashtanga yog*.

This is a fact about *ashtanga yog*. However, *ashtanga yog* was established in the *vedic* days of yore. Our present culture is far different from that background. The social and family set-up, the life style, moral, cultural and religious learnings are all different. Our calculations are always in terms of material benefits. Materialism, luxuries and utility are the keywords of our philosophy of life. This is not a proper atmosphere even for preliminary practices of true *yog*. It is doubtful whether we can take up the preliminary stages of *yama* and *niyama* of *ashtanga yog* without difficulty today. We are perplexed while unsuccessfully struggling with the observances of

69

yama and *niyama*. We do not have the appropriate strategy to practise with the code and conduct of *ahimsaa, satya, asteya*, etc. in the same way as we physically perform *asana* and *pranayama*. We are deeply involved in self-gratification. We have become irreligious and pseudo-secular. With such a mind-set, instead of applying ourselves seriously to *yog sadhana* we are actually indulging in its ridicule. Under these circumstances, we are unable to face the rigours of *sadhana*. The practice of *japa, dhyana* and *dharana* further aggravates our problems in *sadhana*. They seem to be unsuited to our dispositions, abilities and capacities. How far is it logical to set out to practise *yogic* principles with our persisting embrace of *shadripus*.

Initially we may be eager to practise *yog sadhana* and determined to embrace the principles of *yama, niyama, shaucha, santosha*, etc. We may try to scrupulously and uncompromisingly adopt a mode of life to inculcate spiritual values under the present circumstances. To take up such a course prematurely and immaturely could be disastrous. We would be hurting ourselves badly in the process. Without a basic conditioning of the mind-set, it would be futile to follow the principles of *yog.*

When *Patanjali* compiled the *yogasutras*, he did so with the *vedic* tradition in mind. He, therefore, directly commenced his scheme of *yog sadhana*, with the fundamental basic stages of *yama* and *niyama*, without the need for any pre-conditioning course. To commence the practice of *ashtanga yog* from the present center-stage of licentiousness, self-centredness and atheistic leanings is well-nigh impossible. In the *vedic* tradition, three valuable principles were posited in the *shaastras*. The entire *Vedic* culture was upheld by these pillars. The *sadhana* and *upaasanaa* of the *vedic* age was based on these principles. It is necessary to acquaint ourselves with these salient fundamental precepts and inculcate them in us to develop the required positive mental frame for commencing the *yama* and *niyama* stages of *sadhana*.

Yajna, dana, tapas

The three principles referred to above are *yajna, dana* and *tapas*, and the establishment of these in the *sadhana* is vitally important. This is the way by which the ethico-religious principles of *yama* and *niyama* become natural and spontaneous as well as organic for us. They remain as mere commandments and mere moral and ethical platitudes in the absence of these principles. *Yama* and *niyama* thus become difficult to practise and continue to remain as mere ideological values. The modern materialistic, pseudo-intellectual and profligate man is un*vedic* minded and he is divorced from the principles of *yajna, dana* and *tapas*. The importance of the influence of this triad of *yajna, dana*, and *tapas* should not be underestimated.

At the foundation of the *yogic* edifice are the three foundational blocks of *yajna, dana* and *tapas*. Over the foundation there is the structure of *ashtanga yog* consisting of *yama, niyama, asana, pranayama, pratyahara, dharana, dhyana* and *samadhi*. This ground floor gets raised up to the first floor, transmuting itself into *kriya yog* comprising of the integrated *tapas, svadhyaya* and *Ishvarapranidhana*. This *kriya yog* has the foundational components of the four main *yogas*, viz. *jnana yog, karma yog, dhyana yog* and *bhakti yog*. Any one of these *yogas* can lead one to the apex point of the edifice of *Kaivalya*, the final accomplishment, and *Nirvana*, the final liberation. The entire *yogic* edifice is thus founded on *yajna, dana* and *tapas*. One who believes in, imbibes and practises the principles of *yajna, dana* and *tapas*, which is not different from real

71

Manava Dharma, qualify for *ashtanga yog*. Without this, man remains only as a bi-footed animal, human in form, animal in conduct. Therefore it is natural and perfectly appropriate that he cannot succeed in the practice of *yama* and *niyama*.

Yajna

Yajna is the principle of sacrifice. It does not merely consist of pouring oblations into the sacrificial fire. It is based on our acknowledgement of our indebtedness to Nature. We are immensely indebted to Nature and have to express our gratitude to Nature's bounty. We must sacrifice something for Nature and that is the principle of *yajna*. It is because Nature has provided us abundantly with air, water, food, plants, etc. that we are living in this world. The environmentalists today are rightly emphasizing importance of the natural resources like trees, rivers, mountains, forests. It is true that they support life on the earth. We are also beholden to Nature's creatures such as animals, birds, insects and other living beings. They are responsible for the balance in the environment.

The love, affection, warmth and the sense of protection and security that the family showers upon us is invaluable. All these factors keep us indebted to the family for ever. A calf stands on its feet almost as soon as the cow gives birth to it, whereas the child takes so many days for it, and so many years to be self-supporting, but the role of the mother, father and other family members is invaluable even in this. The family roots lie in the mother whose role in the family is indispensable. All the wealth of the three worlds would be inadequate to repay the debt to the mother. The love, affection, warmth and sense of protection and security that she bestows on us is beyond measure. One should be grateful even to remain permanently indebted to the mother. There is thus no doubt that the role of the mother, father and other members of the family is immeasurable. Expression of our indebtedness to the family contributes to cultural richness. Imagine the plight of a child born in Siberia, isolated and parentless under the open sky. Our heritage, lineage and culture provide us a lofty platform in the world, at the time of our birth.

We have inherited wisdom, culture and conduct from our ancestors. Had they remained in the caves in jungles, we would have done the same. Our dazzling material progress today is a result of their continuous efforts with thirst for knowledge. We should be proud of our culture, heritage, legacy and tradition. All this contributes to our cultural richness. So we are indebted to our ancestors for the inheritance of wisdom, culture and conduct from them. Also the social system offers us affection and security through relationships, health services, education and so many other things to elevate us above the status of being merely 'a social animal' and become persons. We owe our gratitude to society for this. The *vaidic*, therefore, has a sense of indebtedness towards society.

Our feeling of indebtedness to family, ancestors and heritage, eliminates the selfishness and selfcentredness in us. As a result the practice of *ashtanga yog* becomes smooth. The *shadripus* of *kama, krodha, lobha, mada, moha* and *matsara* are kept at bay due to the virtue acquired under the influence of the above principle of *yajna*. The *Manava Dharma* of *Manusmriti* makes us aware of the need for the *panchayajna*, five-fold sacrifice for Nature, for our family, for society, for our ancestors and for our culture and heritage. One becomes noble, modest and sublime in tendencies by being influenced by these principles of *yajna*. We have to acknowledge our indebtedness to them. Acknowledgement of indebtedness controls our natural propensities in our lives and selfishness is kept at bay. For the *vaidic*, this sense of indebtedness is quite spontaneous, and is none other than *yajna*.

According to *vedism*, each element of Nature has a presiding deity. Oblations are offered during sacrifice to the presiding deities or *devatas* of the five physical elements of Nature, viz. air, water, fire, space and earth. All the elements of nature are energized by the *devatas* like *Varuna Devata, Indra Devata*, etc. We are indebted to the constituents of Nature, and we owe all the deities for their celestial grace and support. The celestial grace of *Prithvi Devata, Vana Devata* or deity of forests, *Rudra Devata, Vasu Devata, Varuna Devata, Mano Devata*, the *Navagrahas*, bestow on us natural wealth for our existence and nourishment. The concept of *yajna* or sacrifice on the part of man has come up in the *vedic* tradition. *Deva yajna, manushya yajna, bhuta yajna* are some types of *yajnas*. The celestial grace of these *devatas* descends on us by our offering of oblations.

The acceptance of the principle of *yajna* takes precedence over the perfunctory performance of the rituals. The principles of *yajna*, all *sattvik* qualities of nobility, modesty, sublimity, gratitude, selflessness, *tyaga*, distaste for sense gratification, generosity, etc., qualify the *sadhaka* for the practice of the principles of *yama* and *niyama*.

Dana

The second feature of the *Vedic Samskriti* is *dana*. *Dana* is the nature, tendency and action of gifting. One develops the sublime nature of parting with what one possesses to someone who needs it. Gifting away something not wanted by us is not real *dana*. When one is influenced by the principle of *dana*, petty-mindedness and selfishness are kept aside. The tendency of our age is towards possessiveness. Man's avarice is unending. To restrain this tendency,

74

a portion of our earnings should be given in charity. Our *Dharma* and tradition have laid stress on this noble principle. It is pertinent to recall an anecdote from the *Upanishads*.

Prajapati Brahma, the Creator, was approached by his three descendents, gods, humans and demons. All three of them sought his counsel. *Brahma* initiated them into the word *'Da'*. All the three construed the word rightly. The gods felt that they were required to subdue or effect the *da-mana* of their craving for the enjoyments of Heaven, and that the word meant *damana*. The demons thought that since they behaved like wicked brutes, the word *'Da'* meant *daya* or compassion for them. Humans felt that since their selfish desire to amass wealth was to be controlled by gifting a part of their earnings, the word meant *dana*.

Thus *dana* has great significance for man. It is natural to accumulate wealth for one's own sake, but it is obligatory to gift at least 10% to 20% of our earnings. The practice of *dana* enables one to overcome selfishness, petty-mindedness and possessiveness, thus providing a good antidote to the modern self-centredness.

At this juncture one has to bear in mind the words of the *Gita*. The *Bhagavadgita* has mentioned three classes of *yajna* and *dana*. These are the *sattvic*, *rajasic* and *tamasic* types. It is the *saattvic yajna* which is required to be inculcated. In the 11th *shloka* of the 17th chapter, the Lord says:

अफलाकांक्षिभि: यज्ञ: विधिदृष्ट: य: इज्यते ।
यष्टव्यम् एव इति मन: समाधाय स: सात्त्विक: ।।

In the *sattvic yajna* nothing is aimed at in return. This is in accordance with the injunctions of the *vedas* and the *shastras*. The sacrificial ritual has to be performed with selflessness and single-minded devotion. This attitude bestows nobility, loftiness, contentment, peace and tranquillity of mind to the *yajamana*, the propitiator or patron. In the 12th *shloka* of the same chapter, are described the characteristics of the *rajasic yajna*:

अभिसंधाय तु फलं दम्भार्थम् अपि चैव यत् ।
इज्यते भरतश्रेष्ठ तं यज्ञं विद्धि राजसम् ।।

The Lord tells *Arjuna* that *raajasic yajna* is showy and ostentatious. It is performed with the aim of obtaining material fruits of the sacrifice. *Tamasic yajna* is of a still inferior type. The 13th shloka in the same chapter describes *tamasic yajna:*

विधिहीनम् असृष्टान्नं मंत्रहीनम् अदक्षिणम् ।
श्रद्धाविरहितं यज्ञं तामसं परिचक्षते ।।

This *tamasic yajna* is not according to the injunction of the *shastras.* It is performed without oblations for the sacrificial fire. Due gifts are not given to the *brahmanas.* There is no sanctity, *shraddha* or devotion. This description will give an idea of the spirit with which a *sattvic yajna* has to be performed.

Coming to the principle of *daana*, this is also of three types, *sattvic, rajasic* and *tamasic.* Chapter 17, *shloka* 20, of the *Bhagavadgita* speaks of *saatvic daana* as follows:

दातव्यम् इति यद् दानं दीयते अनुपकारिणे ।
देशे काले च पात्रे च तद् दानं सात्त्विकं स्मृतम् ।।

That *dana* arising out of a sense of duty-mindedness, which is given in a proper place and time to a worthy person from whom no reciprocation is expected, is held to be *sattvic. Chapter* 17, *shloka* 21, describes *rajasic dana.*

यत् तु प्रत्युपकारार्थं फलम् उद्दिश्य वा पुन: ।
दीयते च परिक्लिष्टं तद् दानं राजसं स्मृतम् ।।

The *dana* done by causing agony, intimidation or offence to the beneficiary and also with expectation of reciprocity is *rajasic*. The 22nd *shloka* of the same chapter describes the *tamasic dana*.

अदेशकाले यद् दानं अपात्रेभ्य: च दीयते ।
असत्कृतं अवज्ञातं तत् तामसम् उदाहृतम् ।।

The *dana* done without bestowing due honour, which is wrongly timed, wrongly placed, wrongly conditioned, wrongly situated and done to the undeserving persons is *tamasic*. The beneficiary is demeaned or insulted here.

Tapas

Having noted the characteristics of the *vedic* principles of *yajna* and *dana*, we will turn our attention to *tapas*. *Tapas* or austerity, restrains the animal tendencies in man. Man is usually sub-human in his tendencies, and his conduct is brought to the normal plain of human qualities, where he is expected to be. This is accorded by the practices of *tapas*. *Tapas* works like a sculptor for carving man out of the subhuman. *Tapas* develops the mind as well as the body. The mind and senses are restrained, purified and sublimated by *tapas*. In chapter 17 of the *Bhagavadgita* there are three means of pursuing the practice of austerities. The 14th *shloka* explains and describes the *sharira tapas* :

देवद्विजगुरुप्राज्ञपूजनं शौचं आर्जवम् ।
ब्रह्मचर्यं अहिंसा च शारीरं तप उच्यते ।।

Revering, honouring, worshipping gods, preceptors and the wise and virtuous is *tapas* of the body. So also, practising candidness and celibacy, purity and piety in conduct and character is *sharira tapas*. *Shloka* 15 describes *vangmaya* or *vachika tapas* :

अनुद्वेगकरं वाक्यं सत्यं प्रियहितं च यत् ।

स्वाध्यायाभ्यसनं चैव वाङ्मयं तप उच्यते ।।

Our speech should be pacifying, soft, truthful, affectionate and soothing. We should perform *vedashastra adhyayanam* and practise *nama japa* ceaselessly. So the organ of speech must be involved in righteous deeds. This is *vangmaya tapas* i.e. *tapas* of speech.

The *manasic tapas* is mentioned in the 16th *shloka* :

मन:प्रसाद: सौम्यत्वं मौनम् आत्मविनिग्रह: ।

भावसंशुद्धि: इति एतत् तप: मानसम् उच्यते ।।

Manasic tapas is to try to make the mind placid, pleasant, sober and mild. Performing *Bhagavadchintanam,* that is meditation on God, with controlled and pure mind for attaining peace and tranquillity is *manasic tapas. Mauna*, abstaining from speech helps this *tapas*.

Lord *Krishna* says in the 24th and 25th *shlokas* of the 17th chapter, about *yajna, dana and tapas;*

तस्मात् ओम् इति उदाहृत्य यज्ञदानतप:क्रिया: ।

प्रवर्तन्ते विधानोक्ता: सततं ब्रह्मवादिनाम् ।।

तत् इति अनभिसंधाय फलं यज्ञतप:क्रिया: ।

दानक्रियाश्च विविधा: क्रियन्ते मोक्षकांक्षिभि: ।।

It is essential that the direction and endeavour of the *sadhaka* must be towards attaining the values of life based on the *yajna, dana* and *tapas* and only then would it be possible to commence *ashtanga yog.*

Sadhana

We will now examine the different stages in *sadhana*. The beginning stage known as the *arambhavastha* has to be understood by the neophyte who is eager to start practice. The neophyte must ideally take up an extensive and elaborate scheme of practice so that it is *sarvasparsha* (omni-dimensional), comprehensive and circumspect. The teacher or the preceptor must schematize the instruction so that a firm, extensive, deep, comprehensive and elaborate foundation is provided to the *sadhaka* for the practice of *ashtanga yog*.

The *sadhana* must essentially be *sattvic*, consisting of

(1) *Kayika* (of the body)

(2) *Vachika* (of the speech)

(3) *Manasika* (of the mind)

The endeavour must comprise of bodily and mental involvements. It should be noted here that the involvement of mind is primarily of the nature of thought and we are conversant with the expression 'thoughtful practices'. Thoughts are a subtle form of speech itself. Rather, our tradition divides speech in four parts—*para, pashyanti, madhyama* and *vaikhari*. Thoughts are *madhyama,* as a form of silent speech. Thus it is expected here that one should intently and consciously apply the speech to *sadhana* apart from body and mind. This will ensure complete involvement in practices. This complete involvement is composed of physical, psychological, mental, emotional and intellectual nature. This entails an integral approach which is consistent with the precepts of the *Gita*.

The neophyte has a *sadhana* of three aspects, viz.,

(1) *Satsanga sadhana*   (2) *Sadhanasanga sadhana*

(3) *Shastrasanga sadhana*

These are the three instruments each of which comprises the *kayika, vachika* and *manasika* aspects, in which the *sattvic* content is the most important. These three instruments must be influenced by association and application of the principles of *yajna, dana* and *tapas*. It further implies *sadhusanga* or *santasanga* which is association with saintly and wise people, as such persons augment *the sattva guna*. *Satsanga* also demands *sattvic ahara, sattvic vihara, sattvic achaara* and *sattvic vichara*, thus resulting in a large inflow of *sattva guna*. If such saintly people are not around, their books are treasures of their life blood and spirit in the form of gospels. They are *satsanga* itself.

Sadhanasanga consists in practising the principles of *yajna, dana* and *tapas*. *Sadhana* comprises of *shama sadhana, dama sadhana, tapas sadhana, japa sadhana, dhyana sadhana, titiksha sadhana, abhyasa sadhana, vairagya sadhana* and *uparati* (abstinence from sexual acts) *sadhana*. After having been influenced by the principles of *yajna, dana* and *tapas* one should assimilate and practise these principles.

In *shastrasanga* one gets influenced by the Scriptures which refer to *yajna, dana* and *tapas*. The *sadhaka* is presumed to be a student of the *shastras*. *Shastrasanga* comprises of the study of *vedic Dharmashastra, Vedas, Vedashastra, Dharmashastra, Karmashastra, Yogshastra, Puranas, Upanishads, Gita, Santasahitya* and *Adhyatmashastra*.

We will now take up a detailed study of *kayika, vachika and manasika sadhana*. First, we will discuss *satsanga*.

Shri Krishnaarpanam astu.

80

Discourse 7

Patanjala Sadhana 2

Satsanga

We will now try to understand the meaning of *satsanga*, and also what one needs to do for developing *satsanga*. The modes of *satsanga* are *sadhusanga, sattvic ahara, sattvic vihara, achara* and *vichara*. *Satsanga* helps to develop the disposition of *yajna, dana* and *tapas*. The mind starts gravitating towards these principles with an intrinsic motive. Normatively these principles are hard to practise. They would become severe disciplines but with *satsanga* the process is naturalized. We require to develop contact with the principles of *yajna, dana* and *tapas*. It implies contact with noble and saintly people, which should be constant and lasting. These principles instil and augment noble principles in our lives.

The *vaidic* culture recognizes the importance of *satsanga*, which is the first aspect of *sadhana*. The literature of saints can also be viewed as *satsanga*. Thus, there is no dearth of means for acquiring *sattvic achara*. *sattvic vihara* also becomes possible by visiting various holy centers of pilgrimage. The importance of *sattvic ahara*, too, cannot be overstressed. Marathi people chant a *shloka* before starting to eat their meals, 'उदर भरण नोहे । जाणिजे यज्ञकर्म ।' "Food is godly. So eating is not just filling the belly. It is a kind of *yajna*." This food is an offering in the altar of the gastric fire or *jatharagni*. Just as in a ritualistic sacrifice substances are offered with consecration and bounties are received from heavens, so here, too, the food is offered in the gastric fire and then nutrients, energies and powers required for sustenance are attained. Thus the ingested food must be like offering in *yajna* and should not be devoured gluttonously.

This is a lofty concept in our culture. The discrimination between what to eat and what not to eat can be found in this concept. The food that we eat does not merely consist in the usual two meals of the day. This concept includes the nourishment not only of the body but also of the mind, emotion and intellect. Through *satvika ahara* the mind is flooded with *satva*, i.e. "an influx of *sattvaguna*" takes place. Hence the *sattvic* characteristic is augmented by the *satsangasadhana*.

Sadhana - Sanga

The second aspect of *sadhana* is *sadhanasanga*. It may be noted here that *satsanga* puts a seed of disposition in the mind which is required for *yajna, dana* and *tapas* while *sadhanasanga* evolves and enriches it. One is expected to exercise a sacrifice, *tyaga*-the act of giving up something with reverence and in the light of indebtedness for the sake of something considered more worthy, for the sake of Nature or society or family or race or cultural heritage or humanity or God. The sacrifice itself is a *sadhana*. For this, one needs to practise *yajna, dana* and *tapas*. The *sadhana* in *sadhanasanga* also means the practice of the integrated *ashtanga yog*. The *ashtangas* are *yama, niyama, asana, pranayama, pratyahara, dharana, dhyana* and *samadhi*. There has to be a scheme of *shama sadhana, dama sadhana, Nama, japa, mantra, Omkara sadhana*. These are the *sadhanas* for sense-control and reformation, and control of the mind. Although the path of *sadhana* is always fraught with hurdles this scheme unexpectedly reduces them. The mean, mundane tendencies and fleeting nature of mind is naturally curbed. Thus what at the beginning seemed difficult does not remain difficult when one gets going. Thus the process of the positive transformation commences and the *sadhaka* experiences blossoming of his good fortune and happiness, *shatsampatti*. *Shatsampatti* are *shama, dama, titiksha, uparati, jnana vairagya* and *shanti samadhana*. *Shama* is mental restraint, *dama* is sensory restraint, *titiksha* is tolerance and forbearance, *uparati* is losing taste for sensual pleasures and *jnana vairagya* is spiritual knowledge and thirstlessness. *Shanti samadhana* is peace, tranquility and content. When they are engendered, *sadhana* gets on a fast track. In the light of this description one is expected to look into the concept of *kayika, vachika* and *manasika tapas* of the *Gita*. There should be some volitional restraints like *vairagya*, steadfastness and consistency in practice for reformation and discipline. *kayika tapa- tapa* of the body, *vachika tapa- tapa* of the speech and *manasika tapa- tapa* of the mind are prescribed there. For understanding this practice, the *sadhaka* requires to have an experienced and realized preceptor. *Abhyasa sadhana* is an effort to make the mind quiet. *Vairagya sadhana* overcomes the craze and delirium in the mind and subjugates the sensual tendencies.

Shastrasanga

In the third aspect of *sadhana*, i.e. *shastrasanga*, one must look into the *shastras*, spiritual texts, for *yajna, dana* and *tapas*. The science, rationale and mode of *yajna, dana* and *tapas* are to be traced in the *shastras*. The *sadhaka* should recognize the importance of *Dharmashastra, Karmashastra* and *Adhyatmashastra* as they greatly influence the mind-set. The study of the *Bhagavadgita*, the *Upanishads* and the *Puranas* contribute infinitely to educate and evolve the mind of the *sadhaka*. The lucid and thought-provoking literature of the saints gives us a fountain of *satvaguna*, it offers a double benefit i. e. *satsanga* and *shastrasanga*.

Therefore the trio of *sadhana* consists of *satsanga, sadhanasanga* and *shastrasanga*.

83

All the above *sadhanas* are *kayika, vachika* and *manasika*, of the body, mind and speech, and *prana* constitutes all these *sadhanas*. *Prana* is behind all these aspects. The physiodynamics constitutes the action of the body (*kayika*) and hence comprises of the contribution and involvement of the body in the endeavour. The psychodynamics constitutes the action of the mind (*manasika)* and its faculties are perception, sensation, conception and memory. Mind is involved in the endeavour. The biodynamics involves the action of *prana* and the breath in any of its endeavours which are unique to *yog* and *Adhyatma*.

Thus all these *sadhanas* comprise of:

Physiodynamics [*kayik*]

Psychodynamics [*manasik*] and

Biodynamics. [*pranik*]

Well known saints like Kabir, Gora Kumbhar, Sena Nhavi, Savata Mali performed their daily tasks in the *adhyatmik* way. The devotees integrated their *panch pranas* with their activities. Interestingly, even the moral, ethical, mental, intellectual, volitional and reflective characteristics of their tasks were based on *pranic* dynamics, and biodynamics makes the tasks *pranic*. We have to identify the practices that evolve the *adhyatmic dharana* in life. The same set of practices can evolve all the *yamas*. For instance, the practices for *ahimsa* will also stand good for *satya, asteya, brahmacharya* etc.

Ahimsa in the Yamas

Ahimsa and *himsa* is really a vital subject. The contemporary world is facing horrifying *himsa* or violence everywhere. Certainly the world would be full of immense happiness if only violence is eradicated. The more said about violence, the less would it be.

Ahimsa is normally understood as not hurting any living being physically. This is a gross form of *ahimsa*. However there can be subtle forms of *himsa*. Even a superficial analysis will show that *ahimsa* and *himsa* can be *kayika, vachika* and *manasika*. A *yog sadhaka* has to guard himself from all these forms of *himsa*. *Ahimsa* involves the gradational practice of control of the physical body, control of speech and checking the thoughts of *himsa*. *Himsa* also means showing contempt for others, entertaining unreasonable dislike for or prejudice towards them, frowning at or hating, abusing, speaking ill of others, backbiting are some forms of violence. Vilifying, harbouring thoughts of hatred, uttering lies, trying to ruin somebody in any way whatsoever, are kinds of violence. We should take note of one fact here. The *himsaka* person is sometimes doing *himsaa* by going against his nature, and then he is torturing himself through his conscience. So he is *himsaka* for himself, too. Violence can be suggested and done by movements of the body, facial gestures, eyes even. The sword of the tongue is sharper than a real sword. *Himsaka* words are fiercer than fire itself. Ignoring somebody who wants and needs your attention, it may be intentional or unawares, can be violence for that person. The insulted person's reaction can be furious or malicious. This subtle form of violence can create a vicious cycle of malice in the world. Ignored children in the family who starve for attention prove a menace for the society around. *Ahimsa* is thus avoiding all kinds of killing, offending, injuring, agitating, disturbing, perturbing, ruffling and upsetting others. Hence *ahimsa* is more than a saintly quality.

Of course, it is true that the mind-set of *ahimsa* has to be ingrained. Such a mind does not allow the fire of *himsa* but puts it out with showers of love and affection. The mode of practising *ahimsa* will therefore comprise of *satsanga, sadhanasanga, shastrasanga*. The *satsanga* consists in developing company with *saattvic* people. All associations and intakes of body, mind and senses should be *sattvic*. *Sattvic ahara, sattvic vihara, sattvic achara* and *sattvic vichara* are the *sadhana* for *ahimsa*. It is an amusing thing that we have to do *himsa* of *himsa* so as to bring in *ahimsa*. Even God had to incarnate in human form to do *himsa* of evil people. In the *Gita*, the Lord has said :

परित्राणाय साधूनां विनाशाय च दुष्कृताम् ।
धर्मसंस्थापनार्थाय संभवामि युगे युगे ॥ (4 : 8)

For the proper establishment of *Dharma*, righteousness, and for protection of the saintly, it is necessary to destroy evil and the *shadripus* of the mind. The Lord incarnates Himself as *Rama* and *Krishna* for the destruction of evil in this world. The seed of *ahimsa* lies in cultivating the *sattvic guna* and the avoidance of the *rajo* and *tamo gunas*. *Himsaka* tendencies do not sprout when *shadripus* are eliminated.

We will now try to understand the *sadhanasanga* for *himsa* and the means to counter the *himsa* tendency. The *sadhana* consists of endeavour, effort and a scheme of practice for that effort. Besides the involvement of the endeavour and effort, there should be some sort of restraint. Hence the *ahimsa sadhana* consists of

1.   Endeavour [*prayatna*]

2.   Repeated practice [*abhyasa*]

3.   Observances [*niyama*]

4.   Restraints [*nigraha*]

Ahimsa being a *yogic* principle, is not merely a moral, ethical principle. *Ahimsa*, here, is a step in *yama*, and is to be practised by mitigating the physiology, biochemistry and neurology of *himsa*. There are *asanas* which can work towards this end. *Pranayama, bandhas, kriyas* and *mudras* can work to migitate the tendency and impulse of *himsa* and evolve the nature of *ahimsa*. The *panchaprana* management means management of five pranas viz., *prana, apana, vyana, udana* and *samana* provide a scheme of *pranic* management. Without imbibing the fundamental process for the development of *ahimsa*, i.e. restraining the tendencies and impulses which cause *himsa*, is like taking up swimming with a heavy load tied on the back. *Yogashastra* not only prescribes norms but also gives sets of practices to develop the potential of virtuosity. *Asanas* are one of the ways to counter the *shadripus*. *Yogasanas* such as *halasana, sarvangasana*, and some forward bending postures like *janushirshasan*, can mitigate the aggressive tendencies. The physiology can be softened and cooled down.

Shastrasanga, the third component of practice, which is the same as *mokshashastrasanga*, comprises of the study and reflection of the sacred texts and scriptures, which raise *ahimsa* to greater heights. The *svadhyaya* (self-study), the *shastra adhyayanam*, study of *shastrika* texts, the *shastra vimarshanam*, reflection on sacred texts of *dharmashastra, yogshastra, adhyatmashastra, Gitashastra, karmashastra, Upanishads* and writings of saints, play an invaluable role in infusing nobility, sublimity, contentment, peace and magnanimity of mind.

The other four Yamas

The other four principles of *yama* are *satya, asteya, brahmacharya* and *aparigraha*. The scheme of practice of *ahimsa* so far explained was based on *shanti samadhana*, peace and contentment, *adhyatmadharana* or spiritual mindset and

87

shadripuhananam, destroying the six foes of the mind-*kama, krodha, lobha, moha, mada* and *matsara.*

On the basis of this scheme, one can conveniently have the structure of *satyasadhana, asteyasadhana, brahmacharyasadhana,* and *aparigrahasadhana.* The intensity of *satva* helps these *yamas* to evolve. This makes the role of *satsanga, sadhanasanga* and *shastrasanga* for each of the aforesaid four *yamas* clear for us. The pursuit of the principles of *satya, asteya, brahmacharya,* and *aparigraha* also include *kayika, vachika* and *manasika tapas* as it is in the case of *ahimsa.* Hostile forces make their power felt at all these three levels, which can be described as the "*pathology of vitarkas*" or vicious tendencies. *Patanjali* has cited this notion in the scheme of *yogshastra,* in which the *kayika, vachika* and *manasika* aspects are involved in the steps of *satya, asteya, brahmacharya* and *aparigraha.* In such an endeavour it is possible to achieve the stage of *pranic* management also. Each of the *yamas* contributes mainly to tranquillity of the mind which is a very important desirable condition, and *yogsadhana* is none other than the effort and endeavour to achieve this goal. However, the five *yamas* cannot be accomplished without *vairagya* or dispassion. Every *sadhaka* has to realize that this is a *sine qua non* of the endeavour.

The Five Niyamas

In the next stage of *ashtanga sadhana,* we have the *niyamas* in which the *satva* content requires to be augmented. The *niyamas* comprise *shaucha,* cleanliness and purity, *santosha,* contentment, *tapas,* austerity, *svadhyaya,* self-study, spiritual study and *upasana* and *Ishvarapranidhana,* theism, deism and divinism. *Shaucha* implies both external and internal purity, *santosha* is an attitude of contentment, *tapas* implies control of the senses for *Atmic shuddhi,* svadhyaya is *mantropasana* and other devotional practices, and *Ishvarapranidhana* is faith in the Almighty and involves the worship of *Ishvara*.

Shuddhi and *pavitryam* is *shaucha*. *Shaucha* is to be practised on the three fronts of *kayika*, on the plane of the body, *vachika*, on the plane of speech and *manasika*, on the plane of mind. *Shaucha* is not merely practice of hygiene of the body but also working for *shuddhi* and *pavitrya*. Water and soap can cleanse the body and also give purity to the mind, which is *shaucham*. *Nama sadhana*, *japa sadhana* and prayers bestow sacredness both to body and mind. The *asana kriya, pranayama kriya, bandha kriya* and *prana kriyas* help cleanse the body and confer organic cleanliness and purity.

Yog technology has an excellent practical scheme of *pranic* cleansing. All the *pranic* channels, the gross, subtle and the causal bodies are cleansed, purified and consecrated by the *Omkara mantra*, *namasadhana*, and *japasadhana*. The *shastras* declare :

अपवित्र: पवित्रो वा सर्वावस्थां गतोऽपि वा ।
य: स्मरेत् पुंडरीकाक्षं स बाह्याभ्यंतरशुचि: ।।

Remembrance of *Pundarikaksha, Krishna*, purifies one internally and externally. In short, *shaucha niyama* is attained by proper *achaara, vichara* and *ahara* involving *kayika shaucha, vacha shaucha* and *manasika shaucha*.

Santosha is the second *niyama*. The organic biochemical aspect of *santosha*, too, like *shaucha*, is evolved by the three modes of *satsanga, sadhanasanga* and *shastrasanga*. It is psychomentally developed by devotional *puja* and *archa*. The literature of saints such as *Jnaneshwari, Dasabodha* is full of noble qualities. Saints love all living beings without any kind of discrimination. So the reading of it pacifies our minds and greatly contributes to *santosha*. Regular practice of this *niyama* makes the mind lofty, sedate and sublime. *Santosha* acts like a catalytic agent in *yogsadhana* whereas *asantosha* acts like a warping agent.

The third *niyama* is *tapas*. *Tapasadhana* is at the centre of *adhyatmasadhana* as it empowers man for any accomplishment. *Tapas* is a *niyama* basically for *kamajaya*, i.e. for controlling our passions. The life of sage *Vishwamitra* relates to us the glory of the conquest of *kama*. Although not a *Brahmana*, *Vishwamitra* attained *Brahma Teja*, glory of a true *brahmana* because of *tapas* and *kamajaya*. He conquered *kama*, passion and later *krodha* or anger and that is how he became a *Brahmarishi*. *Tapas* as described in the *Mahabharata* befits the *niyamanga tapas*. A story in the third *parva*, which is *vanaparva* in the *Mahabharata*, defines tapas as follows:

इंद्रियाणि एव संयम्य तपो भवति न अन्यथा ।

Restraint of the *indriyas* is a major factor of *tapas*. Austerity is of the nature of *indriyasamyama*. It is controlling the sensory and sensual tendencies. *Tapas* is described in the *Mahanarayanopanishada* thus :

ऋतं तप: सत्यं तप: शमस्तप: दमस्तप: शांतिस्तप: ।
भूर्भुव: स्व: तप: यज्ञस्तप: दानं तप: ब्रह्म तप: ॥

Rutam is *Tapa*-to follow Reality is austerity.

Satyam is *Tapa*-to follow Truth is austerity.

Shama-restraint of mind, *dama*-restraint of the senses, *Bhurbhuvasvaha-Vyahritis*,mystic words of worship, *Yajna*-sacrifice or *Tyag, Dana*-charity or munificience, *Brahmacharya*-chastity,-all these constitute austerity.

The *Bhagavadgita* gives a beautiful exposition of *Tapas* for the *yog sadhaka* which serves the purpose of the *tapasadhana* of *niyama*. The *tapas* is *sharirika*, of the body, *vachika*, of speech and *manasika*, of the mind. Each of these is *satvika*, *rajasika* and *tamasika*, the relative proportions of which speak of the nature, grade and calibre of the *tapas*. The *satvika tapas* is worthy of praise, supreme in nature and the highest in grade and calibre.

The 14th *shloka* of the 17th chapter of the *Gita*, *sharira tapa*, austerity of the body is thus defined :

देवद्विजगुरुप्राज्ञपूजनं शौचं आर्जवम् ।
ब्रह्मचर्यं अहिंसा च शारीरं तप उच्यते ।।

Sharira tapas involves the worshipping of the noble ones, *Shaucham* is the purity of the external body, organic purity and hygienic purity. It also means celibacy on the physical plane, *ahimsa*, practice of non-violence and non-agitation.

There are also oral and vocal kinds of *tapas*. They are defined in the 15th *shloka* in this way :

अनुद्वेगकरं वाक्यं सत्यं प्रियहितं च यत् ।
स्वाध्यायाभ्यसनं चैव वाङ्मयं तप उच्यते ।।

If speech is soothing, truthful, pleasing and creates well-being, also if it is engaged in studies and *sadhana* it is *vangmaya tapas*.

Jnaneshwar describes a *vak-tapasvi*, an accomplished *sadhaka* of speech, in the 222nd *shloka* of the 17th chapter of *Jnaneshwari*:

ऋग्वेदादि तीन्ही । प्रतिष्ठिजती वाग् भुवनी ।
केली जेवी वदनी । ब्रह्मशाळा ।।

He is one who has learnt the *Rig Veda* and the other *Vedas* by heart so well ,that his mouth seems to be a *Brahmashala*, a resort of *Vedashastra*, a spiritual school.

According to the *shloka* 16 of the *Bhagavadgita*, *manasic tapas*, is as follows :

मन:प्रसाद: सौम्यत्वं मौनं आत्मविनिग्रह: ।
भावसंशुद्धि: इति एतत् तप मानस उच्यते ॥

To attain a peaceful, quiet, placid, sublime state, to observe spiritual and ritual observance of silence, to have the reins of the mind under control, to develop emotional purity and devotion in the mind is *manasa tapa*.

In short, we can say that *tapas* for the *sadhaka* is like fire for gold, it tests him, burns his impurities, makes him precious and leads him to divinity.

In the next topic, we will consider the intrinsic nature of *tapas*, in accordance with the *sattvic, rajasic* and *tamasic* modes.

Shri Krishnaarpanam astu

✛ ✛ ✛

Discourse 8

Patanjala Sadhana - 3

More about Tapas

The *Bhagavadgita* in Chapter 17 describes the *sattvic* mode, the *raajasic* mode and the *tamasic* mode of *tapas* in the following *shlokas* :

श्रद्धया परया तप्तं तपस्तत् त्रिविधं नरै: ।
अफलाकांक्षिभि: युक्ते: सात्त्विकं परिचक्षते ।।   (17 : 17)

The *tapas* which shines with supreme *shraddha,* faith, and performed properly by men without any expectations of fruits or returns is called *sattvic*. It is of three kinds — *kayic, vachic* and *manasic*.

सत्कारमानपूजार्थं तपो दम्भेन चैव यत् ।
क्रियते तदिह प्रोक्तं राजसम् चलम् अध्रुवम् ।।   (17 : 18)

In the *rajasic* mode, *tapas* is done with expectation of some felicitation, returns, honours and worship. The person does it with a view to increase self-importance. It is performed with ostentation. It has no steadiness or firmness.

The *tamasic tapas* is described :

मूढग्राहेण आत्मनो यत् पीडया क्रियते तप: ।
परस्य उत्सादनार्थं वा तत् तामसम् उदाहृतम् ।।   (17 : 19)

When austerities are performed to agonize, agitate, trouble, vex and persecute others, it is *tamasic tapas*. The person is not in the right mind and troubles himself, too.

We see such people who pluck their own hair and torment themselves. *Patanjali* provides an unambiguous direction for *tapas*.

93

He refers to *tapas* as the nature of *dvandva sahanam*, that means ability to withstand dualities such as, honour and dishonour, loss and gain, heat and cold, delight and sorrow. Developing tolerance towards dualities and polarities, developing constancy in dualities and remaining unperturbed is *tapas*. This is the direction given by *Patanjali.* Dualities are on two planes viz., physical and mental. Dualities on the physical plane relate to the body, such as, heat and cold, well-being and diseased state, healthy and unhealthy state. To develop equilibrium in these states of polarities is *tapas.*

Control of food habits is one of the most important modes of practising *tapas,* because food is connected with the body, mind, intellect, senses and organs. Observing strict food habits occupies a central place in the practice of *tapas.* Food greatly influences body and mind. It is said 'आहारशुद्धौ सत्त्वशुद्धि:' Pure food results in pure *satva* in a person. It is further said 'अन्नमयो हि सौम्यमना:' Sattvic food influences the making of a *sattvic* mind. Therefore, the importance of observing control over food habits cannot be overstressed.

The various aspects of *yog sadhana* must be regulated and practised diligently, sincerely and unfailingly. *Tapas* is the best principle for understanding the integral nature of *yogsadhana.* Without *tapas* the *sadhana* cannot be integral. Although *tapas* is only one of the *niyamas* in *ashtangayog,* it is the main constituent of all the other *niyamas,* viz., *shaucha sadhana, santosha sadhana, svadhyaya sadhana,* and *Ishvarapranidhana sadhana.* There has to be discipline, regularity, and an uncompromising will requiring austerity. There is also an element of *tapas,* in the adherence to all the *yamas* – *ahimsa, satya, asteya, brahmacharya* and *aparigraha. Tapas* can therefore be identified as an important constituent fabric in the observance of the aforesaid principles. For example, *satyam* should be *anudvegakara*, i.e., which causes no excitement, and which is truthful, beneficial and pleasant. The adherence to the other aspects of *sadhana* that form a part of *tapas* and that need to be carried out diligently, sincerely and unfailingly are *asana sadhana, japa sadhana, dhyana sadhana,* etc. There is an integration of *yajna, dana* and *tapas* manifested in the *yogsadhana.*

The sense of *yajna*, sacrifice i.e. *tyaga*, the sense of *dana*, generosity, and the sense of *tapas*, austerity, are the constituents of any aspect of *yog.* The sense of *yajna* is *tyagavritti*, renunciation. *Danavritti* is the opposite of accumulation of wealth. *Yajna, dana* and *tapas* should be free from impurity. It is only when these three blocks are involved in raising the structure would the *yogsadhana* be considered genuine and authentic. We have seen that *tapas* is one of the most effective principles of *yog sadhana. Yog sadhana* is a *vrata*, a religious observance, an uncompromising observance or a vow,- a sum total of all the *vratas* or penance. *Vrata* and *tapas* are actually the two sides of the same coin. A *sadhaka* must adhere to vows of *shama, shaucha, santosha, Ishvarapranidhana,* and also of all the *yamas* and *niyamas.* He must also adhere to the vows of *yajna, dana* and *tapas.* These vows reinforce his *sadhana* and introduce substance to it. With *yajna, dana* and *tapas,* the *ashtanga niyama sadhana* is rendered easy for attainment.

Svadhyaya

Many times we are severely distressed with questions. Who am I? Where do I come from? What is all this as it seems? Why am I like this? Why am I here in this world? What is my role here? The questions are endless and without answers. But very soon our questions die down and we forget them in the hustle and bustle of life. Very few are like the *Buddha* who renounced all happiness of this world and set out to the forest in search of answers. A *yog sadhaka* may not give up this world but he pursues these questions. This is known as self-enquiry. Self-enquiry is the basic aspect of *svadhyaya*. *Svadhyaya* pertains to self-study and this questioning is the study of the self.

We shall now consider the *svadhyaya* aspect of *niyama*. *Svadhyaya* is the fourth *niyama*. This *sadhana* comprises of: *Pranava japa sadhana*, or *Omkar sadhana* is also *svadhyaya*. *Ishtadevata upasana* which is worship of one's personal deity is also *svadhyaya*. *Mantra upasana, Nama upasana, devata upasana, dharmashastra adhyayana, karmashastra adhyayana, adhyayana of any of these,- Gitashastra, Mokshashastra, Veda* and *Vedanta* or *santasahitya* is *svadhyaya*.

This is how *svadhyaya* is comprehensively constituted with regard to *ashtanga yog*.

Self-study is the core aspect of *svadhyaya*. Its main objective is to make the individual look inwards and make the mind less outgoing. It helps the *sadhaka* to rise above the tendencies of the flesh. He is influenced by the reality that he is much more than a mere mass of flesh. By *svadhyaya sadhana*, he comes out of the tendencies of the flesh because he realizes that he is the Self, the Soul. I-ness and mine-ness of the mind are given up. Introspection is extremely vital in the practice of *asana, pranayama, bandhas, mudras, kriyas,* etc. Without introspection they are not *yogsadhana*. The *sadhaka* obtains an insight and circumspection with these practices thus giving vital sensitivity and refinement in practice.

The *Pranava upasana* is another aspect of *svadhyaya*. "OM" is the divine touchstone in this *sadhana*. The basic roots in the form of

96

yajna, dana and *tapas*, become meaningful and fruitful when *Pranava upasana* is practised. According to the *Bhagavadgita, yajna, dana* and *tapas* are to be practised with *"Hari Om Tat Sat"*. The *Pranava upasana* is none other than *Ishvarapranidhana*. 'समाधिसिद्धि: ईश्वरप्रणिधानात्', states *Patanjali* in his *yogsutras*. *Ishtadevata upasana* or worship of the personal deity is also a form of *svadhyaya*. Devotion to one's personal deity gives a unique quality of faith and dedication in the *sadhana*. The *sadhaka* becomes noble, august and magnanimous with *Pranava sadhana*. The *Pranava sadhana* develops a keen sense of discrimination between right and wrong and it also develops a feeling for the study of *dharmashastra*. *Dharmashastra adhyayanam* helps develop a right sense of duty or duty-mindedness. *Dharmashastra* involves a study of *karmashastra*, and *Gitashastra*, which is none other than *yogshastra*. This study creates nobleness, sublimity and a tinge of philosophy in our life and conduct. *Mokshashastra* and *Vedvedanta* also work in a similar way. These studies instil essential values in the mind.

Another aspect of *svadhyaya* is : *Prakritishastra adhyayanam* which is the study of the Cosmos or the Universe, *Devdevatashastra* which is the study of the celestial forces which govern the terrestrial conditions. *Devatashastra* is the science of the gods and *jnanavijnana shastra* is the science of spiritual knowledge and spiritual experience.

These are all the salient aspects of *svadhyaya*, which provide versatility to our *sadhana*. In addition, the writings of saints is a significant supplementary incorporating *dharma*, knowledge, morality, *vairagya*, nobleness which are all uplifting and virtuous qualities.

In the *vaidic upasana* we have thirty-three *devatas* viz., the eight *Vasus*, twelve *Adityas*, eleven *Rudras*, *Indra* and *Prajapati*. There are in addition a further thirty-three crores. Why is it that so many

97

gods are worshipped instead of only one? *Yogshastra* tells us that just as man is constituted of the elements and the mind, he is also constituted of the celestial forces. All the senses and organs are governed by the *devatas*.

All these internal and external organs have their presiding deities who reside within man. This is the *yogic* perception. How all these *devatas* are present is beyond the understanding of the human mind. Man may not understand the work of the Almighty in creating these *devatas*. He might have done so because He considered they were indispensable. *Devata upasana* revamps the *sadhana* because of celestial grace. This is how *svadhyaya* works for rapid progress.

There is also the aspect of *Ishtadevata upasana* in *svadhyaya* which takes place with *panchangasevanam* of the personal deity (*Ishtadevata*). The personal deity is worshipped ritualistically, religiously, devotedly and with *panchangasevanam* which includes the following five aspects :

1. *Gita (Bhagavadgita, Suryagita, Shivagita, Devigita, Vishnugita, Ganeshagita.)*

2. *Sahasranam (Vishnu, Surya, Laxmi, Datta, Ganesha)*

3. *Stavana*

4. *Kavacham*

5. *Hridayam* of each *devata*.

The above five aspects represent the traditional method of *devata upasana*. It is the *vaidic* form of worship.

We now come to *Ishvarapranidhana* which is the fifth and last of the *Niyamas*. According to *Patanjali* it is the "all-granting component"- 'समाधिसिद्धि: ईश्वरप्रणिधानात्'. *Patanjali* mentions that *Ishvarapranidhana* can grant *samadhi* to a *yogi*. However, in the

98

sadhaka avastha or stage, it works as an *antaraya abhava* i.e. it works to weaken and remove the obstacles, impediments and limitations in the way of *sadhana.*

Ishvarapranidhaana

There are obstructions and other accompanying factors in the *sadhana* and all these are mitigated and nullified by *Ishvarapranidhana. Ishvarapranidhana* can take place in a particular mode for a *sadhaka.* It could be of one of the following several modes:

1. *Ishvarapujanam* or worshipping God
2. *Ishvarashravanam* or listening to the name of God
3. *Ishvaranamasankeertanam* or singing the glory of God
4. *Namasmaranam* or reciting the name of God
5. *Ishvarachintanam* or *vimarshana* on God, contemplating on God, *mananachintana* on God
6. *Ishvararpanakarma* or surrendering of all our deeds and karmas to God.

Prarthana, prayer is the most popular form of worshipping the Divinity. This prayer becomes a preamble to every auspicious act. Every action of the day is to be consecrated by *Bhagavannama,* name of God. It evolves the religious consciousness in the *sadhaka,* causing the process of *Ishvarapranidhana* to flourish. Thus, finally, it may be said that *yajna, dana* and *tapas* provide the ethos which is of great importance for *yogsadhana,* which becomes genuine, authentic and fructifying.

We now come to the *ashtanga asana sadhana. Asanas* are an extraordinary means of *ashtanga yog. Asanas* appear to be physical exercises. They seem to be mere body contortions, but this is only an appearance. Various psychological, mental, emotional and intellectual aspects are explored in the loci of *asanas*. The scope of *asanas* should not be limited merely to physical therapy. In this context the *yog sutra* '**योग: चित्तवृत्तिनिरोध: I**', becomes extremely pertinent. In all the *yogic* aspects we necessarily have the component of *chitta*, consciousness.

Asanas

We may consider, for example, the visual form of God in the idol. The importance of the idol or icon is usually decided by the external manifestation of its beauty. We check its sculpture, eyes, expression on the face and so on. But the real inner beauty of the visual form can be adjudged only by the devotee. He alone can evaluate the spiritual manifestation of the consecrated idol. In the same way, the *asanas* are to be seen not just as postures but as iconographic positions. The *asanas* thus induct the *sadhaka* to the esoteric physiology. They give lessons in esoteric physiology practically, notionally and experientially, and, therefore, are also considered as archetypal. So *asanas* are not mere postures but in essence they are iconographic and archetypal positions.

Asanas serve as a vast laboratory in exploring the dyad of the human body and mind. The performance of the *bandhas, mudras* and *kriyas* help explore the whole constitution of man. The body is made up of *tattvas* varying from grossness to subtleness, from the phenomenal to the extremely subtle to the suprasubtle. The management of the five elements or the *panchabhautika* management is effected through *asanas*. According to *samkhya* the body is composed of the five elements of *Prakriti*. It is also *panchatanmatrika*. That means it is composed of the five *tanmatras*- the subtle primary elements of *shabda, rasa, sparsha, rupa* and *gandha*. The inner man is formed out of these elements. *yog sadhana* helps a person to investigate the human anatomy and the mind and to understand the science of the esoteric body. According to the esoteric physiology, the psychomental faculties are embedded in the *chakras, nadis* and *panchapranas.* Modern medical science fails to identify these esoteric elements through its instruments. These can only be identified through the faithful practice of *asanas.* The mental conditions such as fear, courage, resilience, decisiveness, indecisiveness, timidity, patience, impatience, tolerance, intolerance and various mental states, whether positive or negative, have their loci within the body. For example, fear is somewhere in the embodiment, resilience is in the embodiment, all these have their loci at some place in the embodiment. *Asanas* assist in overcoming the negative states and conditions of the mind and achieve the positive conditions of the mind. The *asanas* also induct the *sadhaka* to the human body as a mind boggling natural machine. It is a non mechanical machine made up by God. It is a glorious creation of God. The physical and physiological body is a transmechanical machine.

Asanas, therefore, work in giving some basic, fundamental and vital lessons in bio-dynamics, physiodynamics and psychodynamics. Through *asanas* there is also the *saptadhatu* management, *tridosha* management and *panchaprana* management. *Asanas* induct us into the esoteric aspect and help us to explore the loci of the mind, intelligence and various other faculties rooted in the *shatchakras.* All these lessons are extremely fascinating and awe-inspiring.

Asanas also give a very vital lesson and visions in various 'forms of actions' as obviously *asanas* seem to be some actions of the body. Something is done with the body. There are various forms of actions in *karma shastra,* and *asanas* serve as a glorious laboratory to understand these various forms of actions. It is said in the *Gita* 'न हि कश्चित् क्षणमपि जातु तिष्ठति अकर्मकृत् ।', (3 : 5) i.e., verily, none can ever remain even for a moment without performing some or the other action. *Asanas* induct us into another set of actions pertaining to the body, which are motor actions, perceptive actions, sensitive actions and reflex actions. These are:

1. Actions
2. Unactions
3. Inaction
4. Non-actions
5. Reactions
6. Counteraction
7. Complementary actions
8. Supplementary actions
9. Interactions
10. Transcendent actions.

Additionally, each action consists of several secondary effects. There can be no action without inaction. A negative action can contribute to a positive consequence.

Asanas also make us realize the *panchapranic kriya* i.e. *pranakriya, apanakriya, vyanakriya, samanakriya, udanakriya; panchabhutakriya* which means *agneya, jaliya, vayaviya, akashiya, parthiva; tridoshakriya* which means *vata, pitta, kapha;* and *trigunakriya* which are *sattvic, rajasic, tamasic. Asanas* give us a great insight into the relationship between body and mind, mind and *prana*, body and *prana,* body and breath, *prana* and breath. As the aforesaid principles are all interlaced in their manifestation, the

102

sadhaka realizes *prana* as the governor in the embodiment, and how all the other factors and faculties such as body, mind, senses, breath, emotions, intelligence, etc. are governed.

The *sadhaka,* while practising, learning, studying, trying, consolidating and maturing the *asanas,* gains an insight into innumerable aspects of learning, teaching and studying. All these processes in which the body, mind, breath, senses, *prana,* intelligence, emotions, sensations, perceptions and reflections are explored in the *asana* laboratory are thus to be studied in a unified state.

Shri Krishnaarpanam astu

✤ ✤ ✤

Discourse 9

Patanjala Sadhana 4

Scan the mind !

We have seen that *asanas* create an awe-inspiring and exhilarating experience in the unified *asana* laboratory. Here we recognize the difference between *manas* and *chitta*, mind and consciousness. We put our *chitta* in a test tube and examine and assess it. To see the body, as physical matter, is possible anywhere. We can do it before the mirror and we often relish doing it. So also the radiologists see it thoroughly in case there are physical problems. But what about the mind? The psychologist and psychiatrist claim that they can and do it. However, their examination is limited and very scanty when we consider the nature of mind. Mind is more mercurial than mercury. It is the propeller of all physical acts and activities. Everybody knows that conquering the mind is more difficult than conquering the whole world. Even pious and righteous saints admit and declare in their writings that controlling mind is a hard ordeal. A Marathi poetess, *Bahinaabai Chaudhari* has described it graphically. She says that at one moment the mind is as big as the sky and at another moment it is as minute as a poppy seed. Such a mind is un..e. the microscope of *yog*.

Same is the case about the feelings in the mind. We take something as love. One fine morning, we realize, it was not love, just an illusion. We take something as affection or contempt or generosity. It later proves to be something else. True knowledge of these various minute feelings can be available in *yog*. The nature of our emotions is very complex and complicated. Their variety is astounding. The shades are very subtle. The feeling of love has hundreds of shades like regard, affection, attraction, fascination, obsession and so on. Just lack of love may not be indifference or hatred. There are many feelings in between. We cannot assess this rainbow of our emotions without the help of *yog*. A true *yogi* can study breath, senses, *prana*, intelligence, emotions, sensations, perceptions and reflections in an integrated manner. The concepts such as sincerity, diligence, affection, aspiration, spiritedness, inspiration and intent are all laid bare for intrinsic scanning before him. These concepts are familiar to us from the dictionary of psychology, but the in-depth meaning, the implied, thorough and complete meaning is divulged to us only when they are scanned in *asanas*. Similarly, pride, modesty, humility and arrogance are also presented for scanning. *Asanas* give us the great lesson in the *asana* laboratory for all such revelations, and it is also a great laboratory for language or communication. Man understands language subjectively. *Asanas* are a great mine and monitor of *yog* psychology.

The *asanas* begin with a physical endeavour on the skeletal muscular plane for skeletal muscular awareness. Though the *asanas* commence with bodily actions, as the hierarchy grows and maturity blossoms, the *asanas* go through various stages of psychological, analytical, mental, synthesis-related, discriminative, emotional, intellectual phases and they become more iconographic and archetypal. These revelations in the *asanas* unfold and unfurl a great mine of wisdom and understanding.

As we first begin with exercising, *asanas* seem to be physical exercises, but they subsequently head beyond the exercise state or to the trans-exercise state of consciousness. Usually we study our mind subjectively but here in the laboratory we study our mind objectively as well. *Asanas* have a prodigious technology which leads towards *prayatnashaithilyam* or cessation of effort and beyond, towards *anantasampatti,* highest absorption.

One should know the difference between an earthenized posture and an etherealized posture–a *prithvikruta asana* and an *akashikruta asana*. When an *asana* is done under the governance of *apana* it becomes *prithvikruta* or earthenised. Similarly, it can be done by the rest of the three elements. One single *asana* can have five modifications, viz. earthenized, aquified, firized, airified and etherized. Similarly one and the same *asana* can be done with six *kriyas*, technically called *shatkriyas*. In each case, the *asana* will be changing in drive, motive, motion and execution. The same *asana*, when done under the influence of *udana*, becomes etherized. It is indeed amazing to have one and the same *asana* done with a variety of physiodynamics and biodynamics. For a neophyte, *asanas* usually begin on the physical plane with physical needs, a physical endeavour and effort by using the body, joints, muscles, tendons, bones, skin and flesh. The *asana* can then head towards evolution into an astronomical journey, terminating into the infinitude of absorption of *anantasampatti*. With this explanation of *asanas* condensed in a nutshell, an attempt has been made to divulge the implied purport behind their dimensionless expanse.

A neophyte *sadhaka* being a common ordinary person, is rocked, battered, slammed and belted by bodily aches and pains and several other sorrows, pains, diseases and sufferings and humiliations of the mind. This is normally our state before we commence *asanas*. The *sadhaka* is prone to all these aspects from the start, from the plane of the body to the subconscious plane of the mind. *Asanas* come in handy to give solace to the physical, mental, psychological and emotional aspects of the mind as well, such as a person usually turns to *yogasanas* for redemption from physical pain, physical limitations, diseases and sorrows. Since *asanas* are also organic and *pranic* in their exercising, organic diseases are alleviated and mitigated. The various organs of the human system function marvellously in *yogasanas* for correction and reformation. Aspects such as exercising the organs, flooding the organs with blood and filling the organs with *prana,* play a major role in alleviating and mitigating diseases as well as amending and correcting the different systems of the body.

Asanas, therefore, have won an uppermost place in the remedial and therapeutic aspects of human suffering. *Yogasanas* are therefore considered to be alternate therapy which is a science by itself. The *asanas* have their own exercisology for skeletal-muscular and anatomical disorders. There are disorders on account of malfunctioning of *panchaprana, shatchakra, tridosha and sapta dhatus.*

Asanas also work on *panchapranic* management. There is what is known as *panchapranic* therapy. For most of our physical, mental, intellectual, passion-based, emotion-based diseases, there is *panchapranic* therapy of *yog* and this works through *asanas* in conjunction with *chakrology.* There is a connection between *chakrology* and *panchpranology.*

The *pranic* therapy comprises of *chakrology* and *pranology.* It comprises of the *shatchakras* and the *panchapranas.* They work marvellously in this *yogic* therapy through the *asanas, bandhas* and *mudras.* The *yogic* therapy is holistic in the true sense of the term. It works holistically. Thus the beneficiary of this therapy not only overcomes the diseases and disorders but also is able to evolve a *yogic* mind through the *pranic, mantra, upasana, japa, asana, pranayama* practices, with the addition of proper *ahara* and *vihara.*

The *yogic* physician and surgeon makes the *sadhaka* patient not merely to overcome his ailment, but also takes him far beyond, to a transcorporeal, ex-corporeal state of well-being. This is a unique

Chakra	Physical Maladies	Mental Maladies
Muladhara	Excretory problem, piles, fissure	Tendencies of hunger, thirst, sleep, biological fear, sexuality आहार निद्रा भय मैथुन
Swadhi- shthana	Water retentive problem, sex organ जल दोष diseases	Egotism, complexes, inferiority & superiority ego problems
Manipuraka	Digestive problem intestinal problem gastric problem अग्नि दोष diseases	Depression, fear syndrome, work stress, sensuality
Anahata	Pulmonary, coronary problems, chest problems, cardiac problem, कफ दोष phlegm problems, lung problems	Emotional problems, sentimental problems
Vishudhi	Thyroid, throat problem, speech problems, voice problems	Mental stress, anxiety-worry chaotic thought process
Ajna	Cerebral problems problems related to brain, senses	Intellectual problems, lunacy will-volition problems

aspect of *yog* therapy. In all other therapies, the patient, at the most, gets symptomatic relief and is cured of his disease. However if one ailment is cured, another one may crop up another day. Feeling well may be a limited kind of reaction. If a beggar is given bread everyday he will be satisfied for some days but then one day he will demand butter or jam. This is not only a beggarly but human tendency. In *yog* therapy, however, the patient is not merely cured of his disease and is fine, but he will go beyond. His well-being is beyond the body and is on the spiritual plane, and in a sense, he experiences a sense of perfect well-being. Even *pranava sadhana, asanas, mantra* or *japa sadhana* by themselves do not amount to the total *yog* therapy. *Ashtanga yog* therapy alone can be accepted as the one and only genuine total *yog* therapy.

Asana sadhana is comprehensive in nature. Just as the element of *tapas* is typical of *shaucha, svadhyaya, santosha, asana, pranayama*, etc., in the same manner, the *asanas* play a role in evolving the mindset for *ahimsa, satya, asteya, brahmacharya, aparigraha* and *Ishvarapranidhana*. Thus *asanas* can evolve the mindset for all the *yamas* and *niyamas. Aasanas* work in the *pranic* cleansing of the body, mind, senses and organs. *Asanas* work for *shaucha*, innately, intrinsically, essentially. They work for external and internal purity which is *shaucha. Santosha* or contentment is also radiated and generated in various parts of the brain. *Asanas* work beautifully towards self-observation, biochemistry, self-investigation and self-analysis (*svadhyaya*). Essential *svadhyaya* is attained in *asanas. Ishvarapranidhana* requires purity, piety of mind. *Asanas* can help to attain these qualities.

In modern parlance, *asanas* can help evolve the physiology, the biochemistry, the sympathetic and parasympathetic system, to innately, intrinsically evolve the mindset for the assimilation of the *yamas* and *niyamas*. The *sadhaka* attains a quantum leap in the ethico-religious principles through *asanas*, because they work on the biophysics, biochemistry and on culturing the very mindset. A physiology of non-agitativeness is created through *asanas*. There are *asanas* to work for sublimation of the passion zone, to reinforce the emotional zone, for putting in order the ego zone, for providing courage, candidness, unselfishness, modesty, moderation and simplicity. Thus *yogsadhana* contributes to *shantisamadhana* on the *adhyatmic* plane.

Asanas work towards the *pranic* treatment to nullify any imbalances in the *tridoshas* (*vata, pitta, kapha*). In a nutshell it would mean that *yogsanas* work for :

- *Panchamahabhuta* management
- *Saptadhatu* management
- Psychological management
- Psychoneuro management
- Biophysio management
- Psychophysiological management
- *Tridosha* management
- *Triguna* management
- *Prakriti* management.

Asanas work integrally and provide a link between the *yamas* and *niyamas*, and to *pranayama, pratyahara, dharana, dhyana* and *samadhi*.

Ashtanga Pranayama

We shall now turn our attention to *ashtanga pranayama*. *Yogasanas* create a foundational ground for *pranayama*. Some of the sedative, sublimative and introcessive *asanas* and particularly, *shavasana,* are a great support for *pranayama. Asanas* assiduously work for effecting freedom in the *pranic* trafficking. The *prana nadis* are greatly cleansed and accessed by *asanas* and the body and mind become prepared for *pranayama. Asanas* have a scheme of bestowing an insulated and neutralized mind by ridding the mind of polarities and dualities. This is the starting point of *pranayama.* Patanjali describes *pranayama* in this way — 'तस्मिन् सति श्वासप्रश्वासगतिविच्छेद: प्राणायाम:' one should take up *pranayama* only after having attained a neutral, insulated, non-personal mind through *asanas* which is द्वंद्वअनभिघात अवस्था. The duality-free condition, the insulated and neutralized state given by the *asanas* is the pre-condition for commencement of *pranayama* and it is in that state of mind that breath is regulated for *pranayama.*

It should be noted here that merely regulating the breath is not *pranayama,* but regulating the breath after attaining a neutral state of mind – द्वंद्वअनभिघात – is *pranayama* according to *Patanjali,* and this state is achieved in *shavasana* in a wonderful manner. *Shavasana* is an exalted state of body and mind where there is pre-eminence of *udanisation* and etherealisation. The body and mind become *udanibhuta* and *akashibhuta* in *shavasana.* It is only thereafter that breathing is exclusively *pranic* and is to be conditioned through *pranayama* and such a mind is free from conditions given by the initial state of mind and body.

The *sadhaka* is already initiated into some aspects of *pranayama* in the *asanas* themselves. These are *apanika* breathing, *samanika* breathing, *pranika* breathing and *udanika* breathing. All these aspects are learnt in the *asanas.* Anatomically, the patterns can be described as pelvic breathing, gastric breathing, diaphragmatic breathing, thoracic breathing, vocal breathing, nasal breathing, temporal cerebrocortical breathing and spinal breathing. *Asanas* also train the *sadhaka* in *mulabandha kriya, uddiyanabandha kriya* and *jalandharabandha kriya.*

Inhalation and exhalation take place all the time without any particular technology. But the *puraka* and *rechaka* have a methodology as well as a psychology. Normally our inbreath and outbreath do not have a psychology. Both these breaths go on and on whether one is wakeful or dreaming or dormant or unconscious. But for *puraka* and *rechaka* there is a technology and a psychology that is given by *yogsadhana*, and *yogshastra* of *puraka, kumbhaka* and *rechaka*. The *pranayama* later on inducts the *sadhaka* into esoteric physiology. The *nadis* that are used in *pranayama* and *pranayamika* breathing are micro-microscopic. These *nadis* are not to be found in the normal texts of anatomy and physiology from any scan procedure or radiology. That is the esoteric physiology into which the *sadhaka* is inducted and these are the *nadis* that are to be used in *pranayama*. Thus there are :

- *Prana-Vyana* regulated breathing
- *Apana-Vyana* regulated breathing
- *Samana-Vyana* regulated breathing
- *Udana-Vyana* regulated breathing

There are also :

1. *Ida* regulated breathing
2. *Pingala* regulated breathing
3. Alternately regulated breathing starting with either *Ida* or *Pingala*
4. *Sushumna* regulated breathing

These are all the aspects of *pranayama.*

Bandhatraya

The *sadhaka* learns the *bandhatraya*, namely *muladhara bandha*, *uddiyana bandha* and *jalandara bandha*. The *yog sadhaka* learns all these from their basics, to their essence, in *pranayama*. Their techniques, dynamics, nature, essence, role and their functions are all learnt in *yog sadhana* and *pranayama sadhana*. The *sadhaka* realizes the role of *pranayama* on the mindset, in its character, its nature and its constitution. There is a transmutation for the cosmicalisation of the mind. The tendencies in the body, mind, senses, flesh and even in the corpuscular particles of the blood get sublimated. The element of mundaneness of purpose evaporates and there is a quantum leap in the nature and conduct of a *sadhaka* with the practice of *pranayama*. *Pranayama* bestows a glorious experience of the trans-mundane state. There is an incredible change in the *ahara, vihara, achara* and *vichara* of the *sadhaka*, on account of flooding of *satva*. *Pranayama* thus creates a *sattvic* foundation and '*sattvicizes*' the entire being.

In the later stages the *sadhaka* discovers in *pranayama*, the relationship between the breath and *nada,* between *prana* and *nada,* the relationship with ॐ and *prana* and also the syllables of ॐ, which are 'A' *kar,* 'U' *kar* and 'Ma' *kar*. There are three and a half *matras* in, and it may be said for the benefit of the neophyte that A-U-M are the syllables of अणच. The 'A' or 'A' *kara* effects the abdominal contraction of the passion zone and it is *apanic*. The 'U' or 'U'*kara* results in thoracic contraction and emotional purging and emotional purification and it is *pranic*. The 'Ma' or 'Ma'*kara* relates to cerebral contraction and is ego purging and is *udanic*.

The *pranic* geometry is an enchanting *nadatmaka* play of the mind in *pranayama*. This game is not for mere recreation of the mind but for a "re-creation", new creation 'cosmicalisation' and cosmic creation of the mind. This is indeed the cosmic game of the mind.

प्राणायामाय नमो नम:

We will now discuss the next step, *Pratyahara*, in the following discourse.

Shri Krishnaarpanam astu

✢ ✢ ✢

Discourse 10

Patanjala Sadhana 5

Pratyahara

We will now consider the *Pratyahara*,the *laya* or absorption aspect of *ashtanga yog*. The basic aspects of *pratyahara* can be experienced during the practice of particular types of *asanas*. The different poses induct the *sadhaka* in the technique of hibernation. Such an inward withdrawal of the mind leads to peace and tranquility. Some of the *asanas* can electrify and vitalize the body whereas others permeate calmness and placidity. Different stationary poses induct the *sadhaka* into *pratyahara* physiology. *Asanas* such as *halasana, paschimottanasana, viparitakarani, sarvangasana,* etc. result in absorption of consciousness which acquires insulation from attachment to external objects. Such *asanas* are a fountainhead of *pratyahara,* which is a form of *chitta laya.* It is not possible to continue in some poses for a long time whereas we can stay for a fairly long time with ease in certain other poses. It is in these types of *asanas* that the psychological component of *pratyahara* blossoms. They serve as a mine of *pratyaharika* components.

Shavasana greatly influences *pratyahara*. In some *asanas* like *janushirshasana* partial internalization of the senses is achieved. Even though *shavasana* is not perfectly performed, some of the instinctive tendencies and habits are neutralized. *Pratyahara* occurs automatically when we are totally absorbed in the breath during *pranayama.*

Shirshasana has a unique *ajna chakra pratyahara* resulting in withdrawal of the senses and the mind, cutting off all links between mind, senses and external objects. Similarly, *sarvangasana* and *halasana* have a unique *vishuddhichakra pratyahara* which differs from that attained by *shirshasana*. This difference is a result of their corresponding *chakra* technologies. *Janushirshasana* and *paschimottanasana* are benefited by the *anahata chakra pratyahara*. *Asanas* and *mudras* based on *viparitakarani* have *svadhishthana pratyahara* and to some extent the *vishuddhi chakra pratyahara*. *Muladhara pratyahara* is achieved through *suptakonasana* and *suptabaddhakonasana*. *Chakras* are the centres of detachment of the senses. In other words they are the dormancy zones of the *indriyas*. Just as one rests in the confines of one's bedroom, so also the different *chakras* attain corresponding type of *pratyahara* in giving tranquillity and calmness to the organs, senses and mind. Practice of *yogasanas* gives basic knowledge of various components of *pratyahara*. The components of *pratyahara* are gathered from different *asanas* with the help of *shatchakras* and *panchapranas*. Veterans, and the teacher clan, must practise and impart *shatchakra* technology of *pratyahara*.

In modern scientific parlance, it may be said that *pratyahara* is related to the pituitary region. The fabric of *pratyahara* is also formed in the pineal and thyroid regions. These regions are resting places of organs of senses and action. There is also a solar plexus *pratyahara* and a pelvic plexus *pratyahara* and all these are cognized through the *yogic* technique. *Asanas, pranayama, japasadhana, dhyana* ultimately bestow on the *sadhaka* a cosmic metaphysical component of *pratyahara* from the initial stage to the stage of "*tatra pratyaikatanata*" of a *yogi*. The *sadhaka* attains the components of *pratyahara*, viz., the *chakric, granthika, panchapranika* components to a great extent. *Shavasana* is a great mine of the physiological, psychological, glandular, biochemical and emotional components of *pratyahara.* The *pranika, sattvic,* ethereal and *udanic* components of *pratyahara* are also abundantly achieved in *shavasana*. As one gets bottles of chemicals in a chemistry laboratory so the *sadhaka* gets bottles of *pratyahara* in *shavasana*. The core of *yogshastra* is *satvika* and *shavasana* provides not only bottles but a tank of *sattvic* or noble elements. *Udana vayu* is very important in *pratyahara* and it is found here in plenty like an oxygen cylinder. The mine of *shavasana* may not generate precious stones but the physiological, psychological, glandular, biochemical and emotional components are more valuable than everything else.

Pranava

Pranava is an important component of *pratyahara*. *Pranavika* or *Omkara sadhana* is the fountainhead of *pratyahara*. *Pranava* also bestows the *jnana yogic* component, the *karma yogic* component, the *dhyana yogic* component and the *bhakti yogic* component of *pratyahara*. All these are in abundant supply through *ashtanga sadhana,* leading to the building up and enrichment of the *pratyahara* foundation. The *sadhaka* attains a glorious galaxy of *pratyaharika* components bestowed by *ashtanga yog sadhana*. They are as follows:

1. The physical component

2. The physiological biochemical component

3. The psychological component

4. The neurological component

5. The glandular component

6. The sensory component

7. The mental component

117

8. The emotional component

9. The intellectual component

10. The restraintive component given by the *yamas*

11. The observative components given by the *niyamas*

12. The *asanic* components

13. The *pranic* components

14. The *chakric* components of the *shatchakras*

15. The *nadic* components of the *nadis*

16. The *japic* components of *japa*

17. The *mantric* components of *Om*

18. The *namic* components of *nama japa, nama sadhana*

19. The philosophical components of *jnana yog*

20. The *karmika* components of *karma yog*

21. The *pranidhanika* components of *bhakti yog*

22. The *sattvic* components of *ahara, vihara, achara, vichara.*

Having considered the introductory part, we will now make a scientific study of this limb of *ashtanga yog*. The 54th *sutra* of the second *pada* of *Patanjali's yogsutras* states: '**स्वविषय असंप्रयोगे चित्तस्वरूपानुकार इव इंद्रियाणां प्रत्याहार: ।**' When *chitta* retires from contact with external objects of the senses and draws inwards towards the essential consciousness, it is *pratyahara*. *Pratyahara* is not merely physical. We can sit and do *asanas*. We cannot just sit and do *pratyahara* on the same lines. *Pranayama* organization is

118

important for *pratyahara*. *Pranayama* first turns the senses from external objects and subtle *pranayama* turns them inward. For example, while performing an *asana,* the intelligence within the body extends outwards and the senses of perception, mind and intelligence are drawn inwards. The same is the case during performance of *pranayama.* The senses are restrained by depriving them of that which feeds them i.e. the external objective world. *Pratyahara* frees them by withdrawing the supply of nourishment in the form of desires and their satisfaction. However they are not completely devoid of external objects. That would make them sleep. By controlling the senses and mind, the *sadhaka* draws the *chitta* inward. We have to take note of one thing here. The dormancy of the senses during sleep should not be confused for *pratyahara* nor can sleep be equated to *dhyana.* The mind concentrates on the effulgent form of *Ishtadevata* like *Rama, Shiva, Gajanana,* in *dhyana* and the senses are drawn inwards to their source. If *chitta* is drawn completely towards it, senses begin to go in that form. *Japa, pranayama* and techniques of *dhyana* achieve this marvellous result.

It is not easy to steer the consciousness towards *dhyana.* It is normally influenced by the objects of the senses and is drawn outwards towards pleasure. In order to direct the *chitta* from the lower attractions, it should be handled with some tact. Observe a child playing with toys in a basket. He is listlessly going from one toy to another. If we want to take him away from the basket, we have to divert his attention skillfully towards some more attractive matter. We have to use tactics of child psychology here. In the same way, the *chitta* must be given some engaging symbol to be fixed on it. A majestic idol of Lord *Shiva,* a beautiful idol of Lord *Krishna* with his enchanting flute can give the *chitta* a view of the magnificence of the divinity. But, of course, seeds of *yogdharma* have already to be there in the *chitta* for being impressed by these symbols permanently. Without it, the impressions created by the symbols will be temporary. It preserves and augments the *sattvic* nature arising out of *saattvic ahara, vihara, achara* and *vichara*. During the practice of *pratyahara*, the importance of *pranayama* cannot be overstressed. It is instrumental in creating the proper environment and appropriate mindset for *dhyana* and then thereby the *sadhakas* nature becomes lofty. The *sadhaka* is then no longer interested in the objects of the senses. The *yama, niyama, asana, pranayaama*, etc. become cultured and result in *pratyahara*. *Maniprabhakara* has described this state as follows:

'उक्तयमादिभि: संस्कृतचित्तस्य प्रत्याहार: भवति ।'

It is possible for a common man to understand this principle of *pratyahara*. The *Mandala Brahmana* in the 68th *kandika*, subdivision, states:

'विषयेभ्य: इंद्रियार्थेभ्य: मनोनिरोधने प्रत्याहार: ।'

To restrain the mind initially against sense-gratification is to some extent an act of *pratyahara*. A person who is influenced by the rules of right conduct experiences this state. The *Shandilya Upanishad* further states that this type of sense restraint is actually *pratyahara*. A *yogi* attains *pratyahara* through *dhyana, dharana* and *samadhi*. It is also necessary, even normally, to restrain the senses for one's own physical and mental well-being, and not specifically for *yogsadhana*. Self-control is the essence of *pratyahara*. *Pratyahara* also means sensory restraint. It is important not only for the *sadhaka* but also for the common man. Otherwise his health and well-being would be blown to the winds.

120

The following five types of *pratyahara* are described in the *Shandilya Upanishad*:

पंचविधविषयेषु बलाद् धारणेन प्रत्याहार: ।

यत् पश्यति तत् सर्वं आत्मा इति प्रत्याहार: ।

नित्यविहितकर्मफलपरित्याग: प्रत्याहार: ।

सर्वविषयपराङ्मुखत्वं प्रत्याहार: ।

अष्टादशेषु मर्मस्थानेषु क्रमात् धारणं प्रत्याहार: ।

These are the five significant types of *pratyahara*. It is immaterial whether one practises *yog* or not, they are indispensable. The first type helps exercise control over the wayward senses. The second type helps to perceive divinity in whatever we see. वासुदेवम् इदं सर्वम्, वसुधा एव कुटुंबकम् these are the basic tenets of the Hindu view of *pratyahara*. The third type consists in giving up the fruits of daily action. The fourth type consists of weaning away the mind from sensual tendencies and is characterized by dispassion. The fifth type is the highest and is connected with *yogic* technique. It lies in controlling the eighteen vital points of the body. These are :

पादांगुष्ठ गुल्फ जंघा जानु पायु मेद नाभि हृदय कंठकूप तालु साक्षी भ्रूमध्य ललाट मूर्धास्थानानि । तेषु क्रमात् आरोह अवरोह क्रमेण प्रत्याहारयेत् ।

The eighteen locations ascend upwards from the feet to the big toe, from there to the heel, to the shin, knee, thigh and anus, to the generative organ, to the navel, heart, hollow of the throat, to the upper and lower palates, nostrils, eyes, space between the eyebrows, forehead, to the crown of the head; such is the path of the ascent and descent of consciousness in *pratyahara*. This path is followed mainly in *shavasana*.

For attaining *pratyahara* one has to practise *shamasadhanaa* and *damasadhanaa*. 'दमो बाह्येंद्रियनियमनम् – शमो अंत:करणनियमनम्' as the saying goes. *Pratyahara* commences with pacification and restraint of the senses. In the 20th and 21st *shlokas* of Discourse 8 of the 11th *skanda* of the *Bhagavata Purana*, there is a significant reference to *pratyahara*.

इंद्रियाणि जयन्ति आशु निराहारमनीषिण:
वर्जयित्वा तु रसनं तत् निरन्नस्य वर्धते ।
तावत् जितेंद्रियो न स्यात् विजितेंद्रिय: पुमान्
न जयेत् रसनं यावत् जितं सर्वं जिते रसे ।

Going without food, intelligent men may quickly control all other senses but not the palate, which becomes the more demanding, the more it is starved. Man can master the senses at one point but the palate among them is the hardest to control. Whatever his age, the tongue remains rosy. Even the last wish of a criminal to be hanged is often to eat some delicious dish. So we can say that when the palate is conquered, all is conquered.

Pratyahara also means not heeding to the sensual objects. Voluntary detachment from sense desires is also *pratyahara*. By becoming detached to sensual propensities, the senses are subordinated. The more one tries to run away from desires the more one is followed by them if there is no detachment. This is a basic truth. Having sexual enjoyment only for the purpose of reproduction is also *pratyahara*. This action of the detached householder has a spiritual substrate and is also *pratyahara*. The householder may have any occupation like that of cobbler, potter, barber or even butcher.

He can be leading this life in the *adhyatmika* frame. *Tuladhara* in the *Mahabharata* was a butcher but could be better called a butcher *yogi*. Through *yogic* process the mind transcends the base instincts. *Pratyahara* comes naturally, even when mundane pleasures are enjoyed with a sense of detachment and this results in *pratyahara*. Proper *ahara, vihara, achara, vichara,* result in *pratyahara* even in the initial stages of *sadhana*, even without any special *yogic* ability. *Pratyahara* attained in this manner has the same potency as that of *yogic pratyahara*.

So far we have considered the aspects of the fifth *anga*, limb of *ashtanga yog*, i.e. *pratyahara* in detail. We will now turn our attention to the remaining three *angas* viz. *dhyana, dharana* and *samadhi*. After the stage of *pratyahara* one moves on to the inner quest or *antaranga sadhana*. The *ashtanga sadhana* is hypostatized in *Om*. Just as a huge banyan tree exists in a unified form in its minute seed, the entire *yog sadhana* exists in *pranava japa*. It is a *pranava sadhana* or *Omkara sadhana*. It is a *pranika japa*. When this *japa* gets intense engrossment, involvement and concentration, it does not remain oral or mental but becomes *dhyana*. Even a momentary absorption results in a shower of *samaadhi* for the *sadhaka*. The moment of absorption in *Om* becomes a "trancive state" for a *sadhaka*. He is *satvikised* in the body, mind, and senses. The *sadhaka* is *udanised* and etherealized. The whole embodiment is sublimated and ennobled. There is total 'cosmicalisation' and *pranikisation* of body, mind, senses and breath. Such is the process of *dharanaa* and *dhyana*. *Pratyahara, dharana* and *dhyana* for a *sadhaka* is automatically evolved out of the intensity of *pranayama* practice. The profundity of his *dhyana* itself becomes the *samadhi* of the neophyte. The *sadhaka* begins to evolve the *antaranga sadhana* which is *pranika, anahata* or soundless, emotional, religious, *pranava dharma*, respiratory, exhalative and thereby culminates in a glorious *sadhana*. At this stage *ashtanga yog* attains its fulfilment.

We have observed how a systematic plan of action for *ashtanga yog* is evolved. It evolves as a comprehensive base for the higher pursuits in *yog*. In the circumstances, it is implied that *ashtanga yog* has to be accomplished with the basic ingredients of *yajna, dana* and *tapas*.

A cautionary warning !

Today, spirituality has been sadly commercialized. For example, *dhyana,* meditation, is purported to be accomplished within eight or ten days in a meditation camp. Modern man's gullibility and eagerness to find spiritual solace has made him a scapegoat in the hands of such self-proclaimed 'spiritual specialists'. Preposterous claims of awakening *kundalini shakti* of everybody in a huge crowd of eight to ten thousand people are made by them. Certainly everybody has a different mental caliber and will respond very differently to any piece of advice or *kriya*. Even a medicine does not work in the same way on all people. And here all types of *shakti yog, kriya yog,* etc. are offered to the public in the form of ready-made capsules for a price. A self-proclaimed swami in saffron clothing holds a camp for self-realization! Hence the highest caution needs to be exercised by the *sadhaka* before accepting a *guru*. Mere closing of eyes and observing breath is definitely not *yog sadhana*. The highest pursuit of the supreme *yog* is achieved by a systematic and sustained practice of *ashtanga yog*. Similarly, *jnana yog* cannot be attained by mere superficial reading of the *Jnaneshwari, Gita, Upanishadas, Gathas* etc. Also, mere performance of acts of charity is not *karma yog. Ashtanga yog* alone is the life-blood of all these *yogs*.

Today, in the field of formal education, a fifteen year old raw beginner is faced with the very important task of choosing his branch of professional education. This cannot be done in the field of *yog*. The *sadhaka* has to practise *ashtanga yog* intensely along with the principles of *yajna, dana* and *tapas, japa, satsanga* and *shastrasanga* and may be even for decades. In the present world with no *vedic* training and knowledge, practice of *ashtanga yog* as indicated above, is the only path for reaching the Supreme. Even *Yogeshvara* Lord *Krishna* did not teach the science of *yog* to Arjuna within an eight day crash course! He did not get a short cut or by pass invented for this most beloved friend and ardent disciple. He emphatically asserted in the *Bhagavadgita*: 'अनेकजन्मसंसिद्धौ तत: याति परां गतिम् ।' (7 : 45) Several lives need to be expended to attain the supreme stage of *yog*. The *sadhaka* should not forget this instruction of warning. He should also deeply inscribe the fact in his mind... A*shtanga yog is the only path for any form of yog.*

Shri Krishnaarpanam astu

✛ ✛ ✛

125

Discourse 11

From Anna and Annamaya to Anandamaya

Anna

The word *anna* food has special significance in *yogshastra*. According to the *Upanishads,* when we consume food, it is the food that is eating us. Some people eat to live and some people live to eat. Many gluttons live to eat and meet their death by eating voraciously. Food is the substance that constitutes the physical sheath consisting of skin, flesh, fat, bones and filth. This food-body or *annamaya kosha* has a beginning and an end. While discussing the *panchapranas* and *shatchakras*, we have seen that there is another subtle sheath - the *pranamaya* sheath.

Annamaya and Pranamaya Kosha

The state of the *annamaya kosha* determines the physical form of the gross body, its overall health, charm and lustre. The next layer is the *pranamaya kosha*, in which the movement of the *pranic* force directs our physical and mental activities. The type of creativity, mindset, traits and sharpness of mental talents are decided by this *kosha*. These manifestations may be attributed to one's past *karma*. Human consciousness, memories and experiences are founded in the *pranamaya kosha*. This *kosha,* like the *annamaya kosha,* also has a beginning and an end. It comes with the birth and goes with death. Whether there is transmigration into different wombs or not, the *pranamaya kosha* gives us a specific tendency to bear the *prarabdha*, destiny. The *Brahmanandavalli* states that the *annamaya kosha* contains the *pranamaya kosha* but acts as a cover for the *pranamaya kosha* and envelops it completely. We think that the sheaths are like our dressing. We wear one layer of clothes upon the other in winter. We put on a shirt upon a banyan, a sweater upon a shirt, a coat upon a sweater and so on. The sheaths are not positioned in this manner. They are not put on like undergarments. The five sheaths, *annamaya* (food-sheath), *pranamaya* (vital-air sheath), *manomaya* (mental sheath), *vijnanamaya* ('souler' sheath) and *anandamaya* (bliss-sheath), are in the form of concentric circles covering each other. True, *pranamaya* is inside the *annamaya* but *annamaya* occupies *pranamaya*.

Prana is life in the individual. The physiological functions such as movements of hands and feet are controlled by this *pranamaya* sheath. At death, *pranamaya* ends along with *annamaya*. The *pranamaya* effect undergoes a change in every subsequent life. We evolve through this *kosha*, and our nature, consciousness and awareness deepens and expands in the course of our undergoing the *prarabdha*. *Pranamaya* ends with our *prarabdha*. Every *pranamaya* is restricted to the particular life. We have discussed the management of the *pranamaya* in regard to the *shatchakras* of the *sukshma sharira*.

Manomaya Kosha

We will now take a look at the *manomaya kosha*. The *manomaya* exists even beyond the life-span of the individual. The *kosha* is extant from the beginning of Time and in all the previous births. The *manomaya kosha* is the foundation of the mental awareness resulting from past experiences and conditions of life. The *manomaya* harmonizes and balances the *pranamaya kosha*. It is described as the *vasana kosha* or *samskara kosha*. The *samskaras* are stored in the *manomaya* since time without beginning. The imprint of the infinite experience and revelations obtained by man during the 8.4 million births are reflected in this *kosha*. It is, in fact, the archive of mental activities and is the source of *prarabdha*. It endows man with the power of thinking and judgement. At the time of birth, the *karma* of the man during his whole future life is registered in this archive just before his death. All his actions are classified as good or bad and registered accordingly. His evil actions prompt the soul to enter the inferior wombs. The experiences and conditions of life are determined by past *karma*. If the balance-sheet of *prarabdha* shows a positive balance of good deeds, then the soul becomes qualified to enter superior wombs, and vice-versa. The *manomaya kosha* exists in the domain of the subtle layers of the mind. This *kosha* accompanies the soul from one birth to another in its journey through the heavens, the subterranean regions of hell, through the innumerable 8.4 million wombs of insects, animals, birds, etc. in this world and in the other worlds. The *manomaya kosha* functions even after the physical death of the body. In occultism, this is described as the science of transmigration or eschatology. The *manomaya kosha* carries with it the seed of evolution of all the forms of life right from micro-organism to huge creatures like elephant or dinosaur, from the smallest bird to the eagle, from man to Gods, demons, *gandharvas*, and also to the wombs of infernal planes. Man is, therefore, a creature with the potential of transmigration into the lower wombs of animals, insects, etc. depending on his *prarabdha* stored in the floppy disc of the *manomaya kosha*.

The *pranamaya* sheath controls the visible movements of the *annamaya kosha*. The *manomaya kosha* controls the *pranamaya* and *annamaya koshas*. It is also known as the *karma kosha*. Man's bondage is due to his *karma*. This *karma* is influenced by his *vasanas*. Thus the *manomaya* and the *pranamaya koshas* are not mutually exclusive. They are influenced by each other. The *manomaya kosha*, in large measure, constitutes the *linga sharira*. It contains the subtle ingredients for any form of existence. This *kosha* contains the seeds of a man's future lives. It is the internal instrument for storing all the ingredients of past experiences and knowledge.

Just as the *annamaya kosha* consists of physical organs like two eyes, two ears, two nostrils, the *manomaya kosha* also possesses the same characteristics, but these are subtle in nature. These subtle organs have a mental dimension. That is why Lord *Krishna* told *Arjuna* in the *Gita* that he could be perceived only by the inner eye and not by the physical eye. The Lord blessed *Arjuna* with a divine eye for this purpose. The *manomaya kosha* is subtle in nature. It consists of seventeen limbs, the five *tanmatras* i.e. the subtle primary elements of sound, taste, touch, form and smell, the ten senses and organs, the mind and the intellect. These limbs are so subtle in nature that they are not visible to the naked physical eye. The *manomaya kosha* governs the intrinsic tendencies or *vasanas* and the mental activities at conscious and unconscious levels. It is the seat of the five *jnanendriyas,* the five *karmendriyas*, mind, *buddhi, ahankara,* and *chitta.* All this is described in the *Sarvasara Upanishad* in an extremely thought-provoking manner. The *panchakoshas* are described in detail here. The four states of wakefulness, dream state, sleep and *turiya* or the highest consciousness are also mentioned. This *Upanishad* is especially meant for inquisitive practitioners of *yog.* The five *karmendriyas* of the *manomaya kosha* do not have a physical form. The arms, legs, speech organ, the genitals and the excretory organs are not in manifested form but in seed form. In modern scientific parlance the *manomaya kosha* is nominal and the five senses are present here in infra-atomic state. It exists from time without beginning till the time of the final liberation of the soul. The neo-*Vedantins* give a faulty picture of the *manomaya kosha* as made up of the *jnana-karmendriyas* and the mind, and say that the *vijnanamaya kosha* is made up of the *jnana-karmendriyas* and the intellect. The neo-*vedantins* who profess the principle of *Mayavaada* have given undue importance to this view that is basically faulty. The correct approach would be to consider the *manomaya kosha* as the *Lingasharira*.

Vijnanamaya Kosha

The fourth one is the *vijnanamaya kosha*. This *kosha* is the sheath of subtle layers of the human consciousness. It is the source of ultimate knowledge and of self-realization. As mentioned before, the neo-*vedantins* declare that the *vijnanamaya kosha* consists of the ten *jnana-karmendriyas* and *buddhi*, and the *manomaya kosha* consists of the ten *jnana-karmendriyas* and the mind. This is a highly erroneous view and the *Taittiriya Upanishad* is the evidence of it. The *vijnanamaya kosha* is synonymous with the *jivatma* and exists from Time without beginning and is eternal, birthless and deathless. The constituents of the *manomaya* and *annamaya koshas* are *Prakritic* i.e. born out of *Prakriti*. But those of *vijnanamaya kosha* are not like that. The *Taittiriya Upanishad* describes the *vijnanamaya kosha* thus : 'यतो वाचो निवर्तन्ते अप्राप्य: मनसा सह।' It is inconceivable by the mind and speech fails to describe it. It is invisible and not cognizable by the senses and organs. So this *kosha* cannot be known through speech, mind or sense organs. The *Sarvasara Upanishad* says : 'एतत्कोशत्रयसंसक्त: तद्गतो विशेषज्ञ: यदा भासते तदा विज्ञानमयकोश इति उच्यते ।' This *kosha* contains the principle of the finite consciousness. The eternally unchangeable, undecaying, birthless, immutable, formless individual soul has its being in this *kosha*. Since we possess the sheath of intelligence, we know that we are the knower, the discerner, the seer, the feeler, the creator, the conceiver, the enlightened. The constituents of this living consciousness distinguishes the human being from inert mud and stone. The *Taittiriya Upanishad* states : 'विज्ञानं यज्ञं तनुते ।' A knower is the one who performs *yajna karma* or devotional acts. Evidently, an inanimate object is not a performer of any *karma*. Further, the ninth *kandika* of the fourth part of the *Prashnopanishad states* : 'एष हि आत्मा द्रष्टा स्प्रष्टा श्रोता, घ्राता रसयिता मन्ता बोद्धा कर्ता विज्ञानात्मा पुरुष:। Similarly, the *Gita* describes the *Aatma* (15 : 17) : 'मम एव अंश: जीवलोके जीवभूत: सनातन: ।' The life that throbs in this world is my own perpetual particle form. Such is the *vijnanamaya Atma*. It is the secondary incarnation of the *Paramatmaa*.

Anandamaya Kosha

The *Antaryami Brahmana* of the *Brahadaranyaka Upanishad* states that the *jivatma* is the sheath for the *Paramatma*, the *manomaya,* and the *annamaya* for the *pranamaya*. The core of the *vijnanamaya kosha* is *Ishvara* or *Brahman* or *Paramatman*. *Paramatman* is the seat of the Supreme Bliss. He is the Supreme bliss. He is enveloped by the *anandamaya kosha*. He is the Supreme Controller. The *vijnanamaya Atma* is fully detailed in the *Sarvasara Upanishad*. It says of *Paramatman* : "I am birthless, without senses and organs, I am neither the intellect nor the ego, I am the *Prana*, I have no form, I am externally pure, and it is my proximity to the body that charges the body with vital energy. I do not have mind, hence there is no sorrow, no desire for me." Such is the fascinating picture of *vijnanamaya Atma*. This crystal-clear elucidation of the existence of the *jiva* consciousness in the *kosha* directly refutes the principle of *Mayavada* and the confusion created by the neo-*vedantins*.

The body is turned into a temple of God because of the existence of the *vijnanamaya kosha* in man. *Anandamaya Ishvara* is enveloped by the *vijnanamaya kosha* and *yog* is the means of experiencing and attaining his presence. He does not need anything. Lord *Krishna* says in the *Gita*, "There is noting in the world to be achieved by me". However, *yog* is there for us to attain God's blessings. 'आत्मापरमात्मासंयोग: योग इति उक्त: ।' *Yog* is the means of attaining proximity to *Anandamaya*. From the inner mind of *Anandamaya*, we experience the ripples of *Ananda* in the expanse of the mind. *Tukaram* expresses this condition in this way, *Anandache Dohi Ananda Taranga,* The lake of bliss has ripples of bliss. Such a soul can ascend to the spiritual summit. A reference to this topic is found in the *anandamaya adhikarana* of the *Brahmasutras* (1.1.12) : 'आनंदमय: अभ्यासात् ।' The concept of *Brahman* or *Paramatman* who is the support of the *jiva* consisting *anandamaya*, is discussed threadbare. Therein the interpretation of the *Mayavadins* : 'जीव: ब्रह्मा एव न अपर: ।' automatically stands refuted.

The *Mundakopanishad* has mentioned a beautiful metaphor. 'द्वा सुपर्णा सयुजा सखाया' Two birds are sitting on the branch of a tree. One of them is eating a berry and the other is only observing it. Let apart the tremendous rainbow of meanings in this exquisite metaphor. The metaphor itself is the fruit of the *prajna, pratibha* and *sakshatkara,* i.e. genius, creativity and epiphany of our ancient seers. Its interpretation can be a vastly different topic. Here it proves the argument of the *Mayavaadins* to be baseless. There is a distinction between the *Parmatma* and the *jivatma,* the *Paramatman* being treated as an independent entity. Their illustrations of the *panchakoshas* are defective. They presume the *vijnanamaya kosha* to be the *Anandamaya kosha. Brahman* cannot be a part of the self, consisting of bliss, since it is the substratum of the individual soul. *Brahman* is without any limiting adjuncts whatsoever. This fact is reiterated in the *Taittiriya* texts. Those who want more explanation can consult *Anandamaya Adhikarana sutra* 1.1.8 of the *Bhashya* of Shri *Ramanujacharya*. The faulty theory of *Mayavadins* is refuted there and the original theory of *Taittiriya* is established very beautifully. It is explained here now.

Human body – a temple of God

From the above discussion, it can be concluded that the *annamaya kosha* is of the material body, the *pranamaya kosha* has the dimension of the ten *pranic* forces, the *vijnanamaya kosha* is the source of the essential human consciousness, the *manomaya kosha* corresponds to the *sukshma sharira* and the *anandamaya kosha* corresponds to the bliss profuse of Divinity. That is why human body is considered to be a temple of God. We have thus journeyed from the gross to the transcendental. We considered man in each and every minute detail. The Inner Controller or *Paramatman* is at the centre of the heart of every individual. Man's real nature is described thus : 'अंतःप्रविष्ट शास्ता जनानाम् सर्वात्मा' He is not merely the Inner Controller of the inner self, but he is the Lord of the infinite bliss within. The 61st *shloka* of the 18th chapter of the *Gita* says : ईश्वरः सर्वभूतानां हृद्देशे अर्जुन तिष्ठति । भ्रामयन् सर्वभूतानि यंत्रारूढानि मायया ।। O *Arjuna,* the Lord dwells in the hearts of all beings and his delusive power makes them revolve as though mounted on a machine. This *Ishvara* deludes all the beings with his *Maya*. So we revolve on the wheel of Time, seasons and the wheel of life and death. A fly sits on the wheel of a potter and it is moving. Similarly we are revolving with the wheel.

Then we might have a question, is he moving us mercilessly ? Isn't He really Compassion Incarnate ? But the answer is there in the next *shloka*. If we turn inwardly, we attain the *anandamaya* state. As we perceive our inner self, we are again reminded of Saint

133

Tukaraam's words : *Anandache Dohi Anandataranga.* One has to move from the gross to the inner mind for experiencing the infinite mercy of the Lord, otherwise we are extrovert; we move with the wheel and blame Him for our imaginary woes. We say, "O God, give me what You will, when You will, as You will." We generally make this supplication with folded hands but then our hands are inactive, too. It often has selfish motives. Many people say, 'यथा नियुक्त: अस्मि तथा करोमि' That means, I act as I am directed by my fate or God. Seemingly all beings from the dull to the intelligent and saintly, even like *Tukaram*, will agree to this statement. However, there is a world of difference in the sense that it conveys to each one of us. A person like *Duryodhana* will say so with contempt. He will suggest that he cannot stop his wrong and evil behaviour since he is only directed by God to do like that. The saintly person will say so with an awareness of the true nature of the self. Hence, though all of them say the same thing, there will be a difference in the sense with which they say it. The pure and inwardly mind experiences the *anandamaya* state. The *anandamaya kosha,* though it is inside the other *koshas,* still it occupies the outer *koshas.* Do not try to draw its map. You will be confused. It is possible to draw the figure with *annamaya* in the outer layer, then *pranamaya,* then *manomaya and,* then *vijnanamaya* and *anandamaya.* But it is a misleading figure. This holistic view is given in the *Taittiriya Upanishad,* in the *Brahmandavalli* section.

Then follows the *Bhruguvalli. Acharya Varuni* describes the journey to bliss. That is why the *Bhruguvidya* is considered to be *Brahmavidya.* The *Vedanta* describes it as *Brahmavidyopadesha.* What subtle instructions did the *Acharya* give his disciple *Bhrugu* in respect of this *Brahmavidya* ? 'अन्नं ब्रह्मेति व्यजानात् ।' *Bhrugu* realized the *annamaya* as *Brahman,* but was not satisfied with the knowledge. Then he comes to the *Guru* and says : 'प्राणो ब्रह्मेति व्यजानात् ।' Still not satisfied with this realization, he tries further to understand *Brahman*, and comes again to his *Guru* and says : 'विज्ञानं ब्रह्मेति व्यजानात् ।' Subsequently there are amendments starting from *Pranamaya* as *Brahman*. Ultimately he knew **Bliss** to be the *Brahman*, for indeed, from Bliss it is that all beings originate. Having been born, they move towards and merge in Bliss. *Ishvara* is none other than *Brahman*. Bliss is the real form of *Brahman* and it is not merely its attribute. *Anandamaya* thus cannot be *nirguna* or without attributes as claimed by some. We have thus proceeded from the gross body, with the *panchakoshas,* towards the knowledge of the Ultimate Reality. Man is blessed with the knowledge that *Brahman* is Bliss. All this arises because man is constituted of the *panchakoshas.* Experience and understanding of the *panchakoshas* help us to penetrate into the depth of the human mind leading to the Supreme Goal of *Satchitananda Brahman.*

We may study the gross physical dimensions of the corporeal body and relate to its anatomy and physiology. But that will only make us aware of the negative emotions, sufferings and agonies of human beings. *Yogshastra*, through the study of the *panchakoshas*, leads us progressively from the impure, distorted, coloured impressions to the Supreme Consciousness.

Shri Krishnaarpanam astu

 ✛ ✛ ✛

Discourse - 12

Yogic Transformation of the Mind

The corporeal body

The spiritual plane has to be considered from the point of view of various aspects of the corporeal framework of the physical body, mind, senses and organs, the individual soul and finally, the Supreme Soul. We will consider these aspects in the subsequent topic. The corporeal body is formed of four stages : 1 Gross. 2. Subtle 3. Material and 4. Transcendental or metaphysical existence. The mind is characterized by the 1. *Karmendriya* mind 2. *Jnanendriya* mind 3. The thought-*samskara*-desire mind or emotion mind and 4. The metapsychological mind or transmigrating mind. The individual had existed even before he was born into this world. Also, the mind does not die with the death of the individual. Therefore, we have to think of the mind that exists both prior to birth and even after death. These minds are not separate but they are different manifestations of the same mind or its stages during its evolution towards spirituality. Similarly while considering the *indriyas,* we have to take a unified view of their five-fold character.

In the next topic we will be considering different aspects of the corporeal body from the *yogic* stand-point. Generally, for us the study of man is the study of the physical or corporeal body as constituted of the *saptadhatus* and different *indriyas.* Even medical experts with the degrees of M.D. or F. R. C.S. study this science from the same stand-point. They claim that this is a perfect study but this is an illusion. We have to study the body from the point of view of yog*shastra.* We will consider mind or psychology, too, mind in *yogshastra* and psychology in *adhyatma shastra.* We are going to think of *indriyas* from the point of view of organology or *indriya vijnana* of *yogshastra*. We will also study *Atma*. The concept of *Atma* is found neither in the texts of physiology nor in the subject of radiology. So the western neo-sciences are considering man without giving attention to the central point, *Atma*. Isn't this ridiculous against the background of the boasts of modern rational thinking ? Of course, we will not omit technical thinking about human body on the lines of modern sciences but it will be a thorough and comprehensive study because man can be studied almost perfectly only if we think of *Atma* and *Paramatma* along with the body. Therefore, as suggested above, we are going to think of body, mind and *indriyas* on different levels and also of *Atma* and *Paramatma* in the chapter of *yog* physiology or *sharira vijnana*.

We are going to think of body in the beginning in this new chapter There will be some repetition but it is already deemed or expected. We thought of the body structure constituted of *saptadhatus* in the last chapter. This thought may be there in modern physiology too. The chapter of *sharirasthana* in *Ayurveda,* describes various aspects from the bone-ligament arrangement, and the entire arrangement of glands up to the bone-marrow. We can study it. We have already thought about the *sukshma sharira* with its seventeen parts. So we may not go into those details again. So also we will keep aside those parts that are found in modern anatomy and physiology. So we will give attention to an interesting part of *yogshastra* here. It is the science of *sukshma sharira* in *yogshastra*. Therefore, it may not be a repetition as we thought in the beginning.

Body and mind

Please be all ears for this new and novel chapter which will satisfy your curiosity. The sense organs and organs of action, etc are not separate and separable parts of the body but they are inherent and inseparable integral limbs of the body. The limbs like hands, legs, head are not merely parts but are integral parts of our existence. Don't forget the difference between the concepts of parts and limbs. Our external and internal limbs also are our "*angas*". We say these are my "*angas*" or limbs. My "*angas*" - because there is an "I" there. These are "*angas*" of one whom we call I'. And 'I' means my mind. The "*angas*" belong to that I. Why is this I = my mind ? Because we say - I am O.K. if my mind is O.K. We never say, "These are my fingers". Even we do not say, "These fingers are of my hand." When we say "mind" our real intention is to say "of my mind". Thus all the factors are related to the "mind" - they are mental in nature. The ten *indriyas* are mind objectified. They are mind in manifestation, they are of mind, for mind. Whatever we do, we perform it all for the mind and mind only.

If we want to culture the mind there is a way in *yogshastra*, namely, to culture the ten *indriyas, indriyas* of knowledge and of action. *Yogshastra* says, culture the "*angas*" or limb of the mind and you can culture the mind. It is the source of the ten senses and organs. If I want to hurt you, I can hurt you by hurting your "*anga*" or limbs. Suppose, I severe your hand, I am hurting not only your hand but also you, I am hurting your mind. Now look, if I can hurt you by hurting "*angas*", if I can hurt you by hurting these external "*angas*", if I can please you and your mind by forming or reforming your external "*angas*", it is possible to control them by purifying and conditioning the mind. Again, according to *yogshastra*, mind is a mass of the *indriyas*, so we can form a harmonious relationship through a healthy interaction between them. If one wants to cause anguish to another, it is possible to do so by inflicting physical harm, If one's hand is severed, the pain thereby is restricted not only to the body, but is transmitted to the mind as mental pain. Since all the sense faculties are blended in the mind, *yogshastra* can make it possible to develop the mind through *yogic* practices.

We always say that we are helpless before our minds, before our nature. There is a defeatist belief 'स्वभावो दुरतिक्रम: ।' i.e. human nature is hard to change. But this is not right. This helplessness is wrong. All these are "*angas*" of our mind. Reform them and mind shall be reformed or transformed. The technology of *yogshastra* is based on this reality. Culture of the mind can be formed, reformed or transformed by culturing of the body. This concept is the foundation stone of *yog* technology. And so it has succeeded, too. Transformation of mind can be brought about by the joint action of the internal, external, gross and subtle constituents of the human system.

The irony of it is that the very persons who give in to this defeatist belief, have the temerity to advise others in the art of mind control. They even conduct *yog* classes and workshops for this purpose! They are busy telling, "Mr. A, you do this, Mr. B, don't do like this." They indulge in advising others regarding the dos and don'ts, but they find themsleves incapable of making any spiritual progress. They explain how easy it is to spoil the mind or to pervert it. If the negative action is easy, why should the positive action be so difficult? They fail to tell us how the mind is to be controlled. Can this attitude be called logical?

Actually, *yog* physiology helps us to understand the abstruse aspects of the human system. There are numerous techniques in the science of *yog* for transforming the diverse facets of human personality. The entire body structure evolves as a result of the combined action of the active and cognitive *indriyas*. *Yogshastra*

139

describes various techniques and practices which can transform the mind. It has practices pertaining to body, intellect, mind, incantation, austerity, penance; so also practices of speech, mind, thought, emotions and *prana*. Thus, even the ten fingers of the hands, nodes of the fingers, nails, limbs can influence the mind at the macro level and be useful in culturing the mind. The micro mind is dormant even in the little finger as also in the hands and feet. In short, the mind has to be flooded or 'stormed' with vibrations from all the forces running in the body. The *yogsadhaka* can get access to the mind through all these physical channels and he can thereby achieve education, training and refinement of his mind. That is the reason why it has been reiterated in the beginning of this topic that the *indriyas* form the substratum of the mind. Systems like the digestive, respiratory ones and the mind are not mutually exclusive, because the various constituents of the systems are not merely formed out of the physical bodily constituents but they are really the extension of the mind. For example, the liver is the physical constituent of the digestive system, but it has combined physio-mental effect on the human system. Any other type of physical organ such as the stomach also can influence the mind. The liver may be or is a part of the digestive system, but what can it do for the mind ? Let us reflect over this curious profound question.

Shri Krishnaarpanam astu

✤ ✤ ✤

Discourse - 13

Yog Sharira Vijnana

Yogic Knowledge of the Body

The liver is an organ of the digestive system and the lung of the respiratory system. But what is the relation of these physical organs with the mind? We were considering this question. *Yog* has tried to discover reality through this question. The reality is that these organs are directly linked with the mind and are parts of it. We normally say "my belly", "my lungs". We do not say, "the belly of my digestive system" or "the lungs of my respiratory system". Thus the organs, whether external or internal, are limbs of the mind and we can reach iit through them. So, in a way, we possess the combined strength of a thousand hands in the form of all the organs for culturing the mind. We often say that we are unable to master the mind and that we are slaves of our mind. But *yogsadhana* shows the way for reforming this mind. Usually the organs are working for their respective systems but through *yogsadhana* all these organs can be made to work for the mind. This is a valuable thought.

The physical limbs of our body, the *jnanendriyas, karmendriyas,* the *tridoshas,* the *saptadhatus,* the three *gunas,* the *panchapranas,* are so to say *prakritic* in nature. All is *Prakriti,* it is for the *Atma* and the *Purusha Paramatma.* This is the central principle of *Samkhya.* All the above things can act and work to vitalize the mind, *chitta,* the different levels of perception and subliminal experience and help cultivate and develop consciousness. *Yogsadhana* can draw a road map for this purpose. The application of *Pranayama, Japa, Tapa* ennoble the mind since from the gross bone-muscle system to the subtle *panchapranic* state all the parts of the body belong to the mind. *Yogshastra* shows the path for such evolvement. It creates an awareness of the sound principles of the art of living. Clearly, the consciousness of the self is illumined through physical organs. By *yogic* practices of *asanas, mudras, bandhas, japa, tapa* and *pranayama* we are able to apply the actions and sensory inputs of each and every part of the human body for the mind. Right from the tip of the fingers of the hands up to the forehead, including all the limbs, glands, skin can and do take part in this 'operation' of the mind. In this way *we* can evolve consciousness through *yogshastra*. *Asanas* are not just contortions of the body. *Pranayama* is not merely a breathing exercise. *Yogshastra* gives the technique of this application in *yogic* practice. The brain has the centres of activation of all the organs of the body. So does the mind have its centre in every cell of the body in all the states of awareness and experiences of childhood, youth, old age, waking state, dormancy or sleep. That is why every part of the body is factually a part of the mind.

We normally view the limbs and organs merely in their functional form. For example, lungs and belly are recognized only from the point of view of their functional aspect but actually that is not their real nature. Functioning or efficient functioning of these limbs and organs is not the true sign of their state of well-being. The well-being of each physical element of the human system lies in its being in their substantive form [*sva-sthiti*].In substantive form, the senses and organs are able to serve the philosophical and higher purposes of human existence. *Pratyahara* or abstraction of senses through the *yogic* process is the means by which physical organs are brought to their own original substantive form. We generally give attention to their outward action or function, and not this true state. We feel that the function of the eyes or nose is merely to see or smell. However what is their true *'svarupa'*; being?

Unity of body and mind

Patanjali explains how one can understand their real nature:

चित्तस्वरूपानुकार: इव इंद्रियाणां प्रत्याहार: ।

All the limbs are ultimately mental. *Shavasana* can give partial experience of this fact. There we feel that all the features of the body, states of life and awareness are really mental only. We never look at organs from this point of view. We do not use *Pratyahara* but use '*atyahara*'. We feed eyes, ears, stomach, etc. by exceeding their capacity through our immoderate indulgence. We see a lot, hear much, fill the belly fully etc. We regard their efficiency with this limited perception. We should understand their true nature through the *yogic* processes such as *asanas, bandhas, mudras*. The senses and organs should be studied through two-tier analysis i.e. through "exoteric physiology" and the "esoteric physiology".

Western medical science has made an elaborate study of the gross aspects out of these. It has made amazing progress in this regard from the 18th century onwards. The science of anatomy has made great strides in the finer aspects of the human anatomical system and yet there still remains a grave shortfall of knowledge in the subtler esoteric aspects. *Yogshastra* has a holistic approach in the study of the gross body but it also has considered the *sukshma sharira*. One more great qualification of *yogshastra* is that it not only explains the external manifestations of organs and senses but also enables one to modify the gross body mechanism. Modern science explains only the external part of human anatomy. For instance, it gives importance to the heart as a part of the circulatory system. It is studied from that point of view. In *yogshastra* however, the heart center is intimately linked with the mind, emotions, consciousness and the inner self. Actually all languages use the word 'heart' in that way. We say, "heartfelt sympathy, hearty congratulations, yours affectionately, etc." The holistic approach of *yogshastra* does not regard the heart merely as a formation of the auricles and ventricles, the veins and the arteries. The cardiogram or the angiograph merely gives the physical condition of the heart. There is more to be known. There is the Metaphysical element of divinity within. In *shloka* 61 of the 18th chapter the *Gita* says :

'ईश्वर: सर्वभूतानां हृदेशे अर्जुन तिष्ठति ।'

Obviously, this Divinity cannot be made visible through the Doppler test, scan or angiography. There are 101 energy channels with 7.2 million branches which cannot be made visible in the scan. The human navel to all appearances is a mere physical knot in the skin but in reality it is more than that. It is the source of crores of energy channels. The science of embryology explains to us to some extent the mystery of the navel.

Before we turn our attention to the *sukshma sharira* aspect we will take a look at the amazing gross body of the human being. There are many wonderful elements present in human organs. One of them is the presence of fire in the mouth. 'अग्नि: वाक् भूत्वा मुखं प्राविशत् ।' as the saying goes. Our mouth contains froth because there is fire in it. This fire is so powerful in the mouths of all of us that even a fire-fighting squad would not be able to put it out! Once an arrow is released in the form of words from the mouth it is impossible to retract it. The physical constitution of the mouth and tongue is the same in all individuals. However geniuses like *Kalidasa* and *Jnaneshvara* had the divine muse, *Sarasvati* residing on their tongue. There is a vital qualitative difference in the flow of words from the mouths of such men and from those of us, ordinary individuals. There is a similar difference of hands. The hands of personages like *Bhima* of the

Mahabharata or Michael Angelo or Ravi Varma are different from those of ordinary individuals. Their hands are for giving and ours are for taking.

Our legs and their legs have the same physical features, but while our legs lead us to evil, the legs of great men lead them to Heaven! If we want to know the reason behind this, we have to turn to the science of the *sukshma sharira* in *yogshastra,* study it and understand it.

Wonders of human body

Let alone the *sukshma sharira*, we do not even have a clear picture of the gross body. It is amazing to note that nearly eight million of our living cells die every second. We live on account of their destruction. In short, 'जीवो जीवस्य जीवनम् ।'. One life is food of another but at that same instant eight million cells are born. Our life is linked with the birth and death of these cells. Man has a network of blood vessels of sixty-thousand miles in length in his body. In the waking state, blood flows through this entire length every second. In the sleeping state the flow of blood is ten times slower. The eye uses two million million (with 17 zeros after two) cells for reading a normal sentence. The size of the heart is as much as a closed fist but it pumps 340 litres of blood every hour. The lungs require 411 litres of blood every minute. For every word uttered, one makes use of 70 to 75 muscles. The height of man is regulated by nature but not so his girth! A boy attains approximately 40 % of his height on his second birthday whereas a girl attains 52.5% height. Man's brain weighs 3% of his entire body weight. This 3 % of the body controls the remaining 97% of the entire body of man.

Compared to the size of an ant, man is a colossus. He has 650 muscles, 100 joints, 60000 miles of blood vessels and 13000 million brain cells. His bones are tougher than granite stone. These bones have a great capacity of resisting loads. A bone of the size of a match-stick can bear a load of nine tons which means that its resistance is four times that of cement concrete. Thus the bones of even the fattest man can never break under his own weight!

However, as far as consumption of food is considered, the ant is a giant and not man, because it can consume 200 times more food than its own weight. The ant can scale a tree trunk which has no steps carrying a load 200 times its own weight easily. Man requires steps to climb even the attic of his house! Thus to all intents and purposes, an ant is mightier than man.

An elephant consumes on an average 300-350 kg of food material daily. It can consume leaves, bamboos and coconuts along with the shells. It requires this amount of food to maintain the 1000-1500 kg of its weight. It can drink about 450 litres of water through its hose-pipe trunk. As far as man is concerned, even a glutton can hardly eat food 1/3 of his weight. The human heart beats 2000 million times during his life-time. During this period it pumps nearly 500 million litres of blood. This is equivalent to filling completely the petrol tank of a truck every seven minutes. So, imagine the amount of energy provided by nature. If we construct a pipe with the help of the veins and arteries in the lungs this length will be roughly 1500 miles. The digestive fire of the human system is so powerful that it can consume the hardest substances. Even so it does not affect the container stomach on account of the immediate replacement of the cells within the covering of the abdomen, thus leading to the renewal of the covering. The digestive juices thus do not have time enough to settle in the stomach.

There are about one million filters in the urinary bladder of the human system. These filters are even more wondrous than the advanced micro-filters invented by modern science. Every minute 1.3 litres of blood is purified therein. Later, about 1.4 litre of urine is thrown out. The entire human body is supplied with 4.5 litres of blood. The bone marrow manufactures the red corpuscles. Every second one million twenty thousand cells are produced and their life-span is between 100 and 120 days. Approximately half a ton of blood cells are produced from bone marrow. Man sheds his skin like that of a snake. During childhood this shedding process is faster and it slows down in old age. Human skin renews itself in about fifty days. A man sheds about 18 kilos of his tissues during his lifetime. The smallest tendon which is located in his ear is 0.05 inch long. Though there are no veins within this, it is always moist because of the otic fluid pressure in the ear. A man's height increases by .03 inch during his period of resting, but upon waking, due to the force of gravity this increase is nullified. The water content in his body is 80%, in addition to the other life ingredients. The amount of calcium in the body is sufficient to whitewash a small compartment. The total carbon content in the body is enough to produce 12.5 kg of coal. The body contains phosphorus which can provide 2250 matchsticks, it can produce one teaspoonful of sulphur, one inch of an iron nail from the iron content, and in addition thirty grams of other substances. The focussing muscles of the human eye undergo one hundred thousand movements during day-time. The energy required for this is equivalent to walking 50 miles. The eyeball of about the size of one square inch contains 13 crore 7 million minute cells. Thirteen crore of these are used for absorbing black and white colours, and 7 million for other colours. People in rich countries consume 50 tons of solid food and 50 thousand litres of liquids of whatever kind during a lifetime. Human hair consists of 5 million fibres and baldness makes no difference in this number! During sexual activity sperms have to travel a distance of 24'-7". During one ejaculation 50 crore sperm cells are released, though only a few thousand are able to traverse the above distance, and the rest wear out halfway. Out of these 500 million sperm cells only one sperm has the possibility of uniting with the ovum. The human brain has 10,000 million neurons connected with each other. Even if all the telephones in the world are connected together they would not be able to match the capacity of the brain. We must also admit that a so-called illiterate person who has to make his thumb impression on a document is "the wisest of them all" because one has to spend a lot of brain energy while pressing the thumb. The quantum of energy required for this activity of the thumb is the same as that required for the activity of the chest or the stomach. The impulses of the brain have a speed of 180 m/ph which is comparable to that of a racer car!

If such is the organization of the human body, then what can we say about the subtle invisible body! This *sukshma sharira*, as we have seen, migrates through 8.4 million wombs. The mind which has been wandering about since time immemorial is a suitable medium for spiritual tasks. There is a hierarchy of development among the species in the universe. We (conveniently?) suppose that man is at the top in this hierarchy because so far we have not found any other more developed species. In Indian philosophy there is a belief in the species such as *gandharva* or *kinnara* or *yaksha*. The mind is the seat of consciousness in all creatures, right from the bacteria, ants, insects, etc. to *gandharvas*, man, gods, etc. Though we have a specific existence in the present, the mind has been functioning in continuity. From time immemorial, the *samskaras* or mental impressions of the past arising out of our entire past *karma* are stored in the forehead space, like an archive or a floppy. The space between the eye-brows is the storehouse of all the *samskaras.* Thus the body becomes the site for both heaven and hell along with the *shadripus,* which are more ferocious than demons or the evil-minded *Duryodhana.* The *Mahabharata* war is taking place everyday in the mind. The *Dharmakshetra* and *Kurukshetra* are to be found together in this very place. This is the marvellous nature of the human body. So one can imagine what a greatly astonishing marvel the Atma must be. Hence it is said in the second chapter of the Gita,

आश्चर्यवत् पश्यति कश्चित् एनं आश्चर्यवद् वदति तथा एव च अन्य: ।

आश्चर्यवत् च एनं अन्य: शृणोति अपि एनं वेद न चैव कश्चित् ।। (2 : 29)

This description is like that of Lord *Krishna's* 'Vishwarupa darshana'. Nobody can understand the nature of *Atma.* All are only overcome by awe when they try to see or to talk about or hear it. The only truth is that nobody knows it.

The study of man in Yogshastra

Yogshastra studies man in totality. The truth of human nature is found only by *yogshastra.* It has the power of destroying man's angularities and enabling him to reach his innermost self. *Yogshastra* helps pinpoint the causes of diseases. It can help to bring balance in the mind, intellect, consciousness, ego, emotion, etc. It can create true health for body and mind. It shows how to counteract the *shadripus,* and to acquire a treasure of positive qualities through true knowledge of life which is like a *Brahmastra,* the ultimate invincible weapon. All the human *vrittis* can be controlled through *yog.* It can successfully transform man's inner and outer natures. It is panacea for all ailments. Man's physical body is the Lord's most wonderful piece of work. The important task of achieving all-round excellence and eliminating sorrows and further leading one to the blissful state can be done by *yogshastra*. It is the common pathway for both the realized souls as well for the neophyte *sadhakas*.

We have so far discussed various aspects of the the *panchakoshas,* five sheaths or *sthula sharira, sukshma sharira* and *karana sharira.* Mind is a more significant aspect. So the thoughts of inquiry into mind, consciousness, thought process in *yog* and other important characteristics are discussed in the next topic.

Shri Krishnaarpanam astu

✤ ✤ ✤

Discourse - 14

Yog Chitta Vijnana

Yogic knowledge of Consciousness

We will now consider what is known as *Yog Chitta Vijnana*. This is a highly integrated system of knowledge and is the seat of knowledge of the mental, intellectual faculties and the sense of 'I'ness or ego. The *yogsutras* of *Patanjali* explain that the functioning of the consciousness is made up of five planes: 1. *Mûdha* or deluded 2. *Kshipta* or wandering 3. *Vikshipta* or alternating 4. *Ekagra or* one-pointed mind during trance and 5. *Niruddha* or totally restrained. *Chitta Vijnana* comprises of the knowledge and investigation of the above factors. These perpetual mind fluctuations known as *vrittis* can be broadly classified into two categories:

The Vrittis

The *klishta* or defiled consciousness is temporally oriented and supports materialism. The *aklishta* is non-afflictive consciousness. The *klishta vritti* increases worldly attachments along with their consequences. These *vrittis* add to and also create man's afflictions and sorrows. The *aklishta vrittis* on the other hand weaken the effects of the aforementioned *klishta vrittis* and result in spiritual tendencies. These *vrittis* lift the person from materialism and he embarks upon spiritualism. *Yogshastra* considers all the aspects of both the types of *vrittis* in regard to their nature, functions, characteristics and efficacy. The first type of *vritti* is devoid of the sense of discrimination and has sensual propensities, while the other *vritti* induces the sense of discrimination and leads towards the path of *yog*. Each of these *vrittis* has five categories. These are: *Pramana* or valid cognition, *viparyaya* or illusory perception, *vikalpa* or verbal delusion, *nidra* and *smriti* or memory and recollection. These are known as the *panchavrittis* in the *shastras*. Further, there are many subdivisions of these main *vrittis*.

Pramana is the pivot of intellectual inquiry. In modern parlance it iis known as "Epistemology". This branch of inquiry is a science by iitself. It dwells on the sources of valid knowledge, its causes, mode of acquisition, attainment of flawless knowledge and its nature. All this makes a separate branch by itself. *Viparyaya* is also an amazing subject. According to the concept of *viparyaya* one type of human ignorance is effaced only to be replaced by another type of ignorance. This may appear to be strange, but our worldly knowledge is very much so. The 13th chapter of the Gita mentions,

अध्यात्मज्ञाननित्यत्वं तत्त्वज्ञानार्थदर्शनम् ।

एतद् ज्ञानं इति प्रोक्तं अज्ञानं यत् अत: अन्यथा ।। 13.11

Spiritual knowledge is the only true and lasting knowledge. It gives meaning of philosophy. All other knowledge is ignorance only. Our University education conforms to this fact. It is as though one is promoted to the second standard ignorance from the first standard ignorance! The same process is repeated when the student is promoted to the third standard. The so-called worldly knowledge is but *ajnana*. Strangely *vikalpa* or verbal delusion is also a powerful characteristic of *vritti* and is the only means to transmit knowledge about the absolute or *Brahman*. *Vyasamuni* states that *vikalpa* is very realistic and effective, since the transcendental *Brahman* can be defined in words through *vikalpa*. Transmission of knowledge is not possible without it. *Nidra* is elaborately described in *yogshastra*. *Sushupti* is one meaning of *nidraa*. We sleep but we do not know it or about it. The explanation of knowledge of *nidra*, knowledge or consciousness in *nidra* and knowledge about it in *yogshastra* is very interesting.

Two theories also are expounded here. They are *laya* or absorption of the mind and *vishrama* which is rest or repose. This part describes the metapsychology of *sushupti*, too. *Sushupti* has a repository of multiplicity of consciousnesses. Dream state, day-dreaming are very marked states and they are fully explained here. Mental stupor, consciousness and unconsciousness are different states of *nidra* only. Then follows explanation of *smriti*. *Smriti* arises on account of several factors and more than twenty-five of them are mentioned. This part tells us about the nature of *smriti* and the ways of retaining it. The peculiar thing about *smriti* is that it works conveniently for us. We love to do certain things and some things are imposed upon us for doing. For instance, we love to eat and sometimes fasting is imposed on us by the doctor or by religious convention. We do not forget to eat but forget fasting or taking pills, etc! Also, we cannot forget what we want to forget or do forget what we do not want to forget. The analysis of the five *vrittis* forms an independent area of study.

Dimensions of mind

The activities of the mind are uncontrollable, bizarre and haphazard. Sometimes other people do trouble us, but it is also a fact that we are often tormented by our own wavering mind. It imagines forebodings which are perhaps worse than what a real enemy can think of doing. Thus we are afraid more of our own imaginary dangers than the real external ones. Perhaps the reason is our love for ourselves because as Kalidasa said, अतिस्नेह: पापशंकी. Too much of love begets worry and apprehensions. The *Gita* says :
'आत्मा एवं आत्मन: बन्धु: आत्मा एव रिपु: आत्मन: ।' (6 : 5) Our mind

is our friend and our enemy at the same time. This internal enemy, the mind, is more powerful and hostile than the external enemies on account of its unbridled nature. Our consciousness becomes disturbed and agitated. We have commotion of thousands of emotions like worry, tensions, eagerness, desires and cares in our mind. *Yogshastra* shows the way to control the mind with all this. In this respect, the ways and means shown by *yogshastra* are as effective as the *Brahmastra* which is an ultimate lethal weapon. That is why *yogshastra* is known as the science of mind-control and that is why it is a revered science. Once the disturbance of the consciousness is removed, consciousness regains its eternal quiescence. The multiplicity and variety of means of mind control described in *yogshastra* are amazing. They are appropriate for different situations, conditions and levels. All the categories of *sadhakas* from the neophyte to the *siddha purushas* can find means of mind control suitable for each of them.

Most of our hopes, aspirations, desires, *vasanas* are inordinate and naturally they create heavy strain on the *chitta*. *Vairagya* or dispassion is a unique solution for such disturbed consciousness. *Vairagya* is an important topic in the *yogsutras* for managing this state of mind. The topic of *abhyasa- vairagya* is considered jointly at length and it is useful for an accomplished *yogi* as well as for an ordinary person. The S*amadhi Pada* describes the psychology of eternal ecstasy or bliss. This topic unfolds the subtle phenomenon of ultimate revelation, self-realization or self-contentment. One of the sub-topics in this explains the nature of the highest spiritual contentment. It explains how transformation of the consciousness takes place, leading to the experience of spiritual elevation or progress and then the progress towards *Kaivalya* or salvation.

The mind is the storehouse of consciousness. An accomplished *yogi* is either a *jnanayogi, bhaktiyogi, dhyanayogi* or *karmayogi*. All these *yogis* and the characteristics of these different types of celebrated *yogis* are described in the beginning of the *Sadhanapada*. We can see the distinctive, common and different features of *jnanis* like *Vasishtha, Shankaracharya, dhyanis* like *Patanjali, Yajnyavalkya, karmayogis* like *Janaka* and *bhaktas* like *Namadev, Tukaram*. *Manovijnana* explains the manner in which *kleshas,* suffering or afflictions can be assuaged by adopting any of the four *yogic* paths, namely, *jnana, bhakti, dhyana* and *karma*.

Karma

The next topic is *karma*. On account of *karma* one experiences the dualities -happiness and sorrow, success and failure, fame and ignominy, profit and loss, auspiciousness and inauspiciousness etc. These dualities are caused by *karma* which has different classifications and types. *Yogshastra* in a sense goes further than *Dharmashastra* and culminates into *nishkama karmayog*. We acquire spiritual wisdom by the practice of *yog*. *Kleshas* have five causes: ignorance, pride, attachment, aversion and fear of death. All the impressions of our past 8.4 million lives mould our present and future. The topic of transmigration explains the phenomenon of events happening before birth and after death. This whole explanation is a challenge for our thinking capacity.

Manovijnana

The confusion, aberrations and diseases of the human mind arise on account of the *shadripus* of *kama, krodha, mada, moha, lobha* and *matsara*. These are like poisonous plants in the soil of the *kleshas*. They can convert one's life into a hell. The only way to reduce the effect of the *kleshas* and calm the *chittavrittis* is to deforest the *shadripus*. Our mind is made up of nerves and *shadripus* are active there. The path of *ashtanga yogsadhana* can help us to control them. *Ashtangayog* helps self-purification by gaining control of the *shadripus*. *Ashtangayog* is thus a complete science showing a way for combating afflictions of the mind and enabling it for spiritual development. *Ashtangayog* is constituted of the eight limbs of *yama, niyama, asana, pranayama, pratyahara, dharana, dhyana* and *samadhi*. *Ahimsa, satya, brahmacharya, asteya,* and *aparigraha* are the fivefold extensions of *yama,* while *shaucha, santosha, tapa, svadhyaya* and *Ishvarapranidhana* are aspects of *niyama*. These *yamas* and *niyamas* are formulated with a perfect thinking of *manovijnana*.

The *asana* part of *ashtanga yogsadhana* are not mere physical actions but they have their *manovijnana*. Similarly *pranayama* does not consist of merely holding the nose and breathing. Their subtle aspects are emphasized in *yogshastra*. The finer subtler aspects and mysticism of *pratyahara, dharana, dhyana* and *samadhi* have been churned out in an interesting way. This *manovijnaana* is transcendental. It deals with how the individual mind is developed into the universal mind. The mid-portion of the third *pada* of *yogsutras* discusses the salient aspects of the human mind from a particular point of view. Generally we are engrossed in thinking of our material interests and our actions are directed towards worldly achievements. Thoughts, emotions, desires, fears, worries. All these result in bewildering confusion. This condition of our mind is called *vyutthita chitta* or unbridled nature of the mind which is caused by *vyutthana samskaras* and interests. This begets *vyutthana parinama* which creates *avyagrata* leading to *sarvarthata or anekarthata parinama*. This mind resembles a child sitting before a basket of toys. How his eyes are wandering from one toy to another and his hands are busy touching one toy after another! This is usually the normal frame of our mind. Our mind is always frittering away in several directions.

A *yogi,* however, has an opposite journey of the mind. He has a different order of *parinama.* He has *nirodha samskaras* instead of *vyutthana samskaras.* So he proceeds from *sarvarthata or anekarthata parinama* to *ekagrata parinama.* He can control and overcome the wavering of the mind. His mind becomes steady and one-pointed. These states of mind can be graphically represented by drawing two columns. The left column represents the *vyutthana* excited, activated mind, while the right one is the center of *ekagrata* control and restraint, as shown below:

Vyutthana samskaras/outgoing impressions	Nirodha samskaras/restraining impressions
We	Yogi
Distracted	Restrained
Fluttering fluctuating	Controlled
outwardly	inwardly
wandering	Focussed, one-pointed

The above table shows two different phases of mind, one of the ordinary individual and the other of a *yogi.*

Even between two ordinary individuals the nature of the mind and the *samskaras* or impressions is disparate. Twins may appear similar externally, however, their mental make-up is not perfectly similar on account of their own impressions acquired in the past births. The impressions are mainly of two kinds as shown above and they are present differently in different beings. We behave differently in different circumstances-sometimes logically and sometimes illogically, sometimes calmly and sometimes angrily. A human being is seldom found to be consistently in either of the states i. e. *vyutthita* or *niruddha*. Normally, the mind plays hide and seek between the two extremes of the noble and the bestial tendencies. The same person is saintly and villain, constructive and destructive at different times in his life. The *samskarachakra* revolves incessantly from one type of tendency to the opposite tendency. It is moving as inevitably as the *chakra* of day and night or of wakeful and sleepy states. This shows the difference between the mindset of a *yogi* and that of an ordinary individual.

The third *pada* of the *yogsutras* describes various *siddhis or yogic* powers acquired through *yogsadhana*. A *yogi* possesses clairvoyance, divine vision, he hears divine sounds and has other psychic powers, like *sukshmadarshana, sukshmashravana, viprakrushtadarshana* i.e. vision of remote objects, *vyavahitadarshana* i. e. vision of veiled objects. He has *siddhis* of all the organs, and possesses extrasensory perception, ESP. Modern psychology has to some extent admitted and realized this aspect. Clairaudience, clairvoyance, etc are now accepted traits of human nature.

Manovijnana deals with the questions such as-what is the mind? What are its features? Where do spirituality, egoism, emotions, etc reside? The five *jnanendriyas* and five *karmedriyas* are external and are seen and felt but these are organs of the mind. Spirituality makes man inhibitive of sin. Different people manifest their feelings differently depending upon their emotionality. Thoughts keep on changing according to different states and circumstances of life. The states of infancy, childhood or youth have different ways and directions of thinking. The egoism and individuality of a person keeps on changing in accordance with age, environment, and circumstances. Behaviour is different depending on the kind of company of friends or of elders. We are not the same in the company of children and of respectable persons. *Vasanas* also keep on changing according to age and circumstances. The thinking faculty and the sense of discrimination goes on changing in the same manner. So there is the study of physiology and anatomy of the mental faculties. The third *pada* thinks of and studies the *sukshma sharira* consisting of mind and *samskaras*. The physical and external body has senses, organs and limbs, it possesses a form and shape and it can be studied and grasped. *Yogshastra* looks at the *sukshma sharira* and it can study the *sukshma sharira* just as easily as in the case of this physical body. We have tried so far to summarize in brief the subtle and long description of *manovijnana* in the *yogshastra*.

Shri Krishnaarpanam astu

✦ ✦ ✦

Discourse - 15

Yog Manovijnana 1

Yogic Science of the Mind

We will now take a bird's eye view of *yog manovijnana* which is the *yogic* science of the mind. The nature of man depends upon his mental frame. He is not man just because he has two hands, two legs and one head. He is not man just because he has no tail. Interestingly, the Sanskrit word *mana* for mind is found in all the words for man like *manava, manushya* or human being. The mind is the most important component of the human make-up. It is subtle in nature and indeed the most salient feature of the human system. *Yogshastra* has given it enormous importance and consideration. *Yogshastra,* as a matter of fact, is the science of the mind. It is different from psychology which is just a science of behaviour and treats the mind on the basis of current medical theories. The *yogic* science of the mind is vastly superior to psychology, as it is related to the universal aspect of human existence. The study of the human mind in *yogshastra* is as much as the amount of water in the ocean. *Yogshastra* makes an in- depth study of the mind not forgetting the past, present and future of human existence, whereas psychology restricts its study only to the current or present condition of the mind.

Mind is infinite in nature. 'अनंतं वै मन: I' states the *Shatapatha Brahmana.* *Yogshastra* studies the mind on three levels--*vyashti* mind, *samashti* mind and *parameshti* mind. The *vyashti* level refers to the individual mind or rather the individualized mind and is limited to the span of one life only. It starts existing just at birth and vanishes after death. Modern psychology considers only this limited state and worldly matters. It does not deal with what is auspicious or inauspicious, what is agreeable or disagreeable. The *klishta, aklishta, adhyatmic, paramarthic vrittis* are not described here. The approach of psychology is thus objective only, and it prescribes the means of overcoming and achieving these states. The *yogic manasashastra* studies these things objectively but it also transcends these limited boundaries and shows the maturity of going beyond the individualised mind.

The *samashti* mind is a storehouse of impressions of past lives. The science of *samashti manas* may be referred to as metapsychology, wherein the study of the impressions of an individual's past lives is made. The entire experiences of the lives of nearly 8.4 million life species, the ups and downs of the various lives from time without beginning are manifested in the *samashti* mind. It represents a state beyond that of the subconscious mind and the lower mind. This point has already been discussed in the subject of *linga sharira* or *sukshma sharira.*

The third level or the *parameshti manas* is called the divine mind. It is also known as the cosmic or universal mind. This is the element of divinity in the human mind. In some cases this divinity is revealed to a marked degree. The minds of *Sant Jnaneshvar, Sant Tukaram, Chaitanya Mahaprabhu* are notable examples of this.

Yogshastra has, in fact, described the *manas* in totality and has covered all its aspects. It shows how the mind can be controlled. It does not merely or coldly describe this, but directs the individual in evolving the mind towards perfection and avoid degradation. It describes the *klishta* and *aklishta vrittis*. *Klishta vrittis* are responsible for the downfall of the individual, whereas the *aklishta vrittis* restrain the negative *vrittis* and evolve the mind in the positive direction. These two types of *vrittis* are expressed in five ways. *Yogshastra* has laid down a definite classification of the multifarious *vrittis* into two broad categories with five subject-classifications. These five classifications common to both the *klishta* and *aklishta vrittis* are : (1) *Pramana vritti* is threefold-*pratyaksha- perception- anumana* - which is based on inference. It is said, *yatra yatra dhumaha tatra tatra vanhihi.* Where there is smoke, there is fire. There is a relation between mark and marked. *Agama* is testimony coming from trustworthy persons, authorities and texts. So this is direct perception derived from one's own condition (2) *Viparyaya vritti* - misconception or misperception leading to contrary knowledge, also verbal delusion (3) *Vikalpa vritti* - imagination or fancy, consisting of ideas without factual basis (4) *Nidra vritti*-includes the of dormancy, dreams, day dreams and unconscious states, and (5) *Smriti* - memory, the faculty of retaining or reviving past experiences. There does not exist any sixth type of *vritti.*

Yogshastra has achieved the very difficult task of explaining the functioning of the mind with all its ramifications, and has further spelt out the path of achieving fulfilment in life. It has drawn a map of its origin, structure and journey, and explained its dimensions to help its development. It has devised efficient techniques for controlling the mind. The mind is deeper than the ocean, loftier than the sky and as expansive as the universe. *Arjuna* asks *Shrikrishna* in the *Gita* how the ever unsteady mind could be subjugated. Lord *Krishna* says that this task is difficult but not impossible. *Yogshastra* shows how this is right.

Yogshastra has explained the techniques of restraining the mind and culturing it, by making use of the internal and external limbs and organs of the body. It has considered the contribution of food habits, movements, *satsanga, sadhanasanga, shastrasanga,* and management of *saptadhatus, tridoshas, trigunas, panch jnanendriyas, panch karmendriyas,* etc for this purpose. It has thought of the means of attaining a positive interaction of the mind with external nature. So it has not left out the contribution of the outside world. It has formulated a system of means for mind control with the *yogic kriyas, bandhas, mudras, asana, pranayama,* etc. They are an integral part of *ashtanga yog* and thus *ashtanga yog* is the bedrock of the means.

The *yogic* science of the mind refers to five types of *vrittis*. *Yogshastra* has described two kinds of these *vrittis* viz. *bhog* or the worldly and *apavarga* or the spiritual. The subtle aspects of the *chitta or* consciousness and these five types of *vrittis* associated with the consciousness are also explained. A person's mindset, his *karma, dharma* and *samskaras* have the five *kleshas* at its root. They are described as *avidya* or ignorance, *asmita* or I-consciousness, *raaga* or attachment, *dvesha* or hate and *abhinivesha* or fear of death and clinging to existence. This detailed explanation in the *yogshastra* demands our deep consideration and concern. It provides a comprehensive thinking of the entire psychology related to the external physical body, the science of the physical body, the emotions, senses and organs, human culture, human angularities and perversions, *siddhis* like clairvoyance, the weakening of the *vrittis* and the phenomenon of transmigration from birth to birth. We are now going to learn the science of the senses and organs and also their *manovijnana*. We should understand that each and every, even the minutest, aspect of *ashtanga yog* right from *yama, niyama, asana* to *samadhi* have their *manovijnana* behind it. Just inhaling and

163

exhaling with fingers on the nostrils is a mockery of *pranayama.* *Yogshastra* has expounded the *manovijnana* behind all the *vrittis* and behind their *klishtata* and *aklishtata.*

We cannot study *yogic manovijnana* fully in this chapter, because it cannot be studied without a complete understanding of *yogshastra.* So far we have perused only the introduction to this subject. Many supernatural *yogic* powers, *siddhis,* are described in the *yogsutras.* There is a *manovijnana* behind every *siddhi.* There are different graduation levels of *yogis* like *madhubhumi, madhumati, madhupratika.* The *manovijnana* of these levels varies. There are subtle differences in each of the levels and there are many variations in the actions of *dharana, pratyahara, pranayama, asana* and so on. The mental process behind each of these variations is different. Even a list of the contents of such variations would be too long to mention here. Therefore we must admit that *manovijnana* cannot be explained in a single chapter.

We have only tried to present a blue print or skeleton to explain *yogic* psychology. *Yogshastra* is a science of the mind. Just looking at the list of the contents, we can say that *chitta bhumi* or planes are explained in it. *Yogshastra* has categorized individuals according to the influence of their *chitta vrittis.* It has stipulated five such categories. This is referred to as the principle of *panchabhumi.* We all belong to any one of these *panchabhumis,* five planes of consciousness. Also, an individual can undergo different experiences of his *chitta vrittis,* thus effecting a change in his *bhumi.* Our *chitta* is either scattered, distracted and confused or in an attentive or restrained condition. Therefore, we are in different states of mind at different moments such as tranquillity, unrest, discriminating state, state of fear of committing sin, state of being enticed.

Gulabrao Maharaj on chitta bhumi

The matter of the *panchabhumi* of *chitta* is clearly depicted by *Gulabrao Maharaj,* a Maharashtrian sant, in his **Yogprabhava** in an illuminatingly subtle manner. The *kshipta bhumi* is referred to as affected by *rajoguna,* always flooded by worldly desires. In this regard we remember the following Sanskrit *shloka:*

मर्कटस्य सुरापानं तस्य वृश्चिकदंशनम् ।
तन्मध्ये भूतसंचार: यद्वा तद्वा भविष्यति ।।

One can imagine the behaviour of a monkey drunk with whisky; it is then bitten by a scorpion and later on a ghost possesses it. What could be happening to it --And to the people around, too? This then is the state of the scattered *kshipta chitta bhumi* with *rajoguna.* The same situation is described by *Gulaabrao Mahaaraj.* He says, "This *kshipta chitta* is never stable for a moment. Whether the person is learned or ignorant, he is dreaming of pleasures. His mind has different moods every moment, from romance to sorrow or to bravery. He likes to wander like a fly on the potter's wheel. He would understand this if he were to sit back quietly. For him a quiet and beautiful place is a prison, and solitude like hell."

Gulabrao Maharaj describes the next *mudha bhumi* which is replete with *tamoguna* as follows. "This *chitta* is always sleepy and becomes lazy after waking up. After his snoring is over, he has an idle mood. Naturally, when some difficult situation arises, he behaves like a mad dog. His mind has such inertia that after coming out of sleep, he cannot recognize who is his mother and who is wife. He behaves like a subhuman species. He does not want to work but expects that his wife should earn a livelihood by working hard for him. He is a stubborn fool all the time. "

Then Gulabrao Maharaj describes vi*kshipta chitta bhumi*. Don't we find our own reflection in this mirror? "He follows yog reluctantly and even all his experiences are taken with reluctance. This is vi*kshipta chitta bhumi*. One moment he is saintly like Narada and another moment like a dog. One moment an emperor, another moment a beggar, One moment a Brahmin and another moment a villain, One moment a good disciple, another moment a coward, one moment a generous man, another moment a miser, one moment a sadhu, another moment a hypocrite-such are his changing mindsets. Naturally he has sometimes ecstasy and sometimes agony without good reason. He is a victim of his own instability."

Gulabrao Maharaj depicts the fourth *ekagra chitta bhumi* in a similar manner. But this is not our level. We, ordinary people move between *mudha* and *rajoguna* or *tamoguna*. The person with *ekagra chitta* is able to accomplish *yama, niyama, dharana, pratyahara, pranayama, asana, dhyana* by practice. He obeys *yogis* and controls *rajoguna*. His mind is prepared for *yog* and then it becomes his nature only." So it is clear that this *ekagra chitta bhumi* belongs to an accomplished *ashtang yogi*. We can get only a 'shadow' of this kind of *ekaagrata* while studying for examinations or reading interesting books or listening to enchanting music.

The fifth *chitta bhumi* also is not for us, it is *bhumi* of the *siddha yogi*. Our area is the first three *bhumis*. He has controlled *rajoguna* and *tamoguna*. His *chitta* is naturally full of *sattvaguna*. *Gulabrao Mahaaraj* says that this *siddha yogi* has all his *vrittis* under control and has achieved *asamprajnata samadhi*.

We considered here the nature of the *chitta bhumi* and *manovijnana* of the five *manobhumis*.

Yogshastra takes into consideration an integrated approach to body and mind. It also deals with *papa,* sin, *punya,* merit, *sukha,* contentment, *duhkha,* sorrow, *karma,* action and *dharma* or righteousness in a remarkable manner. Medical science or anatomy describes merely the anatomical arrangement of the physical organs. It describes the *jnanendriyas* like nose, ear, skin and *karmendriyas* like hands and feet, digestive organs, respiratory organs, reproductive organs, circulatory system, bones, muscles, etc. There are specialists for each of these organs. So we get an illusion that these sciences are perfect. However, medical science does not make a study of the *indriyas* in an integrated manner. This topic makes an attempt to remove this misconception.

Five forms of indriyas

Patanjali states in the third *pada* (*vibhuti pada*) :

Grahana, svarupa, asmita, anvaya, arthavattva, samyamat indriyajaya.

He states that there are five forms of the *indriyas.* The first is that of grasping or functional form of senses and organs, the second, substantive form or intrinsic nature, the third the I-consciousness, the fourth collocation of the *sattva, rajas,* and *tamas,* and fifth, the purpose and utilization. If these are perceived, and *samadhi* is attained by restraining them, then it is a perfect conquest of *indriyas.*

Let us take the case of a particular organ e.g. the eye to understand the five levels of the *indriyas.* The eye is the organ of sight. We are able to see various forms by means of the eye. We are able to study its structure and functions in physiological science. When we see an object, its image turns turtle, the nervous system sends impulses to the brain, the respective centres are stimulated and then we 'see' the object–all this process is described in the science of physiology. Though these are physical functions of the eye, they do not demonstrate its intrinsic nature. The function of an organ and its intrinsic nature are not synonymous. *Goroba* was a potter, *Kabir* was a weaver, *Sena* was a barber, but these were their professions, not their intrinsic nature. Their nature was that of a saint. They were devotees of God. Our profession does not signify our real nature. It is hardly logical to equate its functions with nature. The same is the case with the *indriyas*. Seeing with the eye and hearing with the ear are mere actions but they do not really reflect their intrinsic nature. Touch of the skin, smelling of the nose, tasting of the tongue are only sensations or functions but not the real nature of the concerned organs. The same is the case with *karmendriyas*. Speech is the function of the tongue, offering of the hands, defecation of the anus, enjoyment of the genitals, walking of the feet – all these are the functions of the respective organs but they are not their intrinsic nature.

What then really is the intrinsic nature of the various organs of action? But let us first give attention to our confusion regarding other parts of the body, too. Thinking and worrying is the function of the brain but we start thinking that it is the real nature of the brain. It is not so. The function of the brain is not this. We try to pressurize the brain to worry when in a depressed mood. Just as someone is compelled by circumstances to do a work below his capacity and dignity, so also the brain is subjected to different works. The function of the brain is *reflecting* and not *thinking*. We experience a whirlpool of thoughts and turmoil of ideas and passions. At the end we come to some conclusion, establish it, we stay with it. There is quietude of mind. Water is tranquil and can show reflection. We watch it and this is the natural and real function of the brain. It is not meant to produce a train of thoughts. A Mercedes car is not meant for transporting substances like coal.

Instead of attaining this equilibrium, we unnecessarily try to coerce the brain into a tumult of worldly matters, resulting in an injudicious deployment of the brain. Nature has not allotted this work to brain. This is against the laws of nature. We are sending a sadhu to the share market! We do not make positive use of the brain. The nature and function of the other organs such as the liver, tongue or stomach have also to be viewed in this manner only. The same argument holds good for the heart. Circulating blood is its true function, not its nature. Its true nature is to circulate good-heartedness and affection. Its function is to pour out emotions of affection, love and adoration. The heart is, thus, truly the source of celestial feelings and emotions. The real study of the heart cannot be made by any amount of physical cardiological approach. We have to explore the mother's heart. A cardiogram of the mother's heart will enable us to understand the heart with a better perspective. The bliss of life is experienced through the heart. The heart can transform the *vâsanâs* in the blood by vivifying the blood with divine emotions of motherly love and devotion to God. The *Bhagavadgita* says:

'माता अहं अस्य जगतो माता धाता पितामह:'

I am the Mother of this world and I take care of it. I am not only the Mother, I am the Creator of the Mother, too. Further,

'ईश्वर: सर्वभूतानाम् हृद्देशे अर्जुन तिष्ठति'

So the heart is the abode of the Lord in the human embodiment. The Lord is Father, Mother and Grandsire. If you want to know the true nature of the heart, look at the feelings of a mother towards the child. Look at the love of the Lord towards His creation. Have a glance at the vascular test and emotional cardiology of the saints. Their mercy for sinful and meritorious people alike will show you the truth of the heart. This indeed is the *true* nature of the esoteric human heart. It is the repository of compassion towards all living creatures. Hence the physical organs cannot be viewed as mere physical entities but have to be recognized in their psychological and emotional aspects. It is a grave illusion to say that there is nothing beyond functions about the parts of the body. Their nature is far different and we must try to understand it.

Shri Krishnaarpanam astu

✢ ✢ ✢

Discourse - 16

Yog Manovijnana 2

Functions and nature of the organs

The physical organs and limbs of the body like the heart are constantly working. The lungs, spleen, skin, tongue, urinary bladder are always physically active. As it is already discussed, their action or function cannot be considered synonymous with their intrinsic nature. To equate the function and nature of the organs of the body is a mistake as well as an illusion. *Yogshastra* emphasizes this point and enables us to remove the deep rooted illusions in this regard.

Why did *yogshastra* put forth this theory? How and why did they reach this kind of conclusion? Because *yogshastra* and a *yogi* can and do experience the true nature of the various physical organs. They have come to certain conclusions from their experience. We need not agree with them without thinking and should not accept their conclusions blindly. Let us think of these conclusions logically and with reason.

A question may be raised. When are we really close to our true nature? The reply is that we are more in tune with our nature when we retire from our daily chores, our work, domestic as well as professional assignments and commitments. This is a pre-condition. We must be undisturbed in our actions in order to attain peace of mind. We should detach ourselves from the daily activities. In a sense, we are nearer to our true selves when we do nothing. We are far away from ourselves when we indulge in our routine activities. We may be undisturbed while being engaged in any activity, yet we may not necessarily be at peace with ourselves. So also all our *karmendriyas* and *jnanendriyas* are nearer to their selves or intrinsic nature when they are free from their functional activity. When they are functioning, they are in a role but not in their *svarupa*. We can draw this conclusion about any of the *karmendriyas* and *jnanendriyas* and other organs like heart or liver or spleen.

One more important point has to be considered. Even when an *indriya* is inactive, it does not indicate a state of *pratyahara* or absorption in peace. If we order the liver to sit back and rest, it cannot do that. Even if the eyes are closed, it does not mean that they are in their *svarupa* or their intrinsic state. At the back of all the *karmendriyas,* there exists one and the same mind which receives all their signals. The same can be said about the ear which can continue hearing even if the eyes see nothing. The action of one or the other *indriya* must be affecting the common curtain of the mind which is behind all. This means that the real nature of the organs can be attained only if all the organs collectively remain actionless. *Yogshastra* has described this state as the state of *pratyahara*. *Pratyahara* is *prati-ahara*, a subtle *pranic* and *chaittik kriya*. This technique of *yog* can take the physical organs into their real nature. When the mind further progresses towards the thoughtless state (*chittavritti nirodhaha*), of *samadhi,* the organs are finally merged into their real, intrinsic, actionless state. *Shavasana* is a powerful means of stimulating the *sadhaka* to tend towards this state. A proper performance of the *shavasana* or *samadhi* or *pratyahara* leads to calmness of all the physical organs, the five senses, the *chitta,* the *saptadhatus,* the *tridoshas* and the *panchamahabhutas,* the lungs, the abdomen, stomach, liver and all. In *shavasana, pratyahara* and *samadhi* all the above constituents are in an undisturbed and controlled state. What is their svarup then? As the sutra says:

'चित्तस्वरूपानुकार इव इंद्रियाणां प्रत्याहारः ।'

When the senses are withdrawn from the respective objects and drawn towards their essential consciousness, it is *pratyahara*.

All the organs tend to the integrated, homogeneous and united state of the consciousness.

Another facet of the *indriyas* is the *asmita* or I-consciousness. We say, my hands, my feet, etc. i.e. the feeling of "my hands, my feet" is linked with the *indriyas*. Mind is the curtain behind all the *indriyas*, and behind this curtain is the *asmitaa*. The mind stimulates the *indriyas* to action and controls their sensations. Mind is the motivator of the *indriyas* and *asmita* is the motivator of the mind. If the mind is not active behind the *indriyas*, they do not do *grahana*, their function. If the mind is engrossed in something else, even open eyes do not do the function of seeing and ears do not hear anything. A pedestrian does not hear harsh honking of the horn of a lorry, if he is engrossed in some thoughts. So *indriyas* need mind behind them, and mind needs *asmita* or *aham* behind it. *Manovijnana* says this and it needs no more justification. However is it true just because we feel like it or it seems to be so or is there any substantial evidence for it? There must be some science, scientific process to prove this. Then only the conclusions can be valid. It must have a metaphysical basis, and such a basis there is.

Man's corporeal frame is made up of cells. The *karmendriyas* and *jnanendriyas,* veins, nerves and arteries all are made up of cells. The cells constitute tissues of organs of the *panchamahabhutas*. According to the *Samkhya* philosophy, *panchmahabhutas* are produced from the *tanmatras* or the subtle primary elements. *Tanmatras* arise out of *ahamkara*, which is not different from *asmita*. Thus all the elements of the flesh are ultimately created from *asmita*. From the *Mulaprakriti* or primordial matter we have the *mahat* or the cosmic intelligence, from *mahat* arises *ahamkara,* from *ahamkara* we have the *tanmatras* and the inert *panchamahabhutas.* These are one type of elements. The other type consists of mind, senses and organs – of action *karmendriyas* and *jnanendriyas.* If we consider the 24 elements of the *Samkhya* system, it can be concluded that the *indriyas* arise from *asmita.* The body consists of the limbs, *saptadhatus, tridoshas, indriyas,* all of which are constituted of the *panchamahabhutas.* Therefore, *asmita* is the third nature of the organs and limbs. According to metaphysics, if an individual has a cosmic, spiritual, noble and pure *ahamkara,* then all the organs and limbs are in the third form of senses and organs that is *asmita.* This may be achieved through *japa, dhyana* and *pranayama. Asmita* is the third transcendental stage of an organ's form. We therefore see that the first three constitutions of the *indriyas* and limbs are – 1. assuming their physical forms, *grahana* 2. their substantive form, and 3. their being born out of the I-consciousnesss. *Asmita* and mind are the common elements of all the different limbs and organs. The whole body has only one 'I'. The 'I' who suffers from stomach ache is the same who suffers from headache. The perception of sorrow and happiness in all the organs is 'I' only. The I-consciousness pervades all the *indriyas* and their awareness, and perception of the sensations are due to this I-consciousness.

Indriyas have a fourth form. Though the organs and senses have I-consciousness, each and everyone of them is born out of the *trigunas- sattva, rajas* and *tamas.* Metaphysics makes this point. The body is made up of *trigunas.* The entire Universe is *trigunatmaka* i. e. constituted by the *trigunas.* The body is the manifestation of the *trigunas.* This is the fourth form of the *indriyas.* We become *tamasic, rajasic,* or *sattvic* depending on the preponderance of the particular *guna.* These three *gunas* are present in differing proportions in the individual. No individual can possess only one *guna.* For obtaining a predominance of *sattvaguna* in us we should practise *yogsadhana, satsanga, adhyatmasadhana,* and have *sattvic* thinking. This enables us to attain a positive transformation in the physical and the consciousness plane. Through *yogic* knowledge of the *indriyas* a characteristic change can be effected. *Yogshastra* explains how one can acquire a *sattvic buddhi,* right from the level of the physical body to the level of the *chitta.* A genuine approach to the study of the *gunas* is required to understand this. The effect of the *gunas* is realized when one compares the speech of *Jnaneshvara* whose speech would be full of *sattva,* and our speech. The blood of such persons is devoid of the *shadripus.* Doctors take haemograph of blood. If we take spiritual haemograph, we can see the proportions of *shadripus* like *kama, krodha* etc. The persons with *sattva guna* will show very low quantity of the *shadripus.* The functioning of everyone's organs is the same but the *svarupa* is different, proportion of *gunas* is different. Thus though the external actions of the *indriyas* appear to be the same in all of us, there is a vast difference in their internal nature. *Yogshastra* is full of the knowledge of the external and internal characteristics of the physical and subtle organs, their nature and nature of the nature. It explains how spiritual development can be achieved through a *sattvic* nature.

The fifth and final form of the *indriyas* is known as *arthavatva* i.e. the aim and purpose of the *indriyas.* Aim and purpose are synonymous. Nothing in this Universe is devoid of purpose. An object ceases to exist when its purpose comes to an end. '**कृतार्थम् प्रतिनष्टम्**' is the underlying concept of this belief. This principle is found in the subject of teleology, which is a branch of metaphysics. *Indriyas* have two purposes - one is *bhog* for giving mundane and temporal experience and the second is *apavarga*, attainment of the final beatitude, spiritual experience and wisdom. Every *indriya* is involved in the functions of the worldly life of sorrow and happiness. It experiences the dualities which a *jivatma* undergoes i.e., *bhoga*. *Bhog* may be described as "trafficking" of pain and pleasure.

Samkhya describes *bhog* as related to three types of experience such as happiness, misery and delusion. Transcending of these mundane experiences leads to absolution or *apavarga*. Just as the *indriyas* are capable of giving mundane experiences, they can also give *apavarga* or fulfillment. An eye can experience infatuation and it can also discriminate between good and evil. This feature of discrimination of the eye is known as *apavarga* or fulfilment of the function of the *indriya*. A true *sadhaka* or *yogi* is not affected by objects of pain and pleasure but they lift him above the level of mundane existence. All the *jnanendriyas* and *karmendriyas* are retired from experiences of this world and are oriented towards the spiritual path when the *sadhaka* is on the *yogic* path. This is their significant role of the *apvargatva* (fulfillment). This play of *prakriti* is meant for the two purposes- *bhog* and *apavarga*. A *sadhaka* either becomes a *yogbhrashta* (strays from the *yogic* path), or he accomplishes his goal of self-realisation. The Universe is founded on these two objectives- *bhog* (desire for worldly pleasures) and *yog* (seeking after God). This is the root of the philosophy of the *indriyas*. *Prakriti*, via the *trigunas*, gives rise to *asmita* (I-consciousness). The *panchamahabhutas, jnanendriyas* and *the karmendriyas,* have their existence in this. Modern science explains only the physical aspect of the organs,e.g., the eye. The examination of the real esoteric nature of the organs is explained in *yogshastra*.

176

We have seen, while studying the real nature of the *indriyas*, the influence of *adhyatmic*, *adhidaivic* and *adhibhautic* elements. A complete awareness of the *indriyas* is obtained subsequent to the knowledge of all these aspects. *Arthavatva* (purposiveness) is the fundamental nature of the *indriyas*, consisting of the duality of the worldly desires, leading to spiritual fulfillment. The second state is the result of the integration of the three *gunas*. The third state is that of the I-consciousness. The fourth consists of their outward manifestation and the fifth, of action. The integral function of the *indriyas* consists of these five states. In the end, all the *karmendriyas*, *jnanendriyas* and the organs, all are made of the mind or *chitta* stuff. The liver, stomach, the spleen, etc., and also the *saptadhatus*, are the prolongation of the mind. So, for restraining the mind, right conduct, right thinking, character are essential and the *yogic kriyaas* such as *bandhas, mudras, pranayama, japa, tapa*, etc., according to *yogshastra*, vivify every fibre of the human body. The generally mistaken belief is that *yogsadhana* is limited to only the *asanas*, and we go by the external appearances only. All the limbs and organs such as the eye, ear, stomach, heart, have their subtle being as mental entities, and this understanding can only be acquired through a study of *yogshastra*. Each organ satisfies and strengthen the mind and the I-consciousness. By eating, we not only satisfy the palate but also the mind. A *yogi* utilizes his *indriyas* for culturing the mind as a means of attaining the purest bliss.

The second form of the *indriyas* is an important one. Every *indriya* should perform the function appropriate to its substantive form. For an individual this is indeed a difficult task. A person who is fit to be a teacher is normally a misfit in the position of a clerk in an office. Therefore an *indriya* does not experience well-being if this condition is not fulfilled. We cannot pressurize the *indriya* to do something against its nature. It is just like not taking an aptitude test of an individual before assigning his duties. We will have to allow the *indriya* to function appropriately in order for it to be in equilibrium with nature. While we sleep or take rest, it is beneficial only when our mind is really in a peaceful and tranquil state. One should therefore not be taken in by the false glitter of commercial advertisements to achieve tranquillity of mind.

Real rest for the organs

Man requires tranquility in sleep, even so the *indriyas* require calmness. This can be achieved largely through *shavasana.* A tranquil mind gives a sense of well-being to the individual and vice-versa. Thus for the health of both the mind and the body, *shavasana, japasadhana, dhyanasadhana, mantrasadhana* are powerful means for achieving this state of well-being.

Shavasana is an invaluable gift of *yog.* The *indriyas* are stilled through this *asana.* These *indriyas* include not only the stomach but all the organs which are influenced by the mind. There is a constant metamorphosis occurring in these *indriyas* through this *asana.* All the tensions and pressures are relieved through the calmness achieved by *shavasana*, which calmness is a lesser form of that of *samadhi. Shavasana* is a means of progressing towards the ultimate goal of *samadhi.* This *asana* is extremely useful to a *sadhaka* who is in the initial stages of practice. We have thus far noted the principles of the *yogic* science of the *indriyas.*

Mere physical health is different from well-being which is due to the experience of calm. The importance of *shavasana* for achieving this stillness cannot be over-emphasised. Our *indriyas* are controlled by the *chittavrittis* which in turn can be controlled by *yog.* Individual freedom without the necessary constraints can be disastrous. *Yog,* in this regard, is based on self-restraint. The problem is to synchronise individual freedom with *yog.* Whether the so-called individual freedom really exists, or is a mere illusion, is a question. In the next topic we will be considering the relationship between individual freedom and self-restraint.

Shri Krishnaarpanam astu

✤ ✤ ✤

Discourse - 17

Personal Freedom and Self-restraint

Freedom

Man is the slave of his nature. He behaves as his mind dictates but can he control everything about his physical body? No. It is under the control of *prakriti*. He normally does not have any control over the activities of the various constituents of his physical body. The heart continues to beat without anybody's control. Can he ask it to stop beating and go on living? Before the "I" wakes up in a child, the heart has been continuously at work. So the body is under perfect control of something called *prakriti*. And this man is talking vehemently about his personal freedom today! His clamour for demanding freedom is so loud that even a deaf man would hear it. No sooner does he acquire a little knowledge about the world, he starts talking about of his personal freedom. As a baby he is dependent on his mother, he starts lisping the words *Aaee, Maa*. But as soon as he grows up into a boy, he starts using the words like independence and freedom. It apparently seems that *yog* is opposite to his personal freedom since *yog* is restraint and control.

So the self-styled advanced literates regard *yog* as opposite to their individual freedom. But is *yog* really against real freedom? The word *svatantrya* comes from the words *sva* or self and *tantra* or discipline. *Svatantrya* or *sva-tantra* assumes a *tantra* for *sva* or self which means some kind of governance, self-control has to be there, and there is no freedom from *tantra*. *Svatantrya* or freedom does not mean waywardness or indiscipline. Freedom does not suggest that we can conduct ourselves according to our deviations and fancies, and indulge in satisfying all kinds of our desires, expectations and hopes. Our deviations, *vikaras* emerge from the *shadripus* of *kama, krodha, lobha* etc. To imagine that *svatantrya* is to be guided by the impulses of the *shadripus* is against reason. In the previous topic we have studied the real nature of the *indriyas* and we also saw that *sva* or the true self is devoid of *upadhis,* impurities, defects and deviations. The true self is devoid of caste, creed, name, fame. We try to judge an individual from the point of view of his prosperity or adversity, his cleverness or dullness, his caste or creed, gender and we do not view his true self which is unfettered and free from defects. We cannot remain with the *sva* or true self unless we are in the *yogic* state. Therefore, it is meaningless when we ordinary people talk about *svatantrya.* When we get to know about *sva* in the *yogic* state, we can understand what is to be *sva-tantra.* Generally our ideas of *svatantrya* do not go beyond satisfaction of mundane desires and love of pleasures.

The fact is that most of us are troubled by the domestic, social, cultural constraints in our life. Some people are crushed by these constraints and they live like cowards. Many people are influenced by the modern thinking stimulated by the western individualistic thought and they want to revolt against the traditional and religious norms. The so-called socially forward individual feels that real happiness lies in the satisfaction of his materialistic desires. He proceeds to satisfy them at any cost and without any self-restraint. Personal freedom for him degrades itself to the level of licentious behaviour and of submitting to passions. But what is the result of this? Lasting happiness does not come out of this and man is left permanently thirsty and is running after happiness. As it is said in the *Mahabharata,*

न जातु काम: कामानां उपभोगेन शाम्यति ।
हविषा कृष्णवर्त्मा इव भूय: एवाभिवर्धते ।।

Desires are never really satisfied. The more we try to appease them, the more are they hungry. The more fuel we put in the fire, the more it grows. Actually true freedom lies in putting restraints upon us by ourselves. We are not slaves of ourselves. We, however, become the slaves of our *vasanas* incensed by the uncontrolled mind. Real freedom is voluntary self-control. Self-restraint is the foundation of real freedom and also a way towards lasting happiness. It is a pity if they believe that freedom lies in disregarding the principles of righteousness.

Restraint in freedom

Restraint is thus of paramount importance. Do we not prevent a child from sucking his thumb or from eating mud, even though he cries at the top of his voice? The mother's love compels her to be punitive. In the interests of the child she forbids him from eating excess of sweets and chocolates, though the child does not relish this type of restraint. One may appear cruel in order to be kind. Laxity in this regard could lead to serious consequences. A child at least obeys the parents, but when he grows up and enters youth, he feels he knows what is good for him and that no one should teach him what to do. There is a difference between sense and reason, as between nonsense and irrationality. An ignorant child's greatest sign of ignorance is that he believes he is wise. A really ignorant person presumes that he is wise and it is difficult to remove this ignorance. Ignorance is a kind of childishness. Childishness may be there in a young or old person irrespective of the physical age. This ignorance or childishness is manifested differently in different advanced stages of life.

Parents guide a child along the right path. Similarly for people like us, there are the saints, seers, the godly persons to guide us on the right path. They are the real guides, philosophers and friends. Culture and tradition, and the scriptures are our real benefactors, like our parents and they protect us from dangers. They gift us with the faculty of discrimination. They govern us and they have to do this in the interest of society.

In this respect the joint family system had a healthy influence on the members of the family. The head of the family was not an autocratic ruler, but a well-wisher and protector of its members. He was the father but he had the *Dharma* or code of conduct as his father to be followed strictly. There is a strong element of domestic discipline in the joint family system on account of its automatic checks and balances. The self-interest of the individual member is subordinated to the general interest of the entire family. The divided independent or nucleus family does not have the desirable restraint that exists in a joint family. The modern individual reared in this nuclear family tries to shake off these beneficial restraints, showing his sense of ingratitude to the elders of the family. The norms and conventions to be followed in the society are resented by him as they do not cater to his self-interest. He thinks that they are a hindrance to his personal freedom. This ticklish issue requires adept handling.

The question the youth asks loudly is-what does society do for us? Why should we sacrifice our freedom and happiness for it? We have to think of this question carefully. Man is looked after in every way by society around him. Imagine a child's plight if he were abandoned in a jungle or in the desert of Siberia, left to the mercies of the natural forces. Compare a child deserted in a desert and the one born in a private hospital and lying under the care of his parents.

Look at the way he is given a royal welcome at the time of his birth by the family and society in which he lives, as if he is a King or a President. The mother has already knitted a dress for him with loving care as soon as his arrival is announced to her. There is all provision of adequate equipment for his development. In addition, he gets the loving support of his family and this support cannot be counted in terms of material gain. Can we pay off if a mother prepares a bill for all the services she has given her child? It is impossible to value a mother's care of the child in terms of monetary and material considerations. He is provided with a number of facilities and services by society such as public utilities, playgrounds, schools, colleges, health services, medical facilities. We must feel the obligation and indebtedness to our family and culture for our genetic inheritance, our faculties, and our character which is acquired by us without doing any effort. Man is rightly called a social animal as he cannot live stark alone like a Robinson Crusoe. He gets a sense of security being in society which is of prime importance.

It would be relevant here to recall an anecdote told by *Ramakrishna Paramahamsa* during one of his spiritual discourses. A sparsely clad *adivasi* woman was seen by a little boy. He said, "Grandpa, there are two big boils on her chest." Ramakrishna replied, "My child, Nature has provided that for her child so that he can drink the elixir of life." Really this milk provides the child not only with nutrients for his subsistence but also ingrained sentiments of love and affection. The value of this milk is beyond any price. The milk in the market may contain a higher content of proteins and vitamins but not this love. We should realize this and have a sense of gratitude. Even the other members of the family like wife give us so much. Can we not give up something for their sake and limit our freedom (licentiousness)? We should assess the proper nature of personal freedom considering our indebtedness to others. Our personal freedom can then be conditioned appropriately with a sense of balance.

Our *Vedas* are the word of God and we are indeed fortunate to have inherited a lofty culture. Our ancestors possessed and developed a great culture. We do not find such depth, refinement, sophistication and knowledge in non-*vedic* cultures. Which other ancient culture of the world went to think of the origin and purpose of life? Even a comparison of our epics and other epics of the world can show this. Our ancestors did not belong to uncivilized and aboriginal tribes. Actually the real definition of *Dharma* in our culture can be seen in the *Mahabharata*. It is *Dharayati iti Dharmaha*. That means *Dharma* is for sustaining society, so in the course of time some values need to be modified or even changed depending on the changes in the circumstances. Eternal values like love, devotion, compassion, of course, never change but the contingent values are subject to change. The law givers held conferences like *tryavara, dashavara* to bring suitable changes in the governing principles of conservative *Dharma.* The *Manusmriti* was not the only *smriti* or code but they created *smritis* according to the need of society.

So *Dharma* was taken to be a moral code of right and righteous conduct. The goal of *Dharma* was in realizing the highest bliss. However, "kitchen orthodoxy" arose in the Middle Ages. The law-givers lost their broad vision and prescribed pointless restraints on society. Crossing the seas was considered irreligious. Many other irrational prohibitions were inflicted. Now who is to decide upon the mores and morals suitable for the respective society? It is not the job of social scientists and anthropologists to write *smritis.* Only the realized saints and sages can see what is needed for harmony and balance in a society. Only they can suggest the changes to suit the present times. The sages are able to understand the human mind clearly. Great saint-philosophers like *Yajnavalkya, Vyasamuni, Jnaneshvara, Tukaram, Ramdasa,* were the mentors of our world. Such men alone can alter the rigid religious traditions of the past, and give a suitable course to the eternal flow of our *Vedic* culture and traditions. They have the insights to distinguish between conventional and perpetual morality.

The above factors have to be kept in mind to prevent the present generation from developing a tendency to feel that family, society and tradition are obstructions to personal freedom. One must reflect on the true nature of one's self for realizing one's personal freedom. Else, instead of becoming *svatantra,* man becomes *svarthatantra,* self-centred. Real individual freedom is obtained, if one finds the inner self. This "*sva*" or the real self is found only in *yogshastra.* Otherwise one gets the illusory feeling that progress is measured by one's self-aggrandizement and by the satisfaction of lustful desires. The spiritual basis of *yog* enables the *sadhaka* to make true discovery of "*sva*". This "*sva*" cannot be viewed by modern medical technology, such as scanning, ultrasound, sonography, M R I. One can attain real freedom of the self only through *yoga.* If we think that *yogic* discipline is opposed to personal freedom, it is an illusory perception.

Nowadays, a newly married couple resents relatives in their house as intrusion on their privacy. They think only of themselves and of the nurture of their offspring. Father, mother, father-in-law, mother-in-law are considered as strangers (intruders!). But by avoiding these elders aren't they depriving their children of the affection of the grand-parents and the benign ancestral influence? Again isn't it the children's responsibility to take care of the old parents? The grand-parents and the grand-children need the love of each other. Then, the grandparents are sent to old-age homes. This conduct of the young couple is tantamount to unrighteousness.

Senior citizens – Listen !

It is not only the young people who are at fault. The grandparents or the old people have also failed in their role in the joint family system. They, too, became dangerously worldly and self-centred. During their prime, they were motivated by personal gain. Therefore they are equally responsible for the disintegration of the joint family system. If they have not stored any physical, moral or cultural strength they cannot guide the next generation by their examples. They themselves did not feel the importance of values. It was in their days that today's false philosophy of consumerism and of 'only-this-moment-is-important' became popular. They took this wrong message from the new education and modern culture. They thought only of their selfish interests and so decided the criteria in this respect.

This old generation did not prepare themselves in their youth for today. They thought that old age is the right time for thinking of God, when all their faculties are feeble. *Jnaneshvar* has described this kind of mentality in the 13th chapter of the *Jnaneshvari*. People think that they should enjoy all the luxuries of life as long as they are young and they could think of God and spiritual matters when the body would lose its strength, eyesight would blur and hands and legs would be weak. *Jnaneshvar* depicts the pitiable condition of such an old helpless man turning to God when he has nothing to do. He has lost sight of making preparations for his spiritual life. As we have to make material and financial provision for old age, so we have to think of spiritual provision. They did not think of the examples of the stories of the *Ramayana* and *Mahabharata*. They could have gleaned valuable principles of righteous living from there, but this was taken to be irrelevant during youth. They should have earned something noble and valuable when their faculties were active. They could have helped the youth of today with it. They thought of materialism at that time and cared only for what was useful in that way. Now the young generation is not finding them useful and so is dispensing with them.

We two – ours – one ?

Today people are advised to adopt family planning and to restrict the number of children to two, so that adequate health, education and other facilities could be provided for them. If there are many children in the family, it is no doubt difficult to provide proper facilities to all of them. This is the current economics. But there is another side of this issue. You might look at it as mischievous but think of it carefully. In such a small family a child grows up in lonely surroundings. He thinks solely of himself. Such a child could not even share his biscuits with his friends. He cannot become fit as a member of society. His self-centred attitude is good neither for his mental development nor for the well being of society. He cannot think of cooperation. Sociologists must at least give attention to this danger. The person brought up in a wealthy, small family without any monetary tensions cannot be an ideal citizen who shares the resources in the society equitably. Again, there certainly are some greater things of delight beyond this temporal life and being. If he grows to be an intolerant, self-centred and selfish person, his mind may become perverted. He might not be happy in his material prosperity. Can we afford to ignore this cultural fall of the society? Economists and sociologists have to pay attention to the dimensions and far-reaching effects of the one-child family system which they are vehemently advocating. They should take into account this essential cultural aspect of life in addition to socio-economic considerations.

Shri Krishnaarpanam astu

✤ ✤ ✤

Discourse - 18

Jnana Yog

The starting point of *Jnana Yog* is in *svadhyaya* of *ashtanga yog.* *Svadhyaya* means study of or about the self-which ultimately culminates in the study of the Higher Self or the soul. The *niyamas* of *ashtanga yog* are *shaucha, santosha, tapas, svadhyaya* and *Ishvarapranidhana. Svadhyaya* is the root of *jnana yog.* The study of the self starts with the questions- Who am I? From where have I come? Where am I going? And where am I destined to go? What is all this? It is the curiosity and contemplation about these questions. When this type of reflection gives rise to the thinking process, one develops the disposition for *jnana yog. Svadhyaya* is the foundation of *ashtanga yog* which in turn becomes the foundation of *jnana yog.*

Jnana yog is greatly influenced by philosophy. Philosophy in Sanskrit is *tattvajnana* i. e. *tat*=that, the soul or the metaphysical principle, *tva*=being, *jnana*=knowledge. The contemplation, knowledge and understanding of this metaphysical principle is philosophy. The knowledge of the soul is the essence of *jnana yog.* The soul is described as formless, unmanifested and without any attribute, colour, birth, age, death, caste, class, creed, gender, status and stature. It is free from all differences (dualities). It does not have hunger, thirst, sleep or decaying. Such a metaphysical inquiry about the soul commences in *svadhyaya.* This is beautifully described in *shlokas* 23-25 of chapter 2 of the *Bhagavadgita.* Lord *Krishna* says:

Atman –

नैनं छिन्दन्ति शस्त्राणि नैनं दहति पावक: ।

न चैनं क्लेदयति आपो न शोषयति मारुत: ।।

अच्छेद्य: अयं अदाह्य: अयं अक्लेद्य: अशोष्य: एव च ।

नित्यसर्वगत: स्थाणु: अचल: अयं सनातन: ।।

अव्यक्त: अयं अचिंत्य: अयं अविकार्य: अयम् उच्यते ।

तस्मात् एवं विदित्वा एवं न अनुशोचितुम् अर्हसि ।।

No weapon can cut the *Atman*. Fire cannot burn it nor can water drench it or wet it, nor can air dry it. *Atma* is essentially eternal and all-pervasive. It has no beginning and no end.

Arjuna was stricken with grief in the battle-field of *Kurukshetra*. He was to fight against his respected *guru,* teachers, elders, like *Dronacharya*, his dear cousins, and his friends and mates. He was bewildered and confused. Then the Lord thus tells *Arjuna* to know this real nature of *Atma* and not to grieve over the dead. *Arjuna* is told not to feel that he is the doer of the actions and killer of his kith and kin. The Lord tells *Arjuna* that no weapon can injure or devastate the *Atma,* which is unmanifest, immutable and unaffected by sorrow.

Jnana yog follows the above concept of the soul as described by the Lord. A *jnana yogi* is influenced by this principle of *Atma*. The *jnana yogi* thus does not identify himself with his body, mind, caste, creed, status, gender, etc. He is convinced that he is the pure consciousness of the *Atma*. Such a *jnana yogi* conducts the business of his life with this illusion-free knowledge. We tend to identify ourselves as "I am happy. I am sorrowful. I am a woman. I am a man. This is my *vamsha, gotra, varna,* etc. I am the doer of these things, others have or have not done these things." We are thus caught up in this illusion, because the basic "I" in ourselves is itself an illusion, we identify ourselves with this "I". We are falsely conditioned by the notion of "self". As ordinary human beings, we erroneously believe in our so-called social status, individual stature and family name. The interaction of a *jnana yogi* with the world is quite different since the *jnani* is illusion-free. The *yogi* knows that he is not the body but that he is essentially the *Atma*. He has realized the difference between the perishable and the imperishable, reality and illusion, the *Atma* and the gross body and the gross intellect. This spiritual outlook makes him understand that he is not the body, mind and senses but that he is *atma*. This sense of discrimination is of vital importance in *jnana yog,* which is free from the illusion regarding the real self. The *Atma* does not have a caste, creed, gender, status etc. It is only the body and embodiment which has all these external and internal delimiting factors, whereas the soul (*Atma*) does not have any of these conditions. The *Atma* is beyond these notions and mental conditions. The wise man knows "I do not do anything" and that the soul is the non-doer. He knows that all his activities are governed by *prakriti.*

The *Bhagavadgita* in *shloka* 8-9 of chapter 5 beautifully explains this :

न एव किंचित्करोमि इति युक्तो मन्येत तत्त्ववित् ।
पश्यन् शृण्वन् स्पृशन् जिघ्रन् अश्रन् गच्छन् स्वपन् श्वसन् ॥
प्रलपन् विसृजन् गृह्णन् उन्मिषन् निमिषन् अपि ।
इंद्रियाणि इंद्रियार्थेषु वर्तन्ते इति धारयन् ॥

Such a wise man and wise sage, the *jnana yogi*, who is centred in the soul, thinks, "I do nothing at all." Though these various movements and actions of seeing, hearing, touching, smelling, eating, going, sleeping, breathing, speaking, emptying, holding, opening and closing the eyes take place, he is firmly convinced, that the senses move in the midst of sense-objects, and it is not he who is doing all these things. Elsewhere, Lord *Krishna* says that one who thinks "I do it," is *ahamkaravimudhhatma*, -an audacious fool inebriated with pride.

Nature of a Jnaanayogi

The common approach to *adhyatmic jnana sadhana* is to indiscriminately run after the spiritual charlatans for listening to their discourses. We try to understand the *Gita* and the *Jnaneshvari* in the manner of the exposition by these self-styled spiritualists. This is not *jnana yog.* At best it could be an unproductive effort which could perhaps result in some titillating pleasure. A *jnana yogi* conducts himself in a vastly different manner to that of an ordinary individual. The 69th *shloka* of chapter 2 of the *Gita* says :

या निशा सर्वभूतानां तस्यां जागर्ति संयमी ।
यस्यां जाग्रति भूतानि सा निशा पश्यतो मुनेः ॥

When it is night for all other beings, the wise sage is waking and when all beings are awake, it is night for this *muni* who is a seer. Our dos and don'ts do not apply to the *yogi* or *muni*. Our interests and pleasures are not the same for him. The gravity of these is the opposite for him. The *jnani* deems that he does not have the tags and titles of the ordinary individual such as caste, creed, gender, etc., and that he is not a doer of action.

This philosophy of *jnana yog* had a strong influence on *jnana yogis* like *Shankaracharya, Shukacharya, Vamadeva* and *Ashtavakra. Ashtavakra* had a crooked body and people used to make fun of him on account of this, but he was not at all affected. He never felt slighted on this account. On the contrary he felt amused. He had long since realized that he was not the body but the pure unsullied *Atma,* and that it was his body and not his *Atma* that the people were making fun of.

The *Bhagavadgita* is an excellent source of reference for knowing the special characteristics of a *jnana yogi.* Chapter 2 (on *Saamkhya yog*) gives a detailed description of a *jnana yogi. Shlokas* 17, 18, and 19 state :

अविनाशी तु तद्विद्धि येन सर्वम् इदं ततम् ।
विनाशम् अव्ययस्यास्य न कश्चित् कर्तुम् अर्हति ।।
अन्तवन्त इमे देहा नित्यस्य उक्ता: शरीरिण:
अनाशिन: अप्रमेयस्य तस्मात् युध्यस्व भारत ।।
य एनं वेत्ति हन्तारं य: च एनं मन्यते हतम् ।
उभौ तौ न विजानीत: नायं हन्ति न हन्यते ।।

"*Arjuna,* this *Atma* is imperishable. The *Atma* pervades the entire Universe. It is indefinable, eternal and imperishable, even at the time of dissolution of the Universe. During the battle, only the body perishes and not the soul. Therefore, O *Arjuna* fight without fear and misgiving. They are both ignorant, i.e., the one who thinks the soul to be capable of killing, and one who takes the soul as killed, for, verily the soul neither kills nor is it killed."

The soul is diseaseless, eternal and full of infinite bliss. The self-realised soul experiences the highest bliss. ʻआनंदाचे डोही आनंदतरंगʼ - the *yogi* experiences the ripples of bliss in the ocean of bliss (*Sant Tukarama*). आत्मनि एव च संतुष्ट: तस्य कार्य न विद्यते । (3 : 17) Having attained the supreme bliss one does not have to perform any action.

194

In chapter 3, *shloka* 21, the Lord says that even though there is no need for any action (for a *yogi*), one apparently performs action because

यद् यद् आचरति श्रेष्ठो जन: ।
स यत्प्रमाणं कुरुते लोक: तत् एव इतर: अनुवर्तते ।

For, whatsoever a great man or *jnana yogi* does, other people follow and emulate him. The generality of men follow the standards set up by him. That is why the *jnani* opts to be active. In chapter 3, *shloka* 22-23, the Lord says

न मे पार्थ अस्ति कर्तव्यं त्रिषु लोकेषु किंचन ।
न अनवाप्तम् अवाप्तव्यं वर्त एव च कर्मणि ।।
यदि हि अहं न वर्तेयं जातु कर्मणि अतंद्रित: ।
मम वर्त्म अनुवर्तन्ते मनुष्या: पार्थ सर्वश: ।।

"O Arjuna, there is nothing in the three worlds for Me to do, nor is there anything worth attaining or unattained by Me; yet I continue to be active. Should I not engage in action, unwearied at all times, great harm will come to the world; *Arjuna*, men follow My path in all the ways."

The nature of an unruffled *jnana yogi* is further described in chapter 2 of the *Gita*. *Arjuna* asks: "How does a man established in spirituality behave?" By this question *Arjuna* shows us his spirit of the *jijnasu*. *Arjuna* asks, "O Lord, what is the mark of a realized soul, established in spirituality?" The Lord describes such a one with his nectar-like words:

य: सर्वत्र अनभिस्नेह: तत् तत् प्राप्य शुभाशुभम् ।
न अभिनन्दति न द्वेष्टी तस्य प्रज्ञा प्रतिष्ठिता ।। (2 : 57)

195

यदा संहरते च अयं कूर्म: अंगानि इव सर्वश: ।

इन्द्रियाणि इन्द्रियार्थेभ्य: तस्य प्रज्ञा प्रतिष्ठिता ।। (2 : 58)

दु:खेषु अनुद्विग्नमना: सुखेषु विगतस्पृह: । (2 : 56)

A *jnani* remains unperturbed in sorrow and happiness. He has no thirst for pleasures. Like a tortoise which withdraws all its limbs inward, he withdraws his senses from the sense-objects. His mind is established in spirituality, he becomes a *sthitaprajna*. A *sthitaprajna* who is unperturbed, is described by the Lord in the *Gita* :

प्रजहाति यदा कामान् सर्वान् पार्थ मनोगतान् । (2 : 55) A *sthitaprajna* is one who totally abandons all cravings of the mind. We ordinary mortals are sometimes, for a moment, in this state of mind of the *sthitaprajna*. We momentarily feel that all our desires are destroyed but it is like fever only. Perhaps this is the reaction of some when there is a bolt from the blue, the death of one's mother, father, or of a near and dear one. Such a state of mind is called *smashana vairagya*, the sense of renunciation at the sight of a cemetery. This is only temporary. Real *vairagya* is referred to as 'आत्मनि एव आत्मना तुष्ट: ' – when one rests satisfied in the self by abandoning all the cravings. An additional characteristic of such a *yogi* is described as follows:

दु:खेषु अनुद्विग्नमना: सुखेषु विगतस्पृह: ।

वीतरागभयक्रोध: स्थितधी: मुनि: उच्यते ।। (2 : 56)

The sage whose mind remains unperturbed in sorrow, whose thirst for pleasures has altogether disappeared and who is free from passion, fear and anger, is the one who is established in spirituality.

य: सर्वत्र अनभिस्नेह: तत् तत् प्राप्य शुभाशुभम् ।

196

न अभिनन्दति न द्वेष्टि तस्य प्रज्ञा प्रतिष्ठिता ।। (2 : 57)

He (the *jnani*) is unattached to everything, meeting with the good and evil neither rejoicing nor recoiling. Ordinary individuals like us rejoice when we get the objects of our desire, and are overwhelmed with grief when we experience disappointment. A *jnani* is unperturbed either way and remains established in spirituality.

यदा संहरते च अयं कूर्म: अंगानि इव सर्वश: ।
इन्द्रियाणि इन्द्रियार्थेभ्य: तस्य प्रज्ञा प्रतिष्ठिता । (2 : 58)

When like a tortoise which withdraws its limbs inward, he withdraws his senses from the sense-objects, his mind is unmoved. Nothing antagonizes or lures him who remains unattached everywhere. Everything in him is in a state of equilibrium. A *jnani* is also described in the shlokas 7-10 of the chapter13 of the *Gita* as:

अमानित्वं अदंभित्वं अहिंसा क्षान्ति: आर्जवम् ।
आचार्योपासनं शौचं स्थैर्यं आत्मविनिग्रह: ।।
इन्द्रियार्थेषु वैराग्यम् अनहंकार एव च ।
जन्ममृत्युजराव्याधिदु:खदोषानुदर्शनम् ।।
असक्तिरनभिष्वंग पुत्रदारगृहादिषु ।
नित्यं च समचित्तत्वम् इष्टानिष्टोपपत्तिषु ।।
मयि चानन्ययोगेन भक्ति: अव्यभिचारिणी ।
विविक्तदेशसेवित्वम् अरति: जनसंसदि ।।

There is absence of pride in a *jnani*, there is freedom from hypocrisy, there is non-violence, forgiveness, straightforwardness, attitude of service for the preceptor, purity of mind and body, steadfastness and self-control. He possesses a distaste towards the

197

objects of the senses, absence of egoism, and a constant revolving in the mind in regard to the pain and evil inherent in birth, death, old age and disease. There is absence of attachment and a consistent balance of mind under all favourable or unfavourable circumstances. The *jnani* is unflinching in his devotion to the Lord, lives in secluded and sacred places in the absence of undesirable company. Such a person according to the *Gita* is called a *gunatita* (one who has transcended the *gunas*).

Now, *Arjuna* while listening to the metaphysical discourse of the Lord becomes perplexed regarding the real nature of a *gunatita*. He asks the Lord:

कै: लिंगै: त्रीन् गुणान् एतान् अतीत: भवति प्रभो ।

किम् आचार: कथं च एतान् त्रीन् गुणान् अतिवर्तते ।। (14 : 21)

What are the marks of one who has risen above the three *gunas*? How does he rise above them?

The Lord says:

प्रकाशं च प्रवृत्तिं च मोहं एव च पांडव ।

न द्वेष्टि संप्रवृत्तानि न निवृत्तानि कांक्षति ।। (14 : 22)

He is one who feels neither engaged nor disengaged because of attachments or aversions. He feels no gravity of the three *gunas*. He does not long for them. He is not moved by the *gunas*.

उदासीनवत् आसीनो गुणै: यो न विचाल्यते ।

गुणा वर्तन्ते इति एव य: अवतिष्ठति नेङ्गते ।। (14 : 23)

The *yogi* who sits like a neutral witness, is not moved by the *gunas,* and who knowing that only the *gunas* act, remains firmly established in *Paramatmaa*, and is never shaken from that state.

समदु:खसुख: स्वस्थ: समलोष्टाष्मकांचन: ।

तुल्यप्रियाप्रियो धीर: तुल्यनिंदात्मसंस्तुति: ।। (14 : 24)

मानापमानयो: तुल्य: तुल्यो मित्रारिपक्षयो: ।

सर्वारंभपरित्यागी गुणातीत: स उच्यते ।। (14 : 25)

A *yogi* takes sorrow and joy alike, is established in the self, regards a clod of earth, a stone, a piece of gold, as equal in value, receives both pleasant and unpleasant things in the same spirit and views censure and praise alike. The *yogi* has equanimity about honour and dishonour, is equal to friend and foe, and has renounced the sense of doership in all activity. He is said to have transcended the three *gunas*.

Further, in the *Gita* the Lord says:

क्लेश: अधिकतर: तेषां अव्यक्तासक्तचेतसाम् (12 : 45)

"Greater is their difficulty, whose minds are set on the Unmanifest." The soul is unmanifest and neomenal, it is very difficult for those whose minds are set on the unmanifest (*nirguna*), for the goal of the unmanifest is very hard for the embodied to reach. Instead, the *yogi* can accomplish *bhakti yog* by concentrating (with devotion) even on one of the auspicious attributes of the *Sarvaguna Ishvara* (the Lord with countless auspicious attributes). These attributes include amongst others, Divine wealth, *Paramavirya* (Supreme prowess), *Paramashakti* (Supreme Power), *Paramavatsalya* (Supreme motherly love), *Paramajnana* (infinite Knowledge), *Paramaishvarya* (Supreme glory), *Paramarjava* (Supreme tenderness), *Paramaoudarya* (Supreme generosity), *Paramakaruna* (Supreme compassion), *Paramachaturya* (Supreme cleverness), *Paramadhairya* (Supreme courage), *Paramavimrityutva* (Supreme immortality), *Paramaparakrama* (Supreme bravery), *Paramagambhirya* (Supreme profoundness), *Paramasauharda* (Supreme friendliness), *Paramasamya* (Supreme equanimity), *Paramashaurya* (Supreme valour), *Paramavijaratva* (etermal youth), *Paramapahatapapatva* (Supreme sinlessness), *Paramamadhurya* (Supreme sweetness), *Paramakrutitva* (doing Supreme deeds), *Paramasthairya* (Supreme firmness and steadiness), *Paramasatyakamatva* (Supreme truth of desires), *Paramasatyasankalpatva* (Supreme accomplishments and resoluteness), *Paramaapipasa*(Supreme thirstlessness).

The celebrated *Vishnu Sahasranama Stotra* describes the thousand divine attributes (*gunas*) of the Lord. This *strotra* most appropriately delineates the Lord's divine qualities. A *bhakta* can achieve *samadhi* by meditating on even one of these *gunas*. A *jnana yogi* who has already reached the blissful states of *dhyana* and *dharana,* can attain *samadhi* by meditating directly on the transcendental *Paramatman*. The *Upanishads* are an important source of *atmajnana*- they contain the total knowledge of the soul. Of the various *Brahmavidyas* therein like *Purusha vidya* (knowledge of the original source of the Universe), *Bhaumavidya, vidya* of infinite bliss, *Aksharavidya, vidya* of the Indestructible, *Antaradityavidya* [*vidya* about the source of animation in the eyes of living beings]., each could lead the *jnana yogi* to *samadhi.* The *jnani* realizes that the soul is a neomenal, unmanifest principle. The *Brihadaranyaka Upanishad* describes the soul as having no shape, form, dimension, caste, creed, colour, status, stature, etc., (i.e. *avyaktam*). 'न तदश्नाति किंचन, न तदश्राति कश्चन.' A *jnana yogi* is capable of meditating on such a formless entity, the Supreme soul, for attaining *samadhi.* The *Mundakopanishad* also describes the attributes of the soul. According to this *Upanishad*, the *Brahman*, is invisible, inaccessible, it cannot be felt, or sensed, and it cannot be seen. Similarly, It is *agotram* or without lineage, *avarnam*, casteless, *achakshuhu* without eyes or organs of perception. The *Shvetashvatara Upanishad*, also, describes the soul as timeless, faultless, unperturbed, free from falsehood. Section 8:7:3 of the *Chhandyogya Upanishad* states: '**एष आत्मा अपहतपाप्मा विजरो विमृत्युः विशोकः अपिपास: सत्यकाम: सत्यसंकल्प:,**' Ordinary mortals cannot fathom the truth behind the soul which is of the nature of *neti, neti,* "not like this, not like this". But the *jnana yogi* alone can perceive the soul bereft of attributes. In this respect, the syllable *Om,* is the key to this type of mystic meditation. Without this meditation on *Om,* one cannot achieve the supreme state of *samadhi.* A *jnana yogi* attains the *dharana* stage by meditating on this syllable and soon thereafter attains *samadhi.* *Jnana yog* is thus founded on the principle of Nature and Soul. It is only when this philosophy of *yog* influences the mind of the accomplished *ashtanga yogi,* that it becomes real *jnana yog.* This *atmajnana* or knowledge of the self is the means of achieving the supreme unmanifest state of *samadhi.*

A *jnana yogi* is not the same as a *jnani* (an exceptionally knowledgeable person), in the ordinary sense of the term. He is not merely the one who is learned and skilled in the scriptures. A true *jnana yogi* is centred on the soul and possesses intense detachment. *Jnana yogic* meditations are extremely difficult. A *jnana yogi* is completely different from the ordinary level of people and is sometimes regarded as a misfit in society. *Jnana yog* is to be regarded as a most advanced postgraduate course in *yog.*

Karma Yog

Having briefly viewed *jnana yog,* we will now have a glance at its ally, the *karma yog. Karma yog* is another specialization branch of *ashtanga yog.* The various types of *yog* such as *bhakti yog* and *dhyana yog* are founded on *karma yog.* Since no one cannot remain actionless even for a moment, one is engaged in the incessant performance of *karma yog.*

The fundamental principle of *karma yog* can be stated as : '**सर्वकर्माणां परमगुर्वार्पणं तत्फलं वा संन्यासो वा I**' Offering of all actions and fruitions to the Lord is *karma yog* and is the most invaluable principle of all *yogs.* In the *Bhagavadgita,* the Lord says

आरुरुक्षो: मुने: योगं कर्म कारणम् उच्यते I (6 : 3)

To the contemplative soul, action without motive is said to be the ladder to rise to the heights of *karma yog.*

Karma yog is firmly established on the highest plane of *ashtanga yog. Karma yog* is necessary for the attainment of success in any field of spiritual *sadhana.* It makes the life of the *sadhaka* noble, sublime, transmaterial, transmundane, and ethereal. It is needless to mention the importance of *karma yog* in the *yogic* pursuit.

Ego, pride, arrogance and self-conceit are the major foes of *yog* and the spiritual life. The *karma yog* principle serves as an indispensible antidote to counter this ego. The spiritual *sadhaka* is not touched by the afflictions of the mundane life. The common man may mistakenly think, that a *karma yogi* is a dispirited individual for not accepting the fruits of his actions. On the contrary, *karma yog* infuses the fervour which helps the *sadhaka* in transcending the stumbling block of delusion.

The spiritual aspirant knows that (*sakama*) *karma* is an impediment in the spiritual path. Worldly activity serves as a wet blanket on the *sadhana,* reducing the spiritual fervour and enthusiasm of the seeker. This is so at least in the initial stages of *yogic sadhana.* Thus the importance of genuine *karma yog* cannot be overstressed. This understanding is especially more important in the initial stages of *sadhana* than even in the final stages when *moksha* is in sight. A true *karmayogi* is unaffected by the results of his actions, though none can remain actionless even for a moment. Each one is helplessly driven to action on account of the qualities born out of *prakriti.* Even the Lord during his incarnation into this world is bound by His *karma.* Lord *Krishna* is an example of the inevitability of the effect of *karma.* He was falsely accused of having stolen the *syamantaka mani* (jewel). He had to undergo severe privations for proving his innocence.

The difference between the *karmas* of ordinary human beings and those of divine beings is that the divine personages are not at all affected by their *karma.* The Lord is the deft magician who has devised the illusion of *karma* in the Universe. However the *karmayogi,* the saints, the realized souls are not affected by the performance of their *karma,* as they favour renunciation in action. They simply behave like actors on the stage playing the part given to them. In spite of their extraneous conduct, the true *yogis* remain in a state of *yog.* The Lord tells *Arjuna*

योगस्थः कुरु कर्माणि संगं त्यक्त्वा धनंजय । (2 : 48)

The *karmayogi* remains even-minded in loss or gain. It is this state of equilibrium that is verily the *yog.* The *yogi* does work with fervour and without attachment. His position is like that of a lotus leaf which remains unattached to the water on it.

Karma affects only the worldly man. A man without discrimination is attached to his *karma,* whereas a *sattvic karmayogi* realizes the ill-effects of bondage. The Lord says

'किम् कर्म किम् अकर्म इति कवय: अपि अत्र मोहिता: ।' (4 : 16)

Even the wise men are confused as to what is action and what is inaction.

'गहना कर्मणो गति: ।' (4 : 17)

Mysterious is the nature of action. The Lord further says

कर्मणि अकर्म य: पश्येत् अकर्मणि च कर्म य: ।

स बुद्धिमान् मनुष्येषु स युक्त: कृत्स्नकर्मकृत् ।। (4 : 18)

He who sees inaction in action and action in inaction is wise among men; he is a *yogi* who has accomplished all action. The Lord then says

तत् ते कर्म प्रवक्ष्यामि यत् ज्ञात्वा मोक्ष्यसे अशुभात् । (4 : 16)

"Therefore, I shall expound to you the truth about action knowing which you will be freed from its binding nature." *Karma* should be performed in a state of mind which is free from any passion, desire, anger, aversion, and jealousy. No doubt, it is very difficult to subjugate these tendencies. It is said that one has to pay for one's *karma* (actions). At times, while performing one action we inadvertently commit another undesirable action. On account of this, we keep on building up a complicated bundle of *karma*. Therefore, what may seem to be a wrong action, may in reality be a *sattvic* action and vice versa. A wise man, however, can see through the veil of superficiality.

In addition to *karma* (action), and *akarma* (inaction), there is also what is known as *vikarma*, performing actions of virtue-coated vice or vice-coated virtue. The result of such a *karma* is a mixture of good and evil. It may result in love-hate relationship; righteousness coupled with unrighteousness, etc. Thus a vicious cycle is formed, often leading one from the frying pan into the fire. The ethical principles of *karma yog* explained above strike a golden mean between the two opposite poles of human disposition. *Karma yog* is the raft which carries one smoothly and easily through life. The illusory *karma* cycle consists of the opposites of *karma* and *akarma, papa* (sin) and *punya* (good deeds), *sukha-dukkha, raga-dvesha.* The common man cannot easily assess the fruits of his *karma*, and he may end up in being disappointed. With this brief connected sequence of *karma yog* along with the preceding *jnana yog,* we will now turn our attention to *karma yog* in detail in the next topic.

Shri Krishnaarpanam astu

✜ ✜ ✜

Discourse - 19

Karma Yog

More about Karma Yog

Man is already tormented by *karmas* and entangled in the cycle of *karma*. So when he faces the terse theorization so as to find solutions he is further frustrated. He becomes confounded when confronted with the concepts of *karma, akarma* and *vikarma* because they are intertwined with each other. An action which appears to be virtuous could be inwardly sinful. On the other hand, some apparently vicious action might be actually virtuous. There is action, inaction, unaction, nonaction, counteraction, reaction, complementary action, supplementary action and so on. All these are actions. Doing is action and not doing also is action. Perhaps man commits sin while trying to avoid sin. So there are many kinds of actions for which the dictionary has no words. Some of these words may not be found in a dictionary. Even the scholars of the *shastras* are perplexed and led to ask:

'किं कर्म किम् अकर्म इति कवय: अपि अत्र मोहिता: ।' (4 : 16)

"What is *karma* and what is *akarma*, the question deludes even a wise man", says the Lord in the *Gita*. The subject of *karma* is thus profound, complex and complicated. The Lord further says that one must understand the concepts of *karma, akarma* and *vikarma*. In the *Gita,* Lord Krishna says :

कर्मणो ह्यपि बोद्धव्यं बोद्धव्यं च विकर्मण: ।
अकर्मणश्च बोद्धव्यं गहना कर्मणो गति: ॥ (4 : 17)

"The truth about action must be known; and the truth about action of virtue-coated vice or vice-coated virtue must also be understood.

Even so, the truth about inaction must be grasped. All these are very terse concepts." The next 18th *shloka* is also worth noting :

कर्मणि अकर्म य: पश्येत् अकर्मणि च कर्म य: ।
स बुद्धिमान् मनुष्येषु स युक्त: कृत्स्नकर्मकृत् ।। (4 : 18)

"One who sees *akarma* in *karma* and *karma* in *akarma* is a wise and intelligent man; and he is the seer among people. Only he is the doer of right and perfect action."

By doing he knows that he is non-doing and vice versa. So he develops scanning eyes for the nature of action, the degree of sin in the action. Such a person is a true *karma yogi* because the only way to come out of the labyrinth of these concepts is *karma yog*. *Karma yog* can solve the puzzle of actions and stop the torment. True, action cannot cease but the frustration is over. In order to understand *karma* and *karma yog,* it is necessary to know that people can be divided in two kinds-1] those who are prone to incessant action and 2] those who are prone to renunciation, i.e., mendicant ascetics.

People of the first type are continuously active and tend to become workaholics. They are obsessed with action. They can be called militant activists. So much of activity is not healthy and it needs moderation.

This excessive activism gets affected sometimes but it is for wrong reasons and in a wrong proportion. So it cannot be called proper. It happens when a near and dear one passes away. A person gets temporarily detached from the world when he loses his mother, father, husband, wife or friend. Then he loses interest in life. He gives up *karma*. Another reason of the momentary detachment is occasional failure or frustration in his occupation. He undergoes fits of depression and his actions become partially or totally paralyzed. These types of reduction of activism are inappropriate. *Karma yog* can bring adequate reduction of activism because this reduction does not smell of disinterest in life. It has no frustration. It is not destructive and depressing but is constructive and motivated. It does not go against a person's own nature.

People of the other kind avoid action. They are either lazy or frustrated. They are inert and disinterested. They assign the work to someone or the other. There are various reasons of inactivity of the people. Sometimes they are afraid of the good or merit or perhaps they resent it. Sometimes their disinterest in it is inborn. These people need boosting of action but this boosting can occur in a wrong proportion and for wrong reasons. Sometimes it occurs for selfish purposes or for some temptation. Sometimes this inactive person is led to action because he is misled by a cheat. This improper kind of boosting can be avoided if *karma yog* is used because boosting of *karma yog* is selfless and does not violate *Dharma*.

So *karma yog* is the golden mean of tendencies of action and inaction. It brings appropriation which is permanent and is for the good. It is strong and constructive. It gives discretion and brings balance between action and inaction. There are controversies among people with different dispositions. They can lead to quarrels. Some people are fatalists and some believe only in human efforts and in no destiny. All of them are trying to defend their views and refute the others. They even go to the extent of hostility. In the field of philosophy also there are controversies between *samkhya* and *yog, karma* and *sanyasa, jnana* and *karma*. In fact, such discrimination is meaningless. Essentially there is no difference between *samkhya* and *karma*. The Lord has quipped at the above critics in the following *shloka* (ch 5) of the *Gita :*

एकं सांख्यं च योगं च य: पश्यति स पश्यति ।

सांख्यं योगं पृथक् बाला: प्रवदन्ति न पण्डिता: ।। (5 : 5)

"He who sees *samkhya* and *yog* as one, so far as their result goes, really is a wise person. It is the ignorant and not the wise who say that *samkhya* and *yog* are poles apart." When the attitude is considered, they are not different and should not be different. Saffron clothes, staff and shaving of head are only outward signs. 'य: संन्यासं इति प्राहु: योगं तं विद्धि पांडव' (6 : 2) "*Arjuna*, know that what they speak of as *sanyasa* is the same as *karma yog*." This advice is deep seated in the heart of the *karma yog*. So *karma yog* stops the debate and brings a dialogue. It is not just a reduction and addition but it has its philosophy. So it ends the dichotomy and a kind of union emerges out of it. It brings *yoga* in the action (*karma*).

Let us consider one point in this debate of *karma.* After all, what is the will for work? We can say it is the restlessness of the mind that makes a person work or do *karma.* He is engrossed in it. This restlessness is of different kinds. Going to sleep is a *karma* and the cause of it is a sort of restless and *tamasic* quietness. In this condition he keeps aside everything else and goes to sleep. At other times his *rajasic* energy makes him do *karma.* As one has to give an outlet for the accumulated steam in a pressure cooker, so he has to give a channel to our energy, or he does not get peace of mind. So he takes up some or the other aim and toils for it till death. Sometimes he pleases himself with unnecessary affairs and indulges in them. He does not rest until the moment of utter exhaustion. Especially the activist puts his intellectual energies at stake for fulfilling his selfish purposes and ulterior motives. All the while he tries to give a justification for his actions and is never at peace. If such a person is shrewd, he engages himself in incessant work for promoting his ideas, takes the garb of social service, altruism, philanthropy and humanitarian work to justify his activities. He gets social recognition, name and fame in this endeavour. People are impressed by his show of services and confer titles upon him such as *karmavir* or *karmasamrat*. His love of work becomes noble in the eyes of the people but the nobility is only skin deep. Actually he is lost in self-love. He tries to show the world that he is working for society.

The other kind of people talk about renunciation. They think that *karma* has noise, tensions and stress. The material side of this life never gives peace. So do not go for it. Renunciation is the sole way to peace. This life is studded only with sorrows. If you are running after the shade of happiness, ultimately you will find yourself thrown in the scorching heat of the sun. Their words have a grain of truth but it happens in case of those who work incessantly. Incessant work blunts the edges of thinking. Ceaseless work fans indiscretion. This thoughtlessness is worse than lack of thinking. It disturbs the peace of mind. We cannot remain introvert and a disturbed mind affects the sense of right and wrong. His concern for values is shaken. If water is being stirred all the while, it cannot be quiet, the dust in it cannot go to the bottom and it cannot become clean and clear. In the same way incessant work does not allow the mind to be clear and quiet. The power of thinking is paralyzed in the turmoil of the work.

Hence the extremes of both the kinds are harmful. A ceaseless worker's brain is active but his emotions and thoughts become blunt whereas the people who admire renunciation may be just hiding their laziness, inertia and frustration under the coating of their renunciation. They find it attractive in some particular phases of life such as infirmity in the old age or some difficult situations because it is convenient at that time. So their supposed renunciation is in fact escapism without anything constructive in it.

Incessant work in the name of altruism and social service, and inertia under the garb of renunciation are the two extremes. It is more than difficult to poise/achieve a balance between them. You are invariably inclined towards one or the other extreme. Only *karma yog* can give you the golden mean of the two because it does not abandon work but it does give freedom from the pride of and attachment to it. The desire for the fruit of work is certainly sacrificed in it. *Karma yog* does make you think comprehensively.

It gives poise by balancing the introvert mindset and the actions. Thoughtfulness and action are blended appropriately. The introvert and extrovert tendencies are appropriated for the right proportion. So there is no conflict between them. By giving up the desire for the fruit without renunciation and sacrifice of work, brings about not only the golden mean but also union of the two tendencies.

Nature of a Karma Yogi

We have to possess certain qualifications so as to accomplish *karma yog*. As long as, the six-fold enemies of *kama, krodha* etc. are dominating our mind, intellect and actions, it is not possible to practise *karma yog*, rather we cannot even entertain the idea of *karma yog*. The *shadripus* are so dangerous. So it is necessary to be well-versed in *ashtanga yog* first and foremost. *Karma yog* is not social service. Opening schools, feeding the poor and such works are useful in society. Uplifting the downtrodden is also a great work but it is not *karma yog* in the spiritual field. Moreover, if this is done for the sake of name and fame, and for limelight, it is Name-*yog* alone. To surrender the fruit of the work to God is imperative for accomplishing *karma yog*.

211

सर्वकर्माणं परमगुर्वार्पणम् तत्फलम् संन्यासो वा ।

So dedicating the fruit of the work to God is the soul and core of karma yog.

The next step that follows naturally is unflinching devotion to God. Unless the devotion is overflowing and genuine, the surrender of the fruit of karma cannot take place. The atheist is ever unable to do this, this is not for him. This devotion is attachment to God and emotional involvement in Him. God is the lover of the yogi. As we do everything for our beloved person, and we do it selflessly without any expectation of returns, so the yogi does his karma for God. He has the same intense longing and attachment for God. The only difference is that his attachment is not for a mortal being.

One more important characteristic of the karma of the karma yogi is his detachment. He does the karma because it is the will and order of God. It is done for Him and in subservience for Him. This detachment is not our detachment in karma. It is yogic detachment. If we do a minute analysis of our detachment, we find that it has a tinge of indifference. It is like a mechanical job. This indifference is missing in that detachment; there is tenderness of devotion and self-surrender there. There is an intense attachment and strong bondage for God. The stronger the bondage, the quicker is the freedom from the worldly matters.

Lord Krishna says;

योगस्थ: कुरु कर्माणि संगं त्यक्त्वा धनंजय । (2 : 48)

"Arjuna, perform your duties dwelling in yog, relinquishing all attachment." This yogic detachment is suggested in the Lord's advice.

Lord Krishna says in the Gita :

सिद्ध्यसिद्धौ समो भूत्वा समत्वं योग उच्यते । (2 : 48)

212

"Disinterest in success and failure, equanimity, is called *yog.*"
This is *yogic* detachment. The *karma* that emerges from devotion to
God along with this equanimity and union with God is *karma yog.*

It is commonly thought that a *karma yogi* should have
extraordinary physical prowess, inherent resources, vibrancy, an
enthusiastic frame of mind, and the external equipments like wealth.
This, however, is not at all real *karma yog.* As mentioned before,
accomplishment in *ashtanga yog,* the resultant sublime state of mind
and control of the *shadripus* can create this surrender to the Lord.
Only a genuine *rishi* can accomplish this and he can become a true
karma yogi. So *karma yog* is a manifestation of *ashtanga yog* in its
highly advanced stages. It may be considered as a post-graduation
course of *ashtanga yog.* A dogmatic activist can never be a *karma
yogi.* If he calls himself a *karma yogi* he is a hypocrite. The self-
styled world reformers belong to this category. They try to present
an inflated picture of their activities and display undue exuberance.
A *karma yogi* can never indulge in such self-aggrandizement.

Vedavyasa defines a *karma yogi* in his commentary on the
yogsutras of *Patanjali* i. e. *yog bhashya.* He puts it beautifully as
follows :

सर्वक्रियाणां परमगुर्वार्पणम् तत्फलं संन्यासो वा ।

"Surrendering of all actions and the fruits thereof, even the
renunciation, to the Almighty. The *karma yogi* of the *Vedic* tradition
has this firm faith. Even if he is not a *karma yogi* the *Vedic* has this
same faith."

कामतो वा अकामतो वा यत्करोमि शुभाशुभम् ।
तत्सर्वं त्वयि संन्यस्तं त्वत्प्रयुक्त: करोम्यहं ॥

"O Lord, whatever I volitionally or otherwise do, all that I

213

passionately or dispassionately do, which may be meritorious or otherwise, I offer all these to You. I do all my actions under your command and under your grace and force. Whatever I do, it may be good or evil, I might have done it willingly or unwillingly, I surrender it to you. There may be many phases of moods between willingness and unwillingness and the *karma* might have been done in any of those phases. The original cause of doing it was your will, O God. So I put it at your feet." Please note that this is not the act of giving something that belongs to us. This is not donating or generosity. The surrendering of *karma* is done because the *karma* was done because of God's will and inspiration only.

We can imagine what kind of *karma* the *karma yogi* must have done. We are doing all kinds of *karma* within the range of ultimate sin and ultimate merit every day. But the *karma* of the *yogi* who is accomplished in *ashtang yog* does not do *karma* like us. Obviously he does not commit sins. He has reached a certain level of spiritual knowledge.

ईशावास्यमिदं सर्वं यत्किंच जगत्याम् जगत् ।
तेन त्यक्तेन भुञ्जीथा: मा गृध: कस्यस्विद् धनम् ।।

The faith that is expressed in this first and very powerful *shloka* of *Ishavasya Upanishad* is firmly rooted in his mind. The seer of the *Upanishad* tells us that all *this* which we have – the body, mind and senses, belong to the Divinity, to *Ishvara*. So it is natural that all the *karma* and the fruits of *karma* should be surrendered to Him. The *yogi* is doing *karma* with this faith naturally rooted in him.

As stated earlier, this *karma yog* can be of two kinds. It may be prone to 1] *Jnana yog* or to 2] *Bhakti yog*.

1] *Karma* takes place through the interaction of the organs of

214

knowledge and the objects. These organs of knowledge belong to *prakriti*. The external objects and God also are *prakriti*. The *prakriti* is the creation born out of His power. All the instruments of *karma*, the will and the ego absolutely belong to Him and He is the ultimate Ruler of everything. Where do I stand in this process? I am not the real doer. So I cannot take the credit of this *karma*, nor can I pride upon its fruit. So I am surrendering all these *karmas* at his feet. This faith is based on *jnana yog* or the knowledge that *prakriti* is the doer and the self is the non-doer.

2] The *yogi* who is doing *karma yog* on the foundation of *bhakti* has the faith that this whole universe in every atom of it belongs to God. All the elements like the sun, wind, water are acting solely with His power. Since the *yogi* is acting like his servant for the sake of the Almighty, he is not proud of doing the *karma*. He thinks that he is only instrumental and so he naturally should surrender the fruits of the *karma* to the Almighty.

The *Gita* declares about the faith and mindset of this *karma yogi*. The 47th *shloka* of Chapter 2 says,

कर्मणि एव अधिकार: ते मा फलेषु कदाचन ।
मा कर्मफलहेतुर्भू: मा ते संग: अस्तु अकर्मणि ।।

"*Arjuna*, thy right is to work only, but never with its fruits; do not claim the right to fruit. Let not the fruits of action be thy motive, nor let thine inclination be to inaction." This also means that one should be careful not to lapse into inaction, thinking that there is no use in performing action if one cannot aspire for and accept rewards from action. As the leaves inevitably are drifted when the wind blows, so everybody has to act inevitably. Since you are a human being, you have this body and your accumulated *karma* behind you. You cannot avoid *karma*; that is your destiny. You belong to the universe of *karma*. How can you avoid karma?

न हि कश्चित् क्षणमपि जातु तिष्ठति अकर्मकृत् ।। (3 : 5)

Lord *Krishna* says in the *Gita*. Nobody can be without *karma* even for a split moment. How can you avoid action and activity, the destined *karma*?

Shri Krishnaarpanam astu

✥ ✥ ✥

Nishkama Karma Yog

The core of Karma Yog

The first rule of the four-fold principle of *karma yog* declares that you have the right only to action. You are surrounded by the *karma yoni*, you are in the *karmic* world. The world is a weft of *karmas*, intrinsic to life, inherent in the creation that is in and around you. Therefore you cannot free yourself from *karma*. As remarked earlier,

न हि कश्चित् क्षणमपि जातु तिष्ठति अकर्मकृत् । (3 : 5)

Since you cannot remain without action even for a moment, you have the right to *karma,* and *karma* alone. 'कर्मणि एव अधिकार: ते ।'. (2 : 47) This the Lord says is the first rule.

Now when we say that we do or have to do *karma,* then why not accept the fruits? Right to *karma* implies right to the fruits. We cannot deny that. But says the Lord,

"Do not claim the right on the fruits of *karma*. Because I am the doer and you are the instrument. You are *Atma,* and it is the force of *prakriti* which makes you perform action because of your *ahamkara*. Prakriti is the cause of all action. It is *prakriti* that acts within itself. 'गुणा: गुणेषु वर्तन्त इति मत्वा न सज्जते' । (3 : 28) Get to know that the *gunas* interact with the *gunas* and knowing : 'मा फलेषु कदाचन' Take note that it is not proper for you to claim the fruits. All this (*karma*) is the play of *prakriti*. The second rule of the fourfold principle of *karma* is 'मा फलेषु कदाचन' Here, it should be noted, 'न फलेषु कदाचन' is not stated. The word मा is used in the sense of prohibition and not न, i.e., negation.

We may ask with good reason, that if we do not have the right to claim the fruits, then why should we do *karma?* To this the third principle of the fourfold *karmasiddhanta* has been stated by the Lord: '**मा कर्मफलहेतु: भू: ।**' Let not the fruit of action be your object , do not perform *sakama karma.* There are several motives behind the performance of our *karma.* We desire to achieve wealth, name fame, riches,etc. We do not do *karma* in a detached manner. Therefore, the third rule says, "do not do *karma* with any motive."

Why then should one perform *karma* if there is nothing to gain? This is our attitude. However we should not remain actionless on this account. We therefore have the fourth rule, '**मा ते संग: अस्तु अकर्मणि**' (2 : 47)

The fourfold principle of *karma yog* as stated by the *shloka* (no 47, ch 2) of the *Gita* is indeed very illuminating. Right to action alone, is the first rule, absence of right to the fruits thereof, is the second rule, do not perform *sakama karma* with any motive, is the third, and since there is no fruit to be aspired for, do not develop the attitude to inaction, is the fourth rule. This fourfold *karmasiddhanta* is stated by the following shloka referred to above, it is the very basis of *karma yog*, and is spiritually elevating. It gives the four principles as follows:

कर्मणि एव अधिकार: ते मा फलेषु कदाचन ।

मा कर्मफलहेतु: भू: मा ते संग: अस्तु अकर्मणि ।। (2 : 47)

The Lord tells *Arjuna,*"Your right is restricted only as far as the performance of action is concerned. You are bound to perform action." Now, *Arjuna* belonged to the *kshatriya* or warrior caste, and it was his duty to engage in warfare. Nevertheless, though he became despondent (to fight against his near and dear ones), to fight was his second nature and being a *kshatriya,* battling in war was his

Dharma. Man is involved in action on account of his past *karma, sanchita, prarabdha,*etc. He could not remain without performing *karma.* One has to perform *karma* in accordance with his *varna.* It is not necessarily forced upon us, but we have a right to perform that *karma.* This right however is not to the fruits. Obtaining or not obtaining the fruits does not rest with us. We understand this from experience. The process of fruition of *karma* is dependent on several factors. Sometimes it is due to natural causes and at other times it may be due to obstacles caused by someone. To aspire for particular fruits of one's actions is not appropriate. To perform *karma* and then to expect the fruits of action is akin to tying a boulder to the back and entering the sea! Because the fruits have not to be acquired and also even if there is no guarantee of obtaining them one should not be attached to inaction. Thus the four rules of the fourfold principle of *karma yog* are in fact supplementary to and blend with each other.

The tree bears the fruits. It would be erroneous to presume that it has the right to its fruits. By chance, one may or may not be able to enjoy the fruits of certain actions. Perhaps it may be possible to obtain them in this very life-span. Sometimes this may not be possible. It is possible for another man's *karma* to be intertwined with one's *karma.* The uncertainty regarding the fruits makes a man resign to fate. Thus, when one does not get the expected returns, he blames his fate or he blames God. With such a mentality it would not be possible to perform *karma* properly. We are generally attached to our *karma,* and are not in a position to avoid expectation of fruits. To perform *karma* sincerely and not to desire its fruits can be made possible through *karma yog.* In order to make it possible to perform *karma* in a detached and disinterested manner, it is the fourfold principle which has to be practised with the requisite approach, outlook and disposition. This itself is known as *karma yog.* This particular frame of mind is described as follows:

योगस्थ: कुरु कर्माणि संगं त्यक्त्वा धनंजय ।
सिद्ध्यसिद्ध्यौ समो भूत्वा समत्वं योग उच्यते ।। (2 : 48)

Thus the Lord states that equanimity of mind is called *yog*. What do we mean by *yogastha*? What is *svastha*? To have equilibrium of one's mind. One who dwells in the Lord, by realizing the oneness of *Atma* and *Paramatma* is *yogastha*. *Yogastha* is the one who is submerged in the devotion to the Lord. To be in the stillness, does not mean to remain actionless. Stillness means being in equilibrium within. It is the successful outcome of the attainment of this knowledge of the self. By moving inwards a man becomes balanced and one-pointed. This frame of mind of the true *karmayogi* is aptly described in this way :

य: तु आत्मरति: एव स्यात् आत्मतृप्त: च मानव: ।
आत्मनि एव च संतुष्ट: तस्य कार्यं न विद्यते ।। (3 : 17)

Atma is the fountain of joy. It is an ocean of bliss. For the man who rejoices only in the self, who is gratified with the self, who is contented in the self alone, there is nothing for him to do and achieve. Such a *svastha, yogastha* state of the mind provides a favourable ground for *karma yog*. The *yogic* frame of mind is really centred in the Lord Himself. Without this *yogic* frame of mind it would not be possible to inculcate the fourfold principle of *karma yog*. In order to be centred in the Lord, *bhakti* is essential. That is why an atheist can never become a *karma yogi*. A *karma yogi* has to be overpowered by selfless *bhakti*. Without the element of *bhakti, karma yog* cannot be realized.

Another aspect of *karma yog* which results in *yogavastha* is the knowledge that *Atma* is the non-doer. Knowing that *prakriti* is the cause of all action, we should surrender to the Lord, realizing the connection of *Atma* and *Paramatma,* we can succeed in *karma yog.* Thus to achieve the fourfold principle of *karma yog* is not possible by a mere theoretical approach. Alternatively, following the difficult path of *jnana* can also lead to *karma yog.* From this point of view, shloka 47 and 48, ch.2 of the *Gitaa* are noteworthy.

It would be pertinent to ask as to why one should have the right only to action and not for its fruits. In our daily life, if we are refused the rewards of the work done by us, we fight for them and may even indulge in litigation for securing them. Then why should we deny ourselves the fruits of our spiritual *karma.* To abandon the fruits under these circumstances could be merely idealistic. Some people may say so but in reality, this is highly practical. We will now examine the truth of these statements.

Karma yog is indeed a highly practical philosophy and not merely theoretical or idealistic. We very often believe that "I" am the doer. I want this or I do not want this, this type of feeling prompts us to search the object of our desire. We may sometimes use honest means to acquire our objective, and sometimes if this is not possible, by hook or crook. The underlying basis of such action is the "I" in us. It is this "I" which excites the desire for action, accompanied with greed, expectation, hatred, pride, jealousy, passion, anger, etc. All these are constituents of the mental frame. They motivate the desire to do *karma.* The "I" impels, and the senses try to find the means to achieve the object through the organs of action. This process is initiated on account of *prakriti* and does not have its source in *Atma.* The Lord says :

प्रकृत्या एव च कर्माणि क्रियमाणानि सर्वशः ।

or

'इंद्रियाणि इंद्रियार्थेभ्य: वर्तन्ते' । (13 : 19)

i.e., In all the actions of *prakriti*, and the senses, the *Atma* is not involved. Because it does not have any limitations. *Prakriti* is the doer, whereas *Atma* is the non-doer. Therefore, the Lord says :

य: पश्यति तथा आत्मानं अकर्तारं स पश्यति । (14 : 29)

The *yogi* sees that the self is actionless. Further on, in shloka 27, ch.3 :

प्रकृते: क्रियामाणानि गुणकर्माणि सर्वश: ।

अहंकारविमूढात्मा कर्ता अहं इति मन्यते ॥ (3 : 27)

All actions are wrought in all cases by the qualities of *prakriti* only (*gunas*). He whose mind is deluded by egoism thinks, "I am the doer". The *yogi* knows the truth, and remains detached.

We know that Particle Physics is the basis of modern science. According to this science, matter is constituted of protons, neutrons and electrons. Thus fire, for example, is composed of protons, neutrons and electrons. Also, water, which is required to extinguish the fire is also constituted of protons, neutrons and electrons. Just as the human anatomy and also the food eaten by human beings, contains these three subatomic particles, in the same way, Nature (*prakriti*), is the common activating principle of *karma*. We are all *prakritivasha* (subject to Nature). We are under the governance of the *gunas* of *prakriti* , which is an ever fleeting flux and keeps us constantly in motion, constantly in action. According to the *samkhya* philosophy, *prakriti* (the female aspect of the Divine), is the motivator for action and thus the fruits of action should automatically go to *prakriti* which is born out of the Lord's *Maya* (or *Shakti*). *Purusha* is however the non-doer. Thus all *karma* resulting from *prakriti* has to be surrendered to God. The surrender should be done willingly and not in a dispirited manner. An action done unknowingly may perhaps give us joy, but when the same action is done with knowledge the joy experienced is multiplied. In the same way the knowledge of the overlordship of the Lord and that all actions are done for attaining His grace, and to surrender the fruits of action to Him, can be the source of infinite bliss. Knowing the importance of *karma yog,* and whatever be the nature of the fruits surrendered, the *ananda* from this is extraordinary. The *karma yogi* is always immersed in bliss because the *karma yog* of his *karma* has already been done. After all what else is there in this world which can give this *ananda?*

Karmayog is an eminently practical philosophy. The common man might present a very candid and straightforward question as to why, if the fruits of *karma* are not to be desired is it that we have the duty only to do our actions. If we think that we should enjoy the fruits of action then it makes us intoxicated with pride (*ahamkara*). The "I"-ness in us, which is the chief motivator, demands one thing after another. How do we perform actions when there is motivation? The conative and the internal organs comprising the mind, or the psyche, are our instruments of action, though we claim that "I did this or that". Actually it is the instruments that do the actions. Secondly, the "I"-ness always comes after the body. At birth, the "I"-ness does not manifest. The "I"-ness comes several months after the birth of the baby. At birth there is only the body, the five conative organs, the five cognitive senses and the mind, but there is no "I"-ness. Therefore, the infant in the mother's lap has the body, the senses and the mind, but it does not have the "I"-ness. So the body comes before the "I"-ness and so the body, mind and senses with which the actions are performed, do not belong to the "I"-ness. They do not belong to us, since the instruments do the actions and the instruments do not belong to us. Even if the "I" (*ahamkara*) which manifests itself later after birth, is an instrument of action, the "I"-ness is not us , it is not we, it is not me. Therefore, the fruits cannot come to me. The fruits may go to the "I"-ness, or the fruits may go to the instruments, and therefore it becomes perfectly proper to reject and refuse and renounce the fruits of action. This obviously explains that the principles of *karmayog* are perfectly realistic and logical, and not merely ideological.

The *Upanishad* declares :

'ईशावास्यमिदं सर्वम् यत्किंच जगत्याम् जगत् ।'

The fruits of every action should go to God (*Isha*). But what should be the frame of mind for such offering? We know how to donate money or some other objects to a particular association. But how have we to offer the fruits to God? The action of offering has to be performed in a particular frame of mind, as we cannot surrender the fruits to God in the same manner as we give donations to a particular organization. That particular frame of mind is described in the *Gita* by the following shloka :

यत्करोषि यदश्नासि यज्जुहोषि ददासि यत् ।
यत् तपस्यसि कौंतेय तत् कुरुष्व मदर्पणम् (9 : 27)

Whatever you do, whatever you eat, whatever you offer in sacrifice, whatever you give, whatever you practise as austerity, do it as an offering unto Me.

A *karmayogi* thus has a profoundly deistic mind as reflected in the above shloka. All that I do O Lord, I humbly surrender to You. The *karma yogi* realizes that whatever he does, it is because of Him alone, because of the strength given by Him. So he says, "I surrender the fruits to you. One cannot underscore the significance of the above philosophy of *karmayog* expounded by the Lord. In this connection, Lord *Vyasa* says in the *Bhagavata Purana* (11th Skandha, ch.2) :

कायेन वाचा मनसा इंद्रियै: वा बुद्ध्या आत्मना वा प्रकृतिस्वभावात् ।
करोमि यद् यद् सकलं परस्मै नारायणाय इति समर्पयामि ।

This well-known shloka in the *Bhagavata Purana* (11th *skandha*, 2nd *adhyaya*) is the foundation of *Bhagavata Dharma*. The devotee says that whatever he does with his body, speech, mind, senses, intellect, soul or with the natural qualities he is born with, he is offering it all unto Supreme *Narayana*. A *karma yogi* has imbibed this principle of *Bhagavata Dharma*.

In accordance with the philosophy of *karmayog*, the *karmaphalas* (fruits of action) are to be renounced. Then how should we go about with the process of surrender (i.e., *karmarpana*)? Many a time we unexpectedly receive a windfall in our fortunes. How then should we give up such fruits.? In case an undeserving person were to receive such a windfall, this may even lead him to evil ways. Thus if one were to receive, say, a crore of rupees, then how could such fruits be dispensed? But according to *karma yog* there are various ways of *karmarpana* and dispensing of such fruits. In the *karma yogshastra (Gita)* is explained the process and mode of *karmarpana* and renunciation of *karmaphalas*. They are *karmaphala anashraya, karmaphalatyaga, karmaphalasanyasa, karmaphalasamarpana,* and *karmaphaladana*. Once it is decided that *karmarpana* has to be made, then the processes of *arpana* have to be understood. Mere uttering of *Krishnarpanamastu* would be futile. In order to eschew the attitude of enjoying the fruits, a successful *karmayogi* has to be a master in the art of *ashtanga yog*. It is the path of motiveless action, and the *karmayogi* at the same time is accomplished in the art of *ashtanga yog.* It is said in the *Gita,*

कायेन मनसा बुद्ध्या केवलै: इंदियै: अपि ।

योगिन: कर्म कुर्वन्ति संगं त्यक्त्वा आत्मशुद्धये ।। (5 : 11)

Karmayogis having abandoned attachment, perform actions by the body, mind and intellect and also by the senses for the purification of the self. A *karmayogi* is unattached to the fruits of his actions. Herein, the Lord says :

युक्त: कर्मफलं त्यक्त्वा शांतिम् आप्नोति नैष्ठिकीम् ।।

अयुक्त: कामकारेण फले सक्तो निबध्यते ।। (5 : 12)

The well-poised *nishkama karmayogi* offers the *karmaphala* to *Bhagavan,* and attains the *Bhagavatapraptirupa shanti* or eternal peace in the form of attaining Divine Grace. He attains that *shanti* by offering his *karmaphala* to the Divinity, while the *sakami,* (as against the *nishkami*) is attached to the fruits that creates the swelling of passion in the mind. A true *yogi* is *nishkaama* (completely unattached). The Lord says :

सर्वकर्माणि मनसा संन्यस्य आस्ते सुखं वशी ।

नवद्वारे पुरे देही नैव कुर्वन् न कारयन् ।। (5 : 13)

Such a *yogi* mentally renounces all actions and conquers all his *vrittis.* He remains contented in the self, in the body with nine gates. He remains still and does not allow the body and senses to act. This is the process of *karmaphalasanyasa.* The next stage is that of *karmaphalanashraya.* The Lord says :

न कर्तृत्वं न कर्माणि लोकस्य सृजति प्रभु: ।

न कर्मफलसंयोगं स्वभावस्तु प्रवर्तते ।। (5 : 14)

The Lord does not create agency or doership. He does press everyone to do action. It is *prakriti* or Nature that does everything. Knowing this the *yogi* remains desireless and detached.

Karmaarpana

Karmarpana is the highest form of *karmayog*. In *karmaphalarpana* there is an element of desire for the fruits and the fruits are surrendered subsequent to their attainment. For example, when one who is not a *yogi* espies a beautiful lotus, he takes it for himself, and then surrenders it to God i.e., he accepts the lotus before surrendering it to God. A *yogi* who does *karmarpana* does not wait for the fruits but surrenders the *karma* itself. Hence *karmaphalarpana* is considered to be of lesser merit. For this *karmaphalasamarpanam,* or *karmarpanam* merely being selfless or desireless is not sufficient. There should also be a profound sense of deism, devotion and *bhakti* towards God, since it is considered to be *Bhagavatarpanam*, which is the highest state of *nishkamavastha*. The real attitude of *arpana* requires an unfailing and sublime *Bhagavatprema.* The process of *karmarpanam* has been beautifully described in the *Kurma Purana*, (third *adhyaya,shloka* 16) thus :

न अहं कर्ता सर्वं एतद् ब्रह्म एव कुरुते तथा ।

एतद् ब्रह्मार्पणं प्रोक्तं ऋषिभि: तत्त्वदर्शिभि: ।।

न अहं कर्ता, I know I am not the doer. 'ब्रह्म एव कुरुते', It is the Divinity which does. Everything in the Universe from the movement of a blade of grass, to the rising and the setting of the sun, is motivated by God. There is alignment of this knowing, and *bhakti*, in the *yogi*. There is the attitude of *Keshavarpanamastu* or *Krishnarpanamastu*. These utterances are not merely verbal, like muttering mechanically *Ramakrishna Hari*, or *Sri Rama Jay Rama Jay Jay Rama*. Of course, saints like *Ramdasa swami* or *Tukarama* would do so with profuse devotion.

The mental frame of such an unattached *yogi* is described in shloka 10, ch.5 of the *Gita* :

ब्रह्मणि आधाय कर्माणि संगं त्यक्त्वा करोति यत् ।

लिप्यते न स पापेन पद्मपत्रम् इव अंभसा ।

The *yogi* does *karmarpana* to God and remains like a lotus in water, untouched by the fruits of *karma*. The *karma yogi's* highest state of self-surrender is known as *sharanagati*. One does *atmarpanam* only once, as, by this, he has already achieved *atmanyasa*. *Shloka* 65, ch.18, describes this state of the *karmayogi*:

मन्मना भव मद्भक्त: मत् याजी मां नमस्कुरु ।

माम् एव एष्यसि सत्यं ते प्रतिजाने प्रिय: असि मे ।।

Fix thy mind on Me, be devoted to Me, sacrifice unto Me, bow to Me. You shall come even to Me, truly do I promise unto you, (for) you are dear to Me. The next *shloka* gives the same profound assurance :

सर्वधर्मान् परित्यज्य माम् एकं शरणं व्रज ।

अहं त्वां सर्वपापेभ्य: मोक्षयिष्यामि मा शुच: ।। (18 : 66)

Abandoning attachment to all *dharma*s, take resort and refuge in Me alone; I will redeem you from all bondage and sin.

The Lord has truly given the highest place to *karmayog*.In *shloka* 12, ch.12 the Lord says :

श्रेयो हि ज्ञानम् अभ्यासात् ज्ञानात् ध्यानं विशिष्यते ।

ध्यानात् कर्मफलत्याग: त्यागात् शांति: अनन्तरम् ।।

Better indeed is knowledge than practice effort of stilling the

228

mind; than knowledge meditation is better; than meditation the renunciation of the fruits of action; peace immediately follows renunciation.

We can now recapitulate, restate the definition of *karmayog* as the surrender of all actions, and the fruits to the Lord. In the process, one has to attain control over the mind and senses and their tendencies. One must become desireless and dispassionate. He must also possess *adhyatmajnana*. Without *jnanayog, karmayog* will be devoid of foundation. One must have excelled in the practice of *ashtanga yog*. He must be well-versed in the *Dharmashastra,*and *Karmashastra* in order to be duty-minded. He must also be skilled in the knowledge of *Karmasiddhanta,* coupled with *viveka vritti* (sense of discrimination) and well-versed in the concepts of *karma, akarma, vikarma* and *nishkama karma.* The *japa* of हरि ॐ *nama* must come naturally. Thus it can again be emphatically said :

कायेन वाचा मनसा इंद्रियै: वा
बुद्ध्या आत्मना वा प्रकृते: स्वभावात्
करोमि यद् यत् सकलं परस्मै
नारायणाय इति समर्पयामि ।।

So, *karma* is to be done in a sublime manner. It should be carried out in a sublime process and it should end with sublimity. Every action should end with a profound sense of surrender.

Shri Krishnaarpanam astu

✠ ✠ ✠

229

Discourse - 21

Bhakti Yog

We will now turn our attention to *Bhakti Yog*. *Bhakti* is the link among the four *yogs* of *karma, jnana, dhyana* and *bhakti*. All these have their foundation in *ashtanga yog*. *Bhakti yog* means *yog* through *bhakti* or *yog* of *bhakti*. The basic question faces us here—what is *bhakti*? The word is so profusely and commonly used in the field of religion, culture, philosophy and *sadhana* that it has become a cliché. It is like ignorance born out of too much familiarity. True meanings of too familiar words and concepts always remain vague and concealed. Curiosity is lost and all kinds of harm are done by taking so much for granted. We have to look at it here with as proper perspective as we can. *Bhakti* is taken to be faith with respect and love. Ordinarily we relate *bhakti* with cymbals, counting of rosary beads, clapping of hands, arati, kirtana, japa with *mala*, smearing of unguents on the forehead and body and reading *Harikatha*. We conveniently suppose that we know the meaning of *bhakti*.

While studying *bhakti*, it is necessary to consider what *bhakti shastra* says about it. The *Narada Bhaktisutra* defines *bhakti* as follows:

'सा तु अस्मिन् परमप्रेमरूपा'

Bhakti is not only love but is utmost great love. This supreme devotion or love manifests itself when it is in relation to God as this supreme form of love cannot be anywhere else than in God. It is of the nature of the highest form of love. This meaning is explained in the *Shaandilya Bhaktisutra* :

'सा परा अनुरक्ति: ईश्वरे ।।'

Psychology of Bhaktishastra –

This supreme obsession, love towards God is *bhakti*.

It surprises an ordinary person that the *Bhakti sutras* never even mention *tala* (cymbals), *mala* (rosary), *kirtana*, (singing praises), *bhajana*, *nama* etc. Another important part of *bhaktishastra* is an analysis of each and every emotion of human beings. Emotions form an essential part of human life. However rational, practical and materialistic he is, feelings and emotions are like the food of every human being's mind. His mind is overwhelmed with a tremendous variety of multitudinous feelings. Sometimes there is noise and chaos of them and sometimes there is peace. But this peace also is never devoid of emotions. In a sense this state of quiet is also emotional in character. These feelings are love, infatuation, affection, pride, faith, friendship, enmity, hatred, compassion, content, indifference, ego, audacity, irritation, care, worry, peace, courage, lust, desire, expectation, rivalry, anger, greed, jealousy. All of these are defined and they are used in *bhaktishastra*. *Bhakti* is taken to be love or affection. According to *bhaktishastra* it is *laukika*, or *alaukika*, either temporal or spiritual. The *laukika* relates to the worldly plane, whereas the *alaukika* to the spiritual one. Temporal love is for this world and spiritual one is for God. *Bhakti* makes affection turn towards God.

In Sanskrit, '*raga*' means attachment, '*anuraag*'a affection and '*viraga*' means detachment. Like love, *raga* and *anuraga* are wrongly used to mean the same thing. Love is used for wife's love as well as for mother's love. This wrong use has created much confusion but according to *bhaktishastra*, *raga* and *anuraga* are two classes of Love. In Marathi '*Rag*' means anger. Keeping in mind all these meanings, we can see that *bhakti* crosses and transcends the two poles of anger and infatuation and ennobles the mind of the *sadhaka*.

The psychology of *bhaktishastra* explains many shades and concepts of love and explains them according to the place, way and time of its application. All these things decide their nature-noble or ignoble. If this explanation and criteria of various feelings are considered the confusion in the field of psychology of love also will vanish, man will be able to give proper direction to his emotions and he can save himself from a mental fall by elevating his mind.

Indian psychology, *yog shastra*, *bhaktishastra* and spiritualism all say that all kinds of emotions have their origin in love. Now look carefully. All the feelings emerge only because we have love for some specific object, person or quality. All the feelings like infatuation, affection, pride, faith, friendship, enmity, hatred, compassion, content, indifference, ego, audacity, irritation, care, worry, peace, courage, lust, desire, expectation, rivalry, anger, greed, jealousy arise out of this love. When the object of love is decided, it is simultaneously decided who is worthy of love, faith or hate and so on. It also decides the objects of enmity, friendship, indifference, cruelty or what. So love for one decides the objects of love and hatred. If there is love for A, the feelings of pride, faith, friendship, affection arise for whatever is favourable for A. Whatever A loves becomes the object of our love, too. On the other hand, feelings of anger, hatred and contempt are seen for those who are not favourable for A. So we can see that our feelings for certain things or persons depend mostly upon the persons with whom they are related. We have to say mostly, because the stars and previous associations also play some role in this connection.

Bhaktishastra makes us aware of one more point. Each and every feeling is born out of the source of love. So when the spiritual *sadhaka* tries to curb the six foes (*shadripus*) of human beings, he has to seek an object of love for himself. If this object is not noble, passion is born which is ignoble. He assesses this object and makes suitable changes in it for his own control of the six enemies. If pride is developing, it is impossible to eradicate passion and anger. The psychology of *bhakti* tells us that if the object of love is material and this-worldly and it is turned to God the mighty enemies are completely defeated and burnt away like camphor. If we set out to fight passion and anger without loving God, the fight is ridiculous and useless. Love for anything else than God causes uncontrollable growth of the weed of passions. Love for God removes love , jealousy and contempt for all other objects. Therefore, saintly people do not hate anybody, whether the person is profane or atheist. Rather they have mercy or pity for him. In the worst case, they keep their distance from such persons. Lord *Krishna* describes the nature and psychology of such persons very lovingly in the 12th chapter of the *Gitaa*. "I love the person who has no ill feeling for anybody, has friendship and compassion for every person. Such a person has no attachment for anything, his mind is stable and full of devotion." So *bhaktishastra* finds the roots of all emotions and feelings in love and recommends love for God as the weapon to fight the six enemies. *Bhaktishastra* suggests the science of love for developing and sublimating all emotions and feelings. The following quote is pertinent for clearer understanding of the subject of *bhaktishastra* :

"Hindu psychologists have traced all emotions to one basic emotion-love. Love is the highest desire and the sweetest attractive force which binds the whole universe into one harmonious existence. What is gravity to physics and capillary action to chemistry, love is to psychology. Human love, reverence, affection, devotion, inclination, veneration, adoration, respect and worship, fear, awe, dismay, anger, annoyance, offence, vexation, displeasure- are all manifestations or mutations of love. Therefore, supreme love is another name of God.

Love is the locus behind all reverence, respect and admiration for powerful, beautiful, holy and virtuous ones. None can revere and admire a being or an object which one cannot love." In this context, we quote Emerson as saying "Love will creep where it cannot go. Love will accomplish that by imperceptible methods being its own fulcrum, lever and power which, no force can ever achieve."

Then *bhaktishastra* gives one interesting, fascinating paradoxical conclusion. Outwardly, the two emotions of love and fear appear to be opposite. Love has the force of attraction whereas fear is a repelling force. Attachment emerges on account of love whereas hatred is produced on account of fear. As stated earlier, fear also has its roots in love. Love for wife, children, parents generates fear out of worry regarding their well-being. As *Kalidasa* says, 'अतिस्नेह: पापशंकी'. Too much of love begets too much worry. If this love is lessened, then the worry and fear also decreases. Thus all the mental states and feelings are the spokes emanating from the same hub of love. Even hatred or contempt is derived from love because a person becomes ferocious when he senses danger to his beloveds and wants to protect them. Love is the primordial emotion. All other feelings are mutations of love. They are all other aspects of love. Since love is the primeval emotion, it is love alone that is intrinsically pure. It is pure, sacred and free from perversions. It is beyond all morbidities. When the refining, purifying and culturing part of love becomes prominent, it leads to *bhakti*. When the sensual part is prominent, it leads to destructive perversions, the six enemies of the mind. If the positive part of love is developed, it takes him to sublimation and the divine path whereas development of the negative part of love makes him morbid and satanic. Refined love culminates into *yog* and sensual and self-centred love is *bhog*.

The *Bhagavata Purana* gives a significant classification of love.

One type of love is the love which is reciprocal. This is only a commercial attitude towards love which is selfish and banal. A slightly higher kind of love has no expectation of returns from the loved one. It is love for the sake of love. The highest kind of love is that which does not accept love or anything from the loved one. But the relationship of love between the devotee and God is exceptional. Even when the devotee surrenders wholeheartedly to God, He does not respond. As a child harasses the mother and exasperates her, so God exasperates the devotee. Of course, this is an aspect of love. And everything is fair in war and love! Indeed the purpose of this harassment is to enhance the devotee's love.

Hindu psychology has looked at all the subtle shades of feelings analytically. It also has divided the qualities of human mind within three *gunas* - *sattva*, absolute purity, *raja*, less purity but not impurity and *tamas*, total impurity. The next *andha tamisra* is (fortunately!) exceptional which is like the chaos before the beginning of the world. There is no awareness of the *tamas* of the self in it. All the shades of hatred naturally belong to *tamas*. If we look at the shades of the blanket term love, we see a spectrum of the feelings of affection, attachment, caring, faith and so on. Further as we differentiate among them from the point of view of the three *gunas*, *raja* is prominent in attachment. Affection, attachment, caring, faith and so on apparently seem to be *sattvic* but, in fact, they are *rajasic* and sometimes even mixed with a tint of *tamas* because of other interests of the person. For example, there may be an expectation of returns, there may be violating norms in the society for the sake of love, there may be discrimination or unfairness and insults towards others while loving one person etc. The subject is very vast and we may not go into details here. But we can certainly say that the attachment for God which is devotion is above and beyond all these feelings. It has no expectation of returns or happiness and so it is *sattva* and absolute purity. The affection for friends, mother, father, brother, etc. is this-worldly and so it binds a person to this world. It can never give liberation as devotion can.

Kinds of Bhakti

Bhaktishaastra considers *bhakti* in two types. (a) *Gauni* and (b) *Paraa*. *Gaunibhakti* is again classified into two types, i.e., (i) *vaidhi* and (ii) *raagaatmika*. We may represent these in the following table:

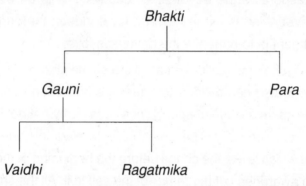

Both the *vaidhi* and *ragatmika* types head towards *Paraa Bhakti*. The *lakshya* or target of both is *Para Bhakti*. *Vaidhibhakti* comes in the beginning, evolves in *ragatmika bhakti* and culminates in *Para Bhakti*.

Now let us consider the first, *vaidhi bhakti*. After all *bhakti* is love only and it comes naturally. Logically and technically speaking, love cannot be learnt or taught. It is an instinctive, natural feeling. How can, then, *bhakti* be *vaidhi* or contain *vidhi* or rituals? How can emotions be with rituals and can these emotions with rituals be flawless? These questions are logical but it is also true that every lover is not able to express his love successfully. He uses some ritual for the expression. The rituals like presenting greeting cards, gifts, flowers, bouquets and loving words and promises are a way of expressing love. Effective rituals make effective expression of love.

Love between men and women is primordial but the ways of its expression have been varying with times, changes in culture and society. Perhaps the dramas, films and novels of today have invented more effective ways of its expression. One can argue that it has become more showy, banal and shallow; but it is a matter for debate. All the same, it is true that appropriate rituals can cherish and express emotions of love. Similarly devotion for God can be cultivated, developed and enhanced through rituals. *vaidhi bhakti* in the *shastras* becomes justifiable in this way.

If young men and women today learn from heroes and heroines how to express and enhance love, devotees learn this art of love from the great devotees like *Pralhada, Narada, Parashara, Pundarika, Vyasa, Ambarisha, Shuka, Shaunaka, Bhishma, Dalbhya, Rukmangada, Vasishtha, Vibhishana, Hanuman, Namadev, Tukaram, Tyagaraja, Tulsidas, Surdas, Kabir, Mirabai. Purandaradasa*, and other countless devotees. *Vaidhi bhakti* is following one's idols of *bhakti* and enhancing one's devotion. *Shravanam* or listening to holy songs, *kirtanam* or singing them, *japa, dhyanam* or meditation, *bahiryaga* or *yajna*, and *antaryaga* or inward worship are some factors of *vaidhi bhakti*. All these aspects have certain observances and restraints which have to be followed very meticulously. In course of time devotion matures and then rituals become less important, gradually even immaterial. Rather, as devotion increases, these *vidhis* are shed like a ripe fruit and emotions overflow. Every action of such a mature devotee shows the devotion. This devotee has transcended all the observances and restraints, religion and morals, and also duties of all kinds. This is also called *ragatmika bhakti*. We ordinary people try to evaluate the behaviour of such a devotee with our own mundane criterion of reasoning which is most irrelevant and inappropriate in this case. Our judgements and verdicts are in fact out of place. We charge the devotee of irresponsible behaviour. We say that he violated social norms and caused suffering for his family. This is like holding a millimeter scale in order to measure astronomical distances! The charges have to be considered with a pinch of salt.

The rituals in *vaidhi bhakti* develop into devotion. The *sadhaka* listens to the greatness of God which is *shravanam*. He does *japa* and *dhyana* in his regular worship. The technical rituals like *Upasthana*, *Dik shuddhi*, *Dig bandha*, *Malachalana* are taken care of. While doing this ritual with the body, he does it with a mind as if he is a servant of God and he is obeying His order as it is his duty. He meditates on God regularly. This daily routine increases his *sattva guna*, purifies his heart and devotion is enhanced. These six parts of *bhakti* move from the level of *kriya* to devotion when they are matured and are unified. This is the acme of *bhakti*. Here the *bhakti* of six parts develops into *bhakti* with nine parts. In the *Bhagavata* sect the same *bhakti* with six parts is explained as *bhakti* with nine parts.

श्रवणं कीर्तनं विष्णो: स्मरणं पादसेवनम् ।
अर्चनं वंदनं दास्यं सख्यं आत्मनिवेदनम् ॥

We will look at this nine-fold *bhakti* with a few examples. The *Bhagavata Purana* was narrated by *Shukacharya* to King *Parikshit*. The king listened to the narration with great reverence and devotion. This is known as *sravana bhakti*. Sage *Narada*, the jewel among the devotees, advocated the *kirtana bhakti* reciting the name *Narayana*. *Draupadi* in the *Mahabharata* was being humiliated very heinously in the court of the *Kauravas*. At that time she invoked Lord *Krishna* and distressfully sought protection from Him. This is *smarana bhakti*. *Bharata*, the brother of *Shri Rama*, performed the *padasevana* of Lord *Shri Rama* by placing His *padukaas*, His footwear, on the throne of *Ayodhya* while ruling this state. *Archana bhakti* is the worship of the idol of the Lord by offering basil leaves (*tulasi*), flowers, fruit and holy water. The *'shodashopachara'* worship is more elaborate and involves sixteen parts. They are *asana,* seat for the Lord, *arghya*, respectful offering of water, *achamana*, sipping of water at the commencement of religious ceremonies, *snana* ceremony of bathing the idol of the Lord, *vastra*, clothing the idol with appropriate raiment, *yajnopavita*, investiture of the idol with the sacred thread, *gandha*, anointing with sandlewood powder, *patram*, offering holy leaves, *pushpam*, flowers, *naivedyam* sweets, *phalam*, fruit, *tambulam*, betel leaf along with areca nut, *dakshina*, gift of money, *dhupam*, incense, *dipam*, lighting a lamp before Him, *pradakshina*, circumambulation from left to right in the form of reverential salutation, and *mantrapushpa*, offering flowers consecrated by *mantra* at the end of worshipping. *Bhishmacharya* and *Akrura* were noted for their *vandana bhakti*, bowing reverentially before the Lord. They never used any other form of worship. The *bhakti* of *Hanuman* was '*dasya*' *bhakti* as he treated himself like a servant of the Lord. *Arjuna* and *Uddhava* possessed *sakhya bhakti*, reverential friendship. *Bali,* a demon king, had the '*atmanivedana*' *bhakti*, full revelation of the self. Our mythologies and history tell us not only about the nine-fold *bhakti* but also about the devotees. The *sadhaka* is expected to perform the *bhakti* according to the best of his ability. *Vaidhi bhakti* purifies his mind and chitta, destroys sins and enhances his *sattva. Sattva Dharma* shines in his heart. This *bhakti* makes his senses also to serve God. Once devotion overflows, rites and rituals lose their priority and even importance. Devotion evolves and expedites the journey towards higher and fuller kind of self-surrender.

This *para* or higher *bhakti* is *samadhi* in the form of *dhyana*. This is an ecstatic state. The ecstasy of *Mirabai, Chaitanya Mahaprabhu,*

239

and *Tyagaraja* is of this nature. It made them forget their duties and commitments towards their families, towards father, mother, son, brother and the society. They gave up their work and were not constrained by the ties of this world. We charge and curse them for this lapse in behaviour. But how can we expect this awareness when they are lost in the emotional ecstasy of *bhakti* of God. From the worldly point of view, they may be wrong but the nature of the object of their *bhakti* should not be overlooked. It is God Himself who is :

"पिता अहं अस्य जगतो माता धाता पितामह: ।"

"गति: भर्ता प्रभु: साक्षी निवास: शरणं सुहृत् ।"

"त्वमेव माता च पिता त्वमेव त्वमेव बन्धुश्च सखा त्वमेव ।"

He is father, mother, protector, goal, creator, master, witness, resort and refuge of the world. Only He is the friend of all.

As He is the *Dharma* for the devotee, in a way he is observing all the *Dharmas*. Apparently it seems his failure in following the ordained duties but the reality is at the other pole. He is following the highest *Dharma* where he is free from the other duties. Their fall, if it can be called a fall, is more sublime than all our observances of earthly rules and duties. We can understand why the Lord says in the *Gita* :

"सर्वधर्मान् परित्यज्य माम् एकं शरणं व्रज ।

अहं त्वा सर्वपापेभ्यो मोक्षयिष्यामि मा शुच: ।" (18 : 66)

"Give up all *dharmas* and take refuge in Me Alone. I will liberate you from all sins. Grieve not on any count." The import of this *shloka* is quite obvious.

Stages of Bhakti

In the *Brihannaradiya purana* various stages of *bhakti* have been nicely described. According to this *purana*, there are ten gradations

240

of Bhakti.

Tamasic bhakti-	(1)	*adhama tamasa*
	(2)	*madhyama tamasa*
	(3)	*uttama tamasa*
Rajasic bhakti-	(4)	*Adhama*
	(5)	*madhyama*
	(6)	*uttama*
Sattvic bhakti-	(7)	*adhama*
	(8)	*madhyama*
	(9)	*uttama*
Gunatita bhakti-	(10)	*uttomottama*

It is interesting and enlightening to know the characteristics of the above classes of *bhakti*. *Adhama tamasa bhakti* happens when one does penance but the purpose is to destroy somebody else even at the cost of one's own life. In the *Mahabharata, Jayadratha* invokes the grace of Lord *Shiva* because he wants to destroy *Arjuna*. Several other similar instances are described in the *puranas* in regard to the *rakshasas* and the *asuras*. Now, what is *madhyama tamasa*? A promiscuous married person is attached to his keep and is unfaithful to his wife. This is *madhyama tamasa*. It is tantamount to cheating. Such a person outwardly professes innocence, but in reality is a villain. *Uttama tamasa* is reflected when a devotee becomes jealous of another sincere devotee, and practises *bhakti* in order to compete with the other to outdo him in his achievements. This type of *bhakti* is present in many individuals. *Adhama rajasa bhakti* is *sakama*, though it can be performed with faith. It is done with expectation of material gain like wealth, food, progeny etc. *Madhyama rajasa bhakti* is performed with desire for fame, name, success, etc. Such a devotee tries to pose as a pious, god-fearing individual. There is an element of pomp in his behaviour. *Uttama rajasa bhakti* is performed with the objective of attaining the kingdom of heaven like *Indra* or Zeus, attaining godhood, (or even being an overlord of gods). It is in fact a subtler type of bargain or 'commercial' *bhakti*. Demons such as *Ravana* and *Bhasmasura* cherished this type of *bhakti*. Human beings also try to perform this *bhakti*.

Now have a look at the three kinds of *sattvic bhakti*. *Adhama sattvic bhakti* is performed with the sincere intention of expiating one's sins, removing the impurities of the mind and weakening the *shadripus*. *Madhyama sattvic bhakti* consists in performing rituals with a detached mind, for the sole purpose of pleasing the Lord. *Uttama sattvic bhakti* is performed with a sense of complete self-surrender to God. God is the ultimate refuge, the near and dear one, the witness, the dwelling place, the Protector. God alone is the mother, father, brother, Creator to the devotee. He is considered to be the Overlord of the Universe. The devotion is unshakeable, unwavering and has full knowledge of God. Devotion overflows with *sattva Dharma*. In the ideal state, God is seen by the devotee even in the gross physical substances like water, earth, wood, stone, etc. The whole Universe is permeated by God and appears to him to be *Vasudeva.* ''**विष्णुमयसृष्टी**'' ''**वासुदेवं इदं सर्वम्**''. Such a devotee is called *Bhagavata* – a true devotee of the Lord. This type of devotion is possessed by great saints. This gradation of devotion in the *Brihannaradiya purana* is pertinent, shows deep insights into human psyche and demands our attention.

Devotion is of great importance in *bhakti,* rather it is at the core of it. The Lord of the Universe hungers for the overflowing *bhakti* in the hearts of his devotees. While praising this intense feeling of devotion, the poet says :

भावेन लभ्यते सर्वं भावेन देवदर्शनम् ।
भावेन परमं ज्ञानं तस्माद् भावावलम्बनम् ॥
भावात् परतरं नास्ति त्रैलोक्ये सिद्धं इच्छितम् ।
भावो हि परमं ज्ञानं, ब्रह्मज्ञानं अनुत्तमम् ॥
भावात् परतरं नास्ति येन अनुग्रहो भवेत् ।
भावात् अनुग्रहप्राप्ति: अनुग्रहात् महान् सुखी ॥
भावेन लभ्यते सर्वं भावाधीनं इदं जगत् ।
भावं विना महाकाले न सिद्धि: जायते क्वचित् ॥
भावात् परमं नास्ति भावाधीनं इदं जगत् ।
भावेन लभ्यते योग: तस्मात् भावं समाश्रयेत् ॥

This is a beautiful exposition of devotion. The shloka explains
the efficacy of devotion comprehensively and totally. Devotion can
give everything along with ultimate knowledge and company of God.
So take support of devotion. Nothing is greater than devotion.
Devotion can give blessings of God that are followed by great
happiness. Nothing is impossible for devotion as the whole world is
subject to devotion. Devotion can give *siddhis* and *yog*. So take refuge
into devotion.

Patanjali, in his *yogsutras*, describes the ritual of
Ishvarapranidhana to be done with *japa* of *Omkara* in his famous
aphorism ईश्वरप्रणिधानाद्वा and

"तत् जप: तदर्थभावनम् ।"

This *japa* is so emotionally profound that it leads one to the highest
samadhi state of *yog*. We have thus observed the classification of
bhakti according to the *bhaktisutras* as well as the classification based
on the three *gunas* according to the *Brihannaradiya purana*.

Type of Bhakti – Padma Purana

The religious sciences also describe certain other gradations. The *Padma purana* classifies *bhakti* as (1) *Laukiki* (2) *Vaidiki* (3) *Adhyatmiki.*

Laukiki is practised through the physical body, speech and mind. *Archana* and *puja* are of body. *Namajapa* is of speech. *Dharana* and *dhyana* of God's *svarupa* are done with the mind. The first type consists of religious rituals and penance having mortification of the body for expiation of sins. It is regulated by the periods of waxing and waning of the moon. The second type includes study of the *Vedas*, the *suktas*, the *Purusha sukta*, offering of consecrated flowers, oblation to the god of fire, sacrifice to the god, *Soma*, ritual sacrifices and penance. In the *adhyatmiki* type of *bhakti*, all the primary and Universal elements are seen as the divine attributes of the personal deity. To this type also belongs the *samkhya* and the *adhyatmika bhakti*. Here all the 24 elements along with the 25th *Purusha* element are seen as the cause of the creation of the Universe. Such is the faith with which *bhakti* is practised. *Pranayama* with *mantras* has an important place and meditation of the Lord is done in the core of the heart. All this description is related to the gradations of *bhakti* found in the *Padma purana*.

Classification of Bhakti - Shankaracharya

Shankaracharya also has made a subtle classification of *bhakti* within five types in his *Anandalahari:*

1. *Sannimitta - Bhakti*, when God is remembered with some *nimitta* or cause, as in times of difficulty and trial.

2. *Sativat* - A *sati* or wife is devoted to her husband during their life-time. Death makes an end to it. Similarly *bhakti* is there as long as the body is there.

3. *Svabhavavasha* - This type is similar to the natural attraction between magnet and iron in case of their proximity to each other. It is like *bhakti* arising in a person when he is in the vicinity of a temple but it vanishes when he goes away from it.

4. *Vrukshalatavat* - Creeper on a tree has no life when it is broken off. But as long as it is integral with the tree it has life. Flashes of bhakti arise in the mind when favourable conditions are there which prompts the devotee to continue with his clapping, counting of beads etc. When conditions become unfavourable to the individual, he withdraws from this state, and may even probably nurse indifference towards God and curse Him.

5. *Nadisagaravat* - Just as a *nadi* or river completely submerges into *sagara* or the sea, the devotee surrenders completely to God.

The eight Sattvic emotions

Knowledge of *bhaktishastra* would be incomplete unless one knows the *ashtasattvic bhaava* or emotions. What are these emotions? When *sattva* reaches the zenith, it manifests in the embodiment in the following ways:

Sharirika bhava - These three types are related to body. (1) *romancha*- hair standing on its ends. (2) *sveda* - dampening of the body. (3) *ashrupata* - tears flow from the eyes. *Sharir-manasa bhavas* — These emotions are psychosomatic. The devotee gets (4) *kampa* i.e. the body trembles under the over-powering effect of emotions. 5) In *stambhana* the body becomes stiff, which could be wrongly seen to be hysteria. (6) *svarabhanga*. In this case, the devotee's voice is choked. The last two types are related to mind. They are (7) *vaivaranam* and (8) *pralayam*. *Vaivaranam* means total vanishing of 'I'-ness. It is a unique state to imagine. *Pralaya* means the *sattvaguna* reaches its zenith taking the devotee to the transcendental state. The student of *bhaktishastra* has to know these *ashtasattvica* emotions.

Four types of Bhakti in the Gita

The student of *bhaktishastra* should also know the four types of *bhakti* described in the *Gita*. They are: *arta, jignyasu, artharthi, jnani*. The *arta* devotee is exasperated by afflictions and so there is poignancy in his prayer and worship. He worships God with remorse. The second type is *jignyasu*. The devotee has a sense of inquiry and performs his *bhakti* on the intellectual plane by studying the sciences. The third type-*artharthi*- does worship for obtaining material prosperity. He firmly believes that God bestows everything for satisfying his desires. The fourth type-*jnani*- is most qualified for *bhakti yog*. He is the one who has revelation of God. He is described as the best of the devotees. *Shlokas* 13-20 of chapter 12 of the *Gita* describe this devotee and the description is worth contemplating. The Lord says that such a one bears ill-will towards none. He looks at all with love and compassion. He entertains mercy towards people in distress. He has equipoise in pleasure and pain, and is ever forgiving. He is always contented, stable in meditation, self-controlled, and possessed of firm conviction. He is one by whom the world is not agitated and who cannot be agitated by the world. He is beyond bubbles of joy, envy, fear and anxiety. He neither rejoices nor hates, nor grieves nor desires. For him censure and praise are equal. He is beyond the dualities of heat and cold, good and evil. Attachment, hate, anger, censure, praise do not touch him. He is free from the fetters of domestic life, relatives and self-interest. He is sacredness, serenity, equanimity and vigilance incarnate. He sees father, mother, brother, protector and all relations in the Lord only.

All the obstacles in the way of fulfillment are destroyed with *bhakti*, known as *Ishvarapranidhana* in *yogic* parlance,. *Shloka* 11 of chapter 10 of the *Gita* says: 'तेषां एव अनुकम्पार्थं अहं अज्ञानजं तम: नाशयामि ।' – and - 'आत्मभावस्थे ज्ञानदीपेन भास्वता ।' The Lord destroys the darkness born of ignorance in the devotees with the luminous lamp of knowledge.

Patanjali has described *bhakti* in this way in the chapter on *bhakti* :

'व्याधिस्त्यान संशय प्रमादावस्था अविरति भ्रान्तिदर्शनम् अलब्धभूमिकत्वानवस्थितत्वानि चित्तविक्षेपा: ते अन्तराया: ।' and also- 'दु:ख दौर्मनस्य अंगमेजयत्व श्वासप्रश्वासा विक्षेपा: सहभुव: ।'

The *Vishnusahasranama* says: 'रोगार्तो मुच्यते रोगात् – बद्धो मुच्येत बन्धनात् ।'

A diseased person gets rid of diseases and a slave is liberated from his shackles. All this indicates that *bhakti* leads one to the ultimate goal, whether it is a gain of one penny or of God-realization. This is the basic principle of spiritual knowledge.

Surrendering is a very important aspect of *bhakti*. It is the vital culminating factor of *bhakti yog*. A surrendering devotee takes complete refuge in God. The *bhakta* is identified by his attitude of surrender. *Shloka* 66 of chapter 18 of the *Gita* says :

सर्वधर्मान् परित्यज्य माम् एकं शरणं व्रज ।

अहं त्वा सर्व पापेभ्यो मोक्षयिष्यामि मा शुच: ।। (18 : 66)

The Lord asks the devotee to give up all other religions and sects and surrender to Him alone. He says, "Do not worry. I will save you from all sins." Generally surrendering is taken to be defeat in life. It is considered to be the end of valour, bravery and exhaustion of courage. Some rationalists also think that *bhakti yog* is for the weak. But in this context surrendering is the limit of courage, bravery and strength. We have to reflect over the concept of surrendering, deeply.

Surrendering is a very important factor in *bhakti*. When a profound devotee surrenders, he is called *'prapanna'*. This word is found in the Gita. *Arjuna* starts his dialogue with the word *'prapanna'*. In the 2nd chapter he says,

शिष्य: ते अहं शाधि मां त्वां प्रपन्नम् ।। (2 : 7)

He says, "I am your disciple and I have approached you. Support me." The end of the dialogue is assurance as follows.

''सर्व धर्मान् परित्यज्य मामेकं शरणं व्रज ।
अहं त्वा सर्वपापेभ्य: मोक्षयिष्यामि मा शुच: ।। (18 : 66)

We have seen the meaning of this *shloka*. Surrendering is difficult because all the other religions are to be given up before it. This will be clearer later.

Surrendering is not defeat or retreat as understood in the ordinary sense. It is the finale reached after a glorious self-effort, and is the peak of fearlessness. It destroys all infirmities and fears in the mind of the *bhakta*. It even transcends the limits of self-confidence, fearlessness and self-effort. Surrendering is undoubtedly of the highest importance in *bhakti yog*. A *bhakta* of the supreme class takes to surrendering and is known as a *prapanna*. *Prapanna* is a word from the *Gita*.

Surrendering makes two kinds of devotees as *bhakta* or devotee, and *'prapanna'*. A *bhagavata* is a mere devotee if he does not surrender and he is a *Prapanna* if he surrenders. *Narayana dharma* describes surrendering or surrendering in this way. *Bharadvaja Samhita* in *Pancha Ratra* says,

"आनुकूलस्य संकल्प: प्रतिकूलस्य वर्जनम् ।
रक्षिष्यति इति विश्वासो गोप्तृत्वं वरणं तथा ।
आत्मनिक्षेप: षड्विधा शरणागति: ।।"

There are six signs of surrendering. It means that whatever is favourable for God is followed in any condition and in whatever way. The foremost sign of surrendering is never to deviate from God even in adverse conditions. The character of *Prahlada* can tell us what bravery and courage is needed for this. His life mainly shows the sign of protection of what is favourable. The life of *Vibhishana* shows abandoning of what is unfavourable. He gives up the side of *Ravana* who was acting against *Dharma*. He left the brother and family to surrender to *Rama*. The third sign of surrendering is the firm faith that God will protect and He will not abandon. It is the faith that He alone is the Saviour. The story (*Gajendra Moksha*) of the elephant *Gajendra* who was saved from the jaws of a crocodile by Lord *Vishnu* shows this sign. *Gajendra* prayed to Him wholeheartedly. Even *Draupadi* supplicated to Him similarly and was saved from dangers. *Ahilya* surrendered to *Rama* in the same way. *Dhruva* protected the *mantra* secretly, which is *goptrutva*. This is the preliminary thinking with regard to surrendering.

The *prapanna* devotee is not tied to any *Dharma* or duty towards his mother, father or anybody else. No duty binds him because God is his mother, father, brother and all. By following God all the duties are performed. Until surrendering he also is caught between dualities like us. Dilemmas in *Dharma* are puzzling him, too. It is like walking on a razor's edge to follow all the commands of *Dharma* and duties at the same time. He has to choose between the orders of mother and wife, father and master and so on because the orders of *Dharma* are not simple and they pose dilemmas like the riddle of the sphinx. The calibre of surrendering solves his problem. In surrendering devotion is more important than rituals. The science of *bhakti* tells us the pertinent sign of '*prapatti*'. We find one in *Narayaniya Dharma*.

"भगवत्प्रवृत्तिविरोधिस्वप्रवृत्तिनिवृत्ति: प्रपत्ति: ।।"

If the devotee retires from his tendency of going against God's orders, this is *prapatti*. We ordinary people do not easily do whatever is favoured by God, but for a devotee this is natural. It is the sign of a *prapanna* to follow whatever God likes. It is a theory in the *Ramanuja* sect that a devotee becomes *prapanna* by surrendering. These concepts are put forth clearly in the books of this sect. For us *prapanna* and devotee or *bhakta* surrendering, and *prapatti* are one and the same. But the *Ramanuja* sect makes the distinction clear. We will consider it in the chapter on knowledge and science of *bhakti*.

The *sadhana* that makes the devotee a true devotee and retains him like that, is *bhakti yog*. We ordinary people associate *bhakti yog* with cymbals, counting of beads, *japa*, recitation of God's name. There are kinds of *bhakti yog* in different states of India. Maharashtra has *bhakti yog* of the *Warkari* sect who are devotees of *Vithoba*. In Gujarat and Rajasthan it is the *Vraja* sect, Bengal has the *Vaishnava* sect of *Chaitanya Mahaprabhu* and in the southern states it is *bhakti yog* of *Vaishnavas*. There is no uniformity among these kinds of *yog*. There are also other sects like *Shri, Ramanandi, Buddhi, Rudra, Shaiva, Ganapatya, Datta, Shakti* sects and there may be contradictions among them. This will create confusion, contradictions and discords. *Bhakti yog* will be replaced by *bhakti vi-yog* i. e. separation from *bhakti*.

250

It is proper to keep aside the *Shri Ramanuja* sect and look at the scientific elucidation given by him. Let us consider this explanation by *Shri Ramanuja*. In fact, the tradition of *bhakti yog* does not exist at present. *Bhakti yog* is not cymbals, rosary, *japa*, recitation of God's name, etc. *Bhakti yog* means *Brahma sadhana* with the *Brahma vidyas* of the *Upanishads*. All these *vidyas* are *dhyana*-oriented. Naturally they are possible during *yog* sadhana. The *dhyana* in it makes it *bhakti yog*. The *Brahma vidyas* in the *Upanishads* are nearly 30 to 35 such as *Sadvidya, Bhruguvidya, Daharavidya, Purushavidya, Antaravidya*. *Bhakti yog* is to get initiation from the master and then to attain *dhyana* in that *vidya*. Absorption in this gives *samadhi* in the *bhakti yog*. This is called *Upaya Bhakti* in the science of *bhakti* because *dhyana* has to be attained with the advice of those who know *Brahman*. That gives success.

This *sadhana* is possible only during *dhyana* according to the principle of *Vedanta* - "आसीनसंभवात्"

Real *bhakti yog* cannot be attained by mere walking, talking, singing and dancing. The ecstasy of *Chaitanya Mahaprabhu* and *Mirabai* cannot reach the heights of real *bhakti yog*, as also the *samadhi* of absorption in music experienced by *Surdas* and *Tyagaraja*. In classical concept of Bhakti yog one must be of a born class and must be innitiated with upanishadic Brahma Vidya. The *Brahadaranyaka Upanishad* says, आत्मनि एव आत्मानम् उपासीत्. This instruction suggests *dhyana* itself. The self should do *sadhana* of self with the self—this means it is *dhyana* only and the ritual for it is only *dhyana*. This is clearly seen in the instructions in *Brahadaranyaka Upanishad* and *Mundakopanishad* such as—

आत्मा वा अरे द्रष्टव्य: श्रोतव्य: मन्तव्य: निदिध्यासितव्य: ।

The self should be seen, heard, listened to, thought about and reflected upon.

Or

आत्मानं तम् एव ध्यायथ Reflect upon the self alone.

Actually it is God who gives salvation but *bhakti yog* directs that *sadhana* of *Brahman* is the way of salvation. That is why it is called *Upaya Bhakti* because *Upaya* means way or solution. Now we will consider the features of *bhakti yog* in the proper order so as to understand it thoroughly.

1] *Bhakti yog* must pertain to some Upanishadic *Brahmavidya* for *Brahma sadhana*.

2] The *sadhana* must be carried out by the meditative process, *yogic dhyana*.

3] The *sadhaka* must be eligible for studying the *Vedas* for *bhakti yog*. This can be done only by the three castes- the *Brahmins*, *Kshatriyas* and *Vaishyas*.

4] The *sadhana* must be carried out only according to the *sutra* of the *Vedas*— *asina sambhavat* and in no other way. The *sadhaka* must know the process of *dhyana* in the science of *yog*.

5] Cymbals, rosary, *japa*, *gomukhi*, ecstatic dancing, ecstatic singing are not required.

6] Even recitation of God's name or *japa* are not required as rituals.

Well, we see that the *Brahmavidya* sect is no longer there now. Initiation by the master on *Brahmavidyas* is not available today. The *varnashrama Dharma* does not exist now. Therefore, the tradition of *bhakti yog* is lost. It compels us to conclude that the *bhakti yog* that shows itself today is not real *bhakti yog*.

It is rightly said in the *Ramanujacharya* sect, that surrendering is markedly different from *bhakti yog*. Let us see why it is justified. The *bhakti yogi* has salvation-oriented attitude but the *prapanna* does not have salvation-oriented attitude in his surrendering. *Dhyana* is the unique and indispensable way for achievement of God in *bhakti yog*, whereas in *prapatti* God is the object of achievement as well as the means i.e. God Himself is the means and God Himself is the end. In *bhakti yog*, '*tailadharavat* [continuous like flowing of oil] *dhyanam* is the highest state in it. But in *prapatti*, *svatma nikshepa* is the highest state. *Svatma nikshepa* means total self-surrender. *Svatma nikshepa* is described as under:

तेन संरक्षमाणस्य फले स्वात्मवियुक्तता ।
केशवार्पणपर्यन्ता हि आत्मनिक्षेप उच्यते ।।

This means that God is taken to be the ultimatum and the devotee submits himself to him. This process presupposes that he is left with nothing before God. All the burdens of his sins, merit and bad and good deeds are surrendered at the feet of God. Even the expectation of salvation does not remain there. God should do whatever He likes to do with the devotee, He may accept or abandon him. This is the attitude of the *prapanna* which is different from the *bhakta* who has a desire of the company, blessings, achievement of God. The *prapanna* is not left with his self-awareness even. This can be illustrated with the example of *Namadev* who was a *bhakta* and not a *prapanna*. *Goroba* told *Namadev* that *Namadev* was a raw beginner in the field of *bhakti*. *Namadev* approaches Lord *Vithoba* and asks Him about his plight. The Lord advises him to meet *Visoba Khechar* in the temple of *Mallikarjuna*. *Namdev* obeys and gets the blessing of maturity. If *Namadev* were a *prapanna*, he would not have tried for maturity. He would have taken his situation as God's will and remained happy with it. The approach of *prapanna* is best described in the *Gita*.

गति: भर्ता, प्रभु: साक्षी निवास: शरणं सुहृत् ।
प्रभवप्रलयस्थानं च निधानं बीजमव्ययम् ॥

God is the last resort, the Master, Omnipotent, Omnipresent, friend, origin of the beginning and ending, ultimate goal and the seed of all. The *prapanna* would be content with his surrendering. Now let us see the difference from scientific point of view.

First and foremost, there is a difference of features between them. *Bhakti yog* has two features of knowledge (*jnana*) and *karma*. *Sadhana* of these two is needed in *bhakti yog* but *prapatti* has surrendering. Its nature was described above

सर्वधर्मान् परित्यज्य मां एकं शरणं व्रज । (18 : 66)

Give up every other religion and surrender to me. No duty or obligation remains for him. *Bhakti yog* is *dhyana* oriented, and *sadhana* is done through *ashtanga yog*. So for the accomplishment of *bhakti yog*, *ashtanga yog* is necessary and success in it is needed. So for *bhakti yog*, pure conscience, pure *karma* and eradication of all impurities is required. We have seen that surrendering is needed for *prapatti* and it has six kinds.

We have seen it in the following shloka-

आनुकूलस्य संकल्प: प्रतिकूलस्य वर्जनम् ।
रक्षिष्यति इति विश्वासो गोमृत्वं वरणं तथा ॥
आत्मनिक्षेप: षड्विधा शरणागति:॥

So the features, strength and scope of *bhakti yog* and *prapatti* are different.

Another factor of difference is the difference of authority. The followers of *Ramanuja* saw the logical meaning of *bhakti yog* as *Brahmopasana* made with the *Upanishadic Brahmavidyas*. So, one should have the right for studies of the *Vedas* and the caste of *Brahmin* for *bhakti yog*. Interested students should remember 'Apashudradhikarana' in the *Brahmasutras*. But there are no such conditions for surrendering.

न जातिभेदं न कुलं न लिंगं न गुणक्रिया ।
न देशकालो न अवस्था योगो हि अयं अपेक्षते ।।

This *yog* does not require any particular caste, family background. It has no difference of gender, qualities, land or situation. In the *Mahabharata, Draupadi* was menstruating when she prayed to *Krishna*. Yet since she had surrendered, she could be *prapanna*. If you have *prapatti*, it does not matter whether you are *Brahmin*, low caste, clean or unclean. Devotion is what all matters. Even it does not matter whether you are human being or not. The story of protection of *Gajendra* is the evidence. Animals and birds can be *prapanna*. There are some requirements for *prapatti*. The *Svetashvataropanishad* says:

मुमुक्षुः वै शरणं अहं प्रपद्ये ।

The above quote makes it clear that the first primary condition is intense desire for emancipation. The *Bhagavata purana* state:

स्त्रियो वैश्याः तथा शूद्राः ये अपि पापयोनयः ।
सर्वे एव प्रपद्येरन् सर्वाधारं अच्युतम् ।।

The *Gita* (9 : 32) states

मां हि पार्थ व्यपाश्रित्य ये अपि स्युः पापयोनयः ।
स्त्रियो वैश्या स्तथा शूद्राः ते अपि यान्ति परां गतिम् ।।

Women, *vaishyas* and *shudras* and sinful people also can get the help of God. If they surrender to me they achieve great and high aim. So, this is the second point of difference. The third one is *sapekshatva-nirapekshatva* (attachment- detachment) *bhakti yog* is subject to *karma* and knowledge. It develops according as and how the inherent factors develop. *Bhakti yog* is subject to knowledge, *dhyana, karma* and *sadhana*. But in surrendering in *prapatti* the object of achievement and the one who achieves is God. Achievement of goal depends on the calibre of the person who is striving. What happens if we apply the same rule to *prapatti*? Achievement of God is as near as the way is efficacious. Therefore *bhakti yog* depends upon the ways and there is no such conditioning in surrendering. *Bhakti yog* has hierarchies, gradations and degrees; knowledge, *karma, dhyana* and *sadhana* have them but surrendering is absolute. It is either there or not there. It has sixteen '*kalas*' – full moon – orbs – all the while. There is no division or breaking point. It cannot be 10%, 20% or the like. Such surrendering is like castles in the air.A *Prapanna* is always, every moment full of God. He is wholly dependent on God's will. He does not entertain the idea of getting salvation with his own efforts. There is no pre-condition or qualification for a *prapanna* as is the case for *bhakti yog* according to *Ramanujacharya*. He is unable even to protect himself. Now this inability may be counted as debility and impotency from a rational point of view, because there are so many weak persons in the world who depend upon God for everything because they either want to avoid their duties or are lazy or insincere. We must use discretion to differentiate between these two kinds of depending upon God.

A *prapanna*, considers *Ishvara* or *Bhagavan* to be the means as well as the end i.e., *Upaya* (means), and *upeya* (end) are both *Ishvara*. In surrendering, there can be no gradation of God as far as means are concerned. However, *bhakti yog* is *upaya sapeksha*. Progress in *bhakti* depends on how intensely one applies the means, whereas surrendering is *nirapeksha* (motiveless). There can be no gradation of the means in surrendering, but in *bhakti yog sadhana*, there is gradation as low intensity, medium intensity, high intensity. Surrendering is *nirapeksha*, hence there can be no gradations, as it is not *sapeksha* as in *bhakti*. In *jnana, karma, dhyana* and *sadhana*, there are. Thus *sapekshatva* and *nirapekshatva* are two distinctly different characteristics. Surrendering is only once. Once you have offered yourself totally there is no way of revoking it or having to do it once again. Since a *prapanna* is *Bhagavata tantra* (dependent), *Bhagavata ayatta*, there is no question of evaluating himself, whether he is capable or incapable, whether he is qualified or unqualified, - as one is required to think in *sadhana*. There is even no desire for *moksha* in him. A *prapanna* relies wholly on God for his protection. His sense of surrender may appear as though he is incapable or unfit for *bhakti*. An incapable person lacks self-effort and is a fatalist. A fatalist says everything is in the hands of God, and a *prapanna* will also say the same thing. There is a difference between the two types, though it is difficult to distinguish between the two.

A mere devotee is a weak person who considers himself to be a defeated person , humiliated and destitute. Therefore he says to himself, "I am totally dependent on God." God is his sole refuge. He has no alternative but to seek His protection. The *prapanna* has God as Omnipotent, Refuge of all, Omniscient, Omnipresent. God is everything, He is Mother, Father, Support for all. He feels himself to be belonging to God. "I am His and He is mine. He resides in my heart and bestows on me knowledge, intelligence and memory. He is the inner Controller. He is full of compassion. He is my Nourisher, Controller and Sustainer." Thus a *prapanna* is in this state of gratitude.

257

Such a *prapanna* is in a supremely sublime state. The surrendering of a mere devotee, however, is negativistic. His surrender to God is not from the heart, while that of a *prapanna* is magnanimous and noble. The first type of surrender is fatalist in nature, while the second type is of absolute gratitude. The first is in a state of supplication of mercy, while the second is flooded with Divine Grace. A *prapanna* has a sense of fulfillment and gratitude. He also feels that the entire Universe is dependent on Him and nothing can be independent of Him. The fatalist feels he is helpless, and therefore dependent on Him. There is thus an ocean of difference between the two surrenders.

The fourth difference between *bhakti yog* and *prapatti* is that the first is gradual, whereas the second is instantaneous. In the *Chhandogya Upanishad* it is said:

'तस्य तावदेव चिरं यावन्न विमोक्षये अथ संपत्स्य इति ।'

God Himself says that He gives salvation immediately. Actually sadhana has to be constant and continuous. *Yog* and *samadhi* might be accomplished in one birth and salvation may come in another birth. The accumulated *karma* might be exhausted but *prarabdha*?? The chain has to be severed and the *sadhaka* has to wait for that. Interested students can consult the *Brahma Sutra* chapter 4.1.1. But in case of *prapanna*, God Himself presses the key for his eradicating his *karma*. In surrendering, the Lord Himself destroys the effects of *prarabdha karma*. How then can there be any delay for liberation when God Himself is instrumental in such a situation?

"अहं त्वा सर्व पापेभ्यो मोक्षयिष्यामि मा शुच:" (18 : 66)

When such an assurance comes from God Himself, how and why should anyone hesitate from becoming a *prapanna*? Thus *bhakti yog* and *prapatti* are different in respect of their operational time for wiping out the *prarabdha karma*.

The fifth difference between *prapatti* and *bhakti* is *sakrutakartavya* and *asakrutakartavya*. What does this mean? Surrendering has to be done once and for all. It can be practiced only once. There can be no repetition. There is no going back because the "I" in the *prapanna* has been completely obliterated. When the "I" does not exist at all there is no question of going back or destroying it. That is why surrendering becomes *sakrutakartavya*. In *bhakti yog*, however, since the meditative process has to be repeated, it becomes *asakrutakartavya*, since meditation is of the nature of continued and constant remembrance. This is the purport of scripture (*Brahmasutra* 4.1.1) ''आवृत्ति: असकृत् उपदेशात् ।'' Also *dhyana yog* gives a similar description of *asakrutatva* nature of the process of meditation. *Yogsutra* 1.14 says,

''स तु दीर्घकालनैरन्तर्यसत्कारासेवितः दृढभूमिः ।''

i.e. the nature of meditation has to be uninterrupted to result in one-pointed concentration.

The *Ramayana* states:

सकृदेव प्रपन्नाय तव अस्मि इति च याचते ।
अभयं सर्वभूतेभ्यो ददामि एतत् व्रतं मम ।।

This is what has been said by *Shri Rama* himself. *Bhakti yog* consists of *asakrutatva*, whereas *prapatti* consists of *sakrutatva*.

In the context of liberation the mental state during the last moments of a man's life are extremely important. This last moment memory is important in spiritualism. The *bhakti yogi* thinks of God at the point of his death. Imagine how difficult it could be to meditate on God at the point of death, when one is in agony of death. To think peacefully of God in the state of death requires assiduous performance of *Dharma* during many past lives. It would not be an exaggeration to say that the object of the *sadhana* of an entire lifetime is to acquire this peaceful condition in the last moment. The moment of death is the apex of turmoil, agony and pain. *Dhyana* is unimaginable at that time. How then can one concentrate on God? We can merely read what the *Gita* says in this context. The Lord says,

अन्तकाले च माम् एव स्मरन् त्यक्त्वा कलेवरम् ।

य: प्रयाति स मद् भावं याति नास्ति अत्र संशय: ।। (8 : 5)

यं यं वापि स्मरन्भावं त्यजति अन्ते कलेवरम् ।

तं तम् एव इति कौन्तेय सदा तद्भावभावित: ।। (8 : 6)

The devotee who leaves this body thinking of Me alone reaches the supreme state. This is certain. Rather a person reaches a state depending upon what he thinks about at the last moment. A *bhakti yogi* has to go through his last moments thinking of God. But God Himself takes this responsibility in case of the *prapanna*. In the *Varaha purana* it is said :

तत: तं क्रियमाणं तु काष्ठपाषाणसन्निभम् ।

अहं स्मरामि मद् भक्तं नयामि परमां गतिम् ।।

I think of this *prapanna bhakta.* And take him to the supreme state.

Prapatti is described in the above *shloka* along with the Lord's assurance of final beatitude to the *prapanna*. The difference between *bhakti* and *prapatti* in the last stage of a man's life is known as *antim smritivailakshanya.* A devotee has to get the ability to exercise his memory to think, whereas in the case of a *prapanna*, God Himself gives this remembrance.

The next characteristic difference between *bhakti* and *prapatti* is *Nishchita Anishchita phaladana*. *Brahma sadhana* has to be completed in *bhakti yog*. In *shloka* 3 of chapter 7, and *shloka* 25 of chapter 7, the Lord says :

मनुष्याणां सहस्रेषु कश्चित् यतति सिद्धये
यतताम् अपि सिद्धानां कश्चित् मां वेत्ति तत्त्वत: ।।
अनेकजन्मसंसिद्धौ ततो याति परां गतिम् ।।

Hardly one among thousands tries for *siddhi*. Out of these *siddhas* also a rare one knows me properly. The devotee can hope to get the supreme state not after one birth but he needs to watch and wait for many births.

So, the moment of fruition is most uncertain. A *bhakta* has to struggle for attaining success, while a *prapanna* easily attains salvation. In short, the differences between *bhakti* and *prapatti* are as follows:

(a) *angavailakshanya*   (b)   *adhikaravailakshanya*
(c) *sapekshatva-nirapekshatva* (d) *vilamba-avilamba vailakshanya*
(e) *sakrutakartavya-asakrutakartavya* (f) *antim-mati vailakshanya*
(g) *phalanishpatti vailakshanya*.

The *bhakta* struggles to meditate on God and tries to retain his concentration, but in case of a *prapanna*, God Himself thinks of him and one cannot imagine that God can forget the *prapanna*. The Lord in *Gita bhashya* of *Ramanujacharya* states this:

अत: तेन विना अपि आत्मधारणं न संभवति ।
ततो मम अपि आत्मा हि स: । (7 : 18)

261

I cannot exist without him. He is like my soul only. In the *prapatti* tradition there are two aspects of surrendering to be considered :

1) *Marjara kishora nyaya* and 2) *Kapi kishora nyaya*

One sect believes that the emotion of *prapanna* is analogous to the nature of the relationship between a cat and its offspring. The cat transports its offspring by holding it in its mouth. In the same way God holds the *prapanna* in His compassion. The second sect holds that this emotion is analogous to the relationship between a monkey and its young one. The baby monkey holds itself to the mother. In the same way the *prapanna* is tied to God. Such are the *prapanna* emotions.

The *yogi*, the devotee, the *prapanna*, the *sharanagata*, the *sthithaprajna*, the one who has reached beyond the *gunas* - all appear like stars in the firmament to the ordinary person. The distances between various stars and planets are not countable for us. Only an expert can say that a dim faraway star is self-luminous, and a seemingly bright star is nothing but a planet illuminated by another star. In the same manner, we are unable to distinguish between the authorities of the great spiritual masters. The difference between a *bhakta* and a *prapanna* is a recognized fact of the sciences of *bhakti*.

Patanjali has described three stages of *Ishvarapranidhana* in the *yogshastra* from the point of view of the *sadhaka*. The neophyte of *bhakti yog* like us is defined as an *adhamadhikari*. He has to follow a prescribed regimen of *niyama* for *Ishvarapranidhana*. Then comes the *madhyamadhikari*, whose bhakti is based on *kriya yog* or technicalities and rituals. Finally the *uttamadhikari* who practises *bhakti* at a higher level. *Patanjali* has thus specified these three stages of *bhakti sadhana* with well-defined procedures along with the *phala* or fruits or benefits of the performance of these procedures. The *sadhaka* should rigidly follow the first procedures of *niyama* to start his *yog sadhana*.

An important aspect regarding *bhakti*, is the difference in the modalities of the *sadhanas* such as *vyaktopasana, avyaktopasana, murtopasana, amurtopasana, sagunopasana, nirgunopasana,* etc. They are not taken to be undistinguishable. Further, on the more subtle plane, the differences between *avyaktopasana, amurtyopasana* and *nirgunopasana*, are not recognized by them. Similarly, the *saguna-vyakta-murta* category is supposed to be inferior to the *avyakta-amurta-nirguna* category. This is a mistaken idea. Let us consider these concepts.

मूर्तामूर्तउपासना

It is stated in the *Brihadaranyaka Upanishad* that there are two aspects of the *Brahmatattva* i.e. God without attributes and God with attributes. *Murta* means perceptible with the senses whereas *amurta* means imperceptible. This is the simple initial understanding of *murta* and *amurta*. *Murta* is suggestive of an embodiment which is finite, limited and perishable. *Amurta* indicates deathlessness, imperishability and infiniteness of *Brahman*. If we consult the *amara kosha*, we find that *murtarupa* is a form consisting of a hard substance, having embodiment, destructible, immobile and finite, and *amurta* is exactly the opposite. That is why *sadhanas* such as *vigrahopasana* , *murtopasana*, and meditation on these forms leads to *murtibhakti*. *Amurtabhakti* is based on the noumenal characteristic i.e., God having no form no shape, infinite and imperceptible to the senses. The fact is that neither one is inferior or superior to the other. The saints and seers described the *murta* and *amurta sadhanas* in different regions of consciousness. Both the regions are noble. Both the *sadhanas* have the same degree of sublimity. Also, *murtopasana* and *vyaktopasana* are not the same. That which is visible is *murtopasana* and that which is not visible but is grasped by the intellect is *vyaktopasana*.

व्यक्तोपासना अव्यक्तोपासना

Vyaktopasana is done when God is not perceptible by the senses but is accepted on the metaphysical plane. When the metaphysical form transcends the intellect, the *sadhana* becomes *avyaktopasana*. The metaphysical aspect is in no way connected with the gross intellect as such, but is attached to the inner consciousness in a very subtle ethereal manner. This path is very hard and arduous since the aspirant does not get the support and attachment to the physical body. The Lord says :

क्लेश: अधिकतर: तेषां अव्यक्तासक्तचेतसाम् । (5 : 12)

The imperishable Self is very hard to reach for those who are attached to their bodies. Further, it is extremely difficult for restless human mind to concentrate on the formless and attributeless Self. That is why the Lord Himself declares that *avyaktopasana* is hard and mind-boggling. We can see that it is not everyone's cup of tea. The Lord's infinite auspicious attributes are planted in the emotional consciousness in *vyaktopasana*. In this *sadhana* there is an abundance of *bhava*, and in *avyaktopasana* there is a diminution of *bhava*. It is difficult for the wretched human mind with the burden of mundane desires and aspirations unfulfilled to grope in the darkness of ignorance for the ethereal principle. It is like extending hands to stars from the ground. As the poet Shelley describes, "It is desire of the moth for the star." Devotion is an extremely important constituent of *bhakti*, and it requires an object which appeals to the mind and this appeal helps evolve the concept of *saguna Brahman*. We can imagine why *vyaktopasana* is prescribed more often and why it is justified.

सगुण निर्गुण उपासना

While considering this class of *sadhana* which is similar to the previous one, it would appear that *saguna* and *nirguna* are two opposing concepts. Though the two words appear to be opposite, it is not so in context of the concept of *Ishvara*. We have seen that the *murta* form of the Lord is not the *amurta* form. That which is *amurta* is also not *murta*. That which is *avyakta* is not *vyakta*. Also that which is *vyakta* is not *avyakta*. But the *saguna* and *nirguna rupas* of *Ishvara* are amazingly identical. God is both *saguna* and *nirguna*. *Saguna* and *nirguna* are both indistinguishable and extraordinary. In the words *Sa-guna* and *nih-guna*, there is a difference between the *guna* in *saguna* and the *guna* in *nirguna*. Mathematically viewed, *sa* is positive and *nih* is negative. The characteristic of the word *guna* is a separate entity in both the *saguna* and *nirguna* terminology, and so there is no room for any difference between the two. Keeping aside the arithmetic of the two types, of *saguna* and *nirguna*, we will first consider the nature of *guna* in the word *saguna*. Now God is full of infinite auspicious attributes. These *gunas* consist of the highest knowledge, glory, prowess, courage, strength, brightness, purity, affection, mercy, gentleness, love, impartiality, compassion, sweetness, serenity, etc. up to infinity. The nature of *guna* in *nirguna* is transcending the three *gunas*. Even a particle of anyone of the above auspicious attributes, manifests itself as pure *sattva* in the common man. But all the above attributes in God are self-created and transcendental. They are not produced on account of *sattva guna*.

In the neophyte stage the seed of *bhakti* is required to be sown in the *sadhaka*. This can be done only when the *sadhaka* is filled with *sattva*. One should therefore take up only that path which increases and enhances the content of *sattva* and reduces the proportions of *rajas* and *tamas gunas*. *Satsanga, sadhanasanga* and *shastrasanga* serve as the alchemy to culture the mind in the path of devotion. In the first stages of *yama* and *niyama, ashtanga yog sadhana* provides for *Ishvarapranidhana* a wonderful assemblage of qualities such as faith in God, *shraddha, shama, dama*. The practice of *yog* increases *sattvashuddhi*, and the seed of *bhakti* is sown in the purified consciousness. *Bhakti* is the natural outcome of the consciousness. The *rajas* and *tamas gunas* produce confusion, and predominance of the six subtle enemies (*shadripus*) in the consciousness or *chitta*. Increase in *sattva guna* diminishes the *rajas* and the *tamas gunas*. *Bhakti* can then be understood to be the true nature of the consciousness and as one gets this perception and one progresses in *bhakti Dharma*. *Bhakti sadhana* evolves with the aid of *ashtanga yog* and *Vedanta sadhana* which is concerned with *saguna* and *nirguna sadhana* which are the highest among the *sadhanas* described above. The starting point of *bhakti* is achieved from the integration of *Dharma*, culture, *sadhana* and the values of life.

Shri Krishnaarpanam astu

✠ ✠ ✠

Discourse - 22

Mantra Yog After Ashtanga Yog

हरि: ओम्, हरि: ओम्, हरि: ओम्

Mantra yog! When the *yogi* is accomplished in *ashtanga yog* and decides to follow the path of *hatha yog* or *kundalini yog*- or rather he is directed to do that-the first stage that he meets is *mantra yog*. The *yog* sciences clearly indicate that there is no *laya yog* without *mantra yog*, no *hatha yog* without *laya yog*, no *raja yog* without *hatha yog* and no *kundalini yog* without *raja yog*. Of course, when the *yogi* is accomplished in *ashtanga yog*, he is directed with his intuition whether he should turn to *jnana yog* or *karma yog* or *dhyana yog* or *bhakti yog*. If his destined path is *dhyana yog*, this accomplished *ashtanga yogi* proceeds on the path of *dhyana yog*. If this path of *dhyana yog* is to go through rising of *kundalini* and for rising of *kundalini shakti*, his way naturally is towards *mantra yog*. After doing penance for *mantra yog*, he is eligible for *laya yog*. So first, *ashtanga yog*, then *mantra yog* of sixteen limbs, then *laya yog* of nine limbs, further *hatha yog* of six limbs, progress of *hatha yog* in *raja yog* and ultimately the culmination of *raja yog* in *kundalini yog*- this is the journey of the *yogi*. Whatever *kundalini yog* is explained today, we should understand that *sadhana* of *raja yog* is already completed there. *Hatha yog sadhana* has been completed before *raja yog* and completion of *laya yog sadhana* has preceded it. *Laya yog sadhana* had started only after accomplishing *mantra yog sadhana*. So it is reasserted that *mantra yog* is the first step for the process of raising of *kundalini* in the path of *dhyana yog*. At the stage of *mantra yog* after *ashtanga yog*, the *yogi* does the journey in the order of *hatha yog, raja yog, rajadhiraja yog, kundalini yog*. A shloka in *Hatha Yog*

267

Pradipika says,

'हठं विना राजयोग:, राजयोगम् विना हठ:
न सिद्ध्यति ।'

Raja yog does not stand without *hatha yog* and *hath yog* has no success without *raja yog*. This is the relationship between *raja yog* and *hatha yog*. They do not oppose each other. They do not stand against each other like two wrestlers. Rather, wrestling has no space in any *yog sadhana*.

There is a wide spread misunderstanding in the spiritual field that *hatha yog* and *raja yog* are far away and different from each other. The *Hatha yogi* and *raja yogi* are taken to be of opposite natures. This is a myth. These are stages in the journey of *dhyana yog* towards raising of *kundalini*. When the *yogi* is accomplished in *ashtanga yog*, his intuition directs him to proceed towards *mantra yog* for *dhyana yog*. We have to understand the place of *mantra yog*. This place is pre-*hatha yog*, pre-*laya yog*, pre-*raja yog*, pre-*kundalini yog*. The process of raising of *kundalini* needs penance of *mantra* and there is no alternative for it. *Kundalini* cannot be raised without *mantra*. *Dhyana* with *mantra* is a must for it. Therefore *tantra* has *beeja mantra* for the six plexii and *upasana* goes on with *beeja mantra*. The process of *kundalini* raising stands on the *upasana* of *mantra yog* and *mantra shastra*.

This is the way how *mantra yog* of sixteen limbs is accomplished after *ashtanga yog*. Tradition does not allow *sadhana* of *mantra yog* without accomplishing *ashtanga yog*. Rather it is impossible to work that way. It will prove to be a false kind of *sadhana*. In a way *mantra yog sadhana* is a post-graduate course after *ashtanga yog*. The *sadhaka* should always remember this fact. We will consider *mantra yog* against the background of this conviction.

The word *mantra yog* reminds us of a *shloka* in a *Smriti*.

''नादरूपो स्मृतो ब्रह्मा, नादरूपो जनार्दनः।
नादरूपा पराशक्तिः, तस्मात् नादात्मकं जगत् ।। हरिः ॐ'

Nada is *Brahma* and *Nada* is *Janardan*. *Nada* is the greatest power in the world and the world is full of *Nada* only. The world is accompanied with *Nada* and it is created out of *Nada*. The creation, construction, maintenance and also destruction of this world is related with *Nada*. *Omkara* is the primordial or primeval *Nada* which is the beginning, middle and the end of this world according to the *Vedas*, according to spiritualism and also according to sciences of *mantra*. The world dissolves in *Omkara Nada*. Poets, sages and saints say this because they have experienced this. We ordinary people do not sense this which is our shortfall. Every situation, action, culmination and everything in this world is related to *Nada*. Every vibration is with *Nada* and this *Nada* is omnipresent. It exists even in silence and peace.

What is *mantra*? *Mantra* is the formula of anything or any happening in the world. It is presented in the shortest form possible but contains optimum meaning. It is pregnant with many possible shades of meaning. The primary, first and perfect *mantra* is *Omkara*. It is like a master key. It is called the King of *mantras*, the *Maha mantra*. The most ancient literature of the world is the *Vedas* and they are perfectly in the form of *mantra*. Rather they are a collection of *mantras*. We can see the greatness of *mantras* here.

We are thinking of *mantra* in the context of *yog shastra* and against the background of *mantra yog*. Sage *Patanjali* also has described the importance of *mantra* in very few words. He says in the beginning of the fourth *pada* that *mantra* can give the *sadhaka* all whatever *siddhis* and power *yog* can give him. Actually *yog* can give *siddhis* to the *sadhaka*. They are *siddhis* related to body, to the five elements, five *pranas* and five senses. *Yog sadhana* can give eight great *siddhis* to him. All these *siddhis* can be achieved with *mantra* as *Patanjali* admits in this first aphorism of the 4th *pada*

"जन्मौषधिमंत्रतप: समाधिजा: सिद्धय: ।"

Siddhis are achieved by birth, with herbs, *mantra*, penance and *samadhi*.

At the outset we have to think of the meaning of the term –*mantra*. We have thought about the meaning and definition of *yog*. So what is the meaning of *mantra* in *mantra yog*? It is created out of the infinitive-*man* (pronounced *mun*), which means to think, reflect plus *tra*. *Tra* means protection. The etymological definition of *mantra* is "मननात् त्रायते इति मंत्र: ।" *Mantra* is whatever protects with thinking, contemplating, meditating. All this delivers one from mundane bondage and sorrows. It is defined in *tantra* as "मननात् सर्वभावनात् त्राणात् संसारसागरात् मंत्ररुपा हि सा शक्ति: मननत्राणरूपिणी" *Mantra* is a power that protects with thinking from this ocean of the material life. *Mantra* itself is a great power. It has dual power of thinking and protecting. The science of *mantra* is a great gift of the tradition of lore, the *Vedas* and ancient mysticism.

We use *mantra* in practical life also in the form of short cut. *Mantra* or short cut makes the way simple, short and easy. *Mantra* never makes things difficult. *Mantra* is a simple way of removing difficulties and solving problems. Whatever is worth achieving is usually far away. *Mantra* can minimize the distance and also the long time required to get it. A definition of *mantra* in *Matsya Purana* tells interestingly :

"देवाधीनं जगत् सर्वम्, मंत्राधीनाश्च देवता:
ते मंत्रा: ब्राह्मणाधीना:, तस्मात् विप्रो हि देवता ।"

The world is under the control of gods. Gods are governed by *mantras* and those *mantras* are in the hands of *Brahmanas*. So *Brahmanas* are like gods. This may not be palatable to all but the fact cannot be denied that the world is governed by gods "देवाधीनं जगत् सर्वम्". The world is subject to gods. These gods are under control of the five elements of earth, fire, water, wind and ether. They have their own gods and these gods are under control of *mantras*. When we worship them with the *mantras*, they are pleased. They give us strength and powers. These *mantras* are possessed by *Brahmanas*. Now the word *Brahmana* does not denote caste but remember the meaning or definition of *Brahmanas* as sages or realized persons. One who knows *Brahman* is *Brahman*. One who knows *Brahman* naturally knows *mantras* and therefore he is taken to be superior. Many people take the meaning in a wrong way and hence the misunderstanding.

Mantra - formula

In this modern age of science, the scientists make use of formulae. Even old sciences like mathematics, algebra, geometry have them at the core. It is their code language to concentrate the matter and to get a short cut for convenience. Aren't they a kind of *mantras* only ? The progressive modern sciences also cannot do without them. Physics, chemistry and other sciences tell their laws with formulae that are like *mantras*. They are understood by the scientists and it is not the cup of ordinary people. The law of social equality and justice does not work in this field and common people have to take knowledge by the word of the scientist. They just have to learn it by heart and use them for solving examples in mathematics

271

and algebra, for presenting a theorem in geometry. *Mantras* are like these scientific formulae and have a similar rational basis. We may not hasten to suppose that they are something belonging to primitive men in caves. As Shakespeare said through Hamlet, there are so many things in reality that are beyond fiction.

As there are problems in mathematics and other sciences, so they are in human life. Perhaps their number is far larger and vaster than in sciences! Rather life is a big and intricate bundle of various problems. These complications of problems are astounding. They are physical, mental, psychological, emotional, intellectual, spiritual and what not. *Mantras* offer us solutions for these problems. They help, solve problems and protect us from difficulties and calamities. *Mantra shastra* asserts this confidently. As the formulae in rational sciences help us in theorems and theories, these *mantras* help us in life in achieving what we long for and in various problems including the material ones.

These *mantras* are in the form of words and sound. To say it properly in the language of modern sciences, they are infrasonic and infra atomic expressions of sound. *Mantras* may not be traditional. The names we have received from our parents are conventional. In the past generations, parents used to give names of gods to their children. But, sadly, how many of them have become gods, or remotely like gods? How many of them tried to behave like what their names suggested? Parents naively believed that their children would behave like Mary or Paul or *Gajanan* but the children did not bother about that. So our names are merely words but they are conventional. *Mantras* are words but they are not conventional.

Why the elements or substances in sciences are named with certain words? Why hydrogen is called hydrogen and oxygen is called oxygen? Why we call carbon as carbon? Why not some other name? These names have come down conventionally. But there are some symbols to denote these names. Oxygen is O and carbon is C. Such symbols are used in *mantras* but they are not just symbolic. They are infrasonic. When the science of chemistry decided the name or symbol C for carbon, there was no particular or logical thinking behind it. It must have been by default that this symbol was chosen. If it were chosen by *mantra shastra*, it would have seen the element or matter of carbon in that C. So whatever words are used in *mantras*, they should be and are related to the specific meaning of the words. They are not just conventional. Why certain meaning has certain word - is the consideration in *mantra*. It is decided because it has something infrasonic. This is followed like a rule.

We can explain *mantra* in one more way. A tree has many parts, such as branches, leaves, flowers, fruits and roots. Now, aren't all these parts inherent and in undifferentiated form in the seed? So the seed has branches, it has leaves and flowers and trunk; it has fruit and roots in it. All these are included in it. So *mantra* is like a seed which has all powers concentrated in it. As the tree contains all the parts in it, so alphabets of the mantra contain powers in it.

Once, a disciple saw a big mango tree. He was amazed to see its vast expansion and he wondered how the tree stood there. Who brought it here? Isn't it a miracle? The trunk is brown, leaves green and the fruit is golden. Now, taste the leaves and they are astringent. And lo, the sweetness of the fruit is just marvellous. It has no parallel. It is such a vast tree but is shapeless and not very beautiful. Yet the fruit is even beautiful to see. When it is raw, it is astringent and is so delicious when it is ripe. How wonderful the whole phenomenon is! He felt fascinated and wished that he should have that tree in his own courtyard. Then he could get those sweet fruits for himself. This was childlike thinking. But he had his Master with him. He understood what was going on in his mind. He said to the disciple, "My child, I know what you are thinking about. You want to take this tree to your courtyard, isn't it so? It is not difficult. Look! Taste and enjoy the gift of nature. Eat the fruit of the tree as much as you want. Then take home the seeds of mangoes. Plant them in your courtyard and then you can get such a tree for yourself." The youth ate mangoes, enjoyed their taste and took the seeds to his house. He planted the seed according to the advice of his Master and later got fruit for himself. So the seed is the *mantra* of the mango. A little seed creates and gives a vast tree. A short mantra can produce great effects with the powers concentrated in it.

Tantra - Mantra - Yantra

Now the next question presents itself. There always is certain way of using the formula in the sciences, whether it is mathematics or physics or algebra. There is some technique for it. The technique makes the formula effective and efficacious. The science that tells how to use this technique is *Tantra*. Our tradition has created science out of *Tantra, Mantra* and *Yantra*. These three are interrelated and interdependent, too. All of them need each other. *Tantra* needs *mantra, mantra* needs *yantra* and so on. All these three elements make this science. The *mantra* in it is the power of formula or we may call it energy formula. So *mantra* is a magic and mystic power. At the same time it is a *tantra* which offers holiness. *Mantra* gives strength, give power, gives holiness. *Mantra* gives life to material and inanimate things. *Mantra* purifies, *mantra* enlivens and *mantra* wakes up dormant powers !! That is why in our *Vedic* tradition everything and every chore is accompanied with *mantra*. It is our practice here to associate every *kriya* with *mantra*, whether it is practical, domestic, cultural or divine.

Every action in the *Vedic* tradition is accompanied with *mantra*. The *vaidic* arises at dawn with a *mantra* which is called '*pratahasmaranam*' or morning prayer. Then first he looks at his hands because he has to do everything with his hands through out the day. He says,

"कराग्रे वसते लक्ष्मी:, करमध्ये सरस्वती,
करमूले तु गोविन्द:, प्रभाते करदर्शनम्"

"You should look at the hand in the morning because *Lakshmi* stays at the tips, *Saraswati* in the middle and *Govinda* at the root of the hands." These are gods of health, wealth, intellect and knowledge. So, all these things are prayed for. The whole day we are working to achieve all these things. *Lakshmi* does not stand here for material wealth only, but also for the glory of all kinds. Physical, psychological, emotional, material glory also is implied here. *Vaidics* are worshippers of knowledge and *Saraswati* is the goddess of knowledge. *Govinda* is God. In this way, the beginning of the day tends to be divinely oriented. The prayers to gods help him work and walk on the right path through out the day.

The next part of the chore is *Shishtanjali*. It is greeting the '*shishta*' people i. e. remembering the great persons who had been like light houses in our tradition. He bows before them. He says,

पुण्यश्लोको नलो राजा, पुण्यश्लोको युधिष्ठिर: ।
पुण्यश्लोका च वैदेही, पुण्यश्लोको जनार्दन: ॥
अहिल्या, द्रौपदी, सीता, तारा, मंदोदरी तथा ।
पंचकन्याम् स्मरेत् नित्यम् महापातकनाशनम् ॥

275

"I think of King *Nala*, King *Yudhishthira*, *Vaidehi* and *Janardana* were great. Also I remember the five noble women of our tradition. They were *Ahilya*, *Draupadi*, *Sita*, *Tara* and *Mandodari*. To remember them in the morning is a way of eradicating sins, however big they are. The *vaidic* is a firm believer in God. So he remembers not only God but also those who believe in and love God. His bliss of thinking of these devotees is perhaps greater than the bliss of God when God is remembered by the devotees. The devotees are so much loved by God that his thinking of them even pleases God. He remembers the devotees as follows. ''प्रल्हाद नारद पराशर पुण्डरीक व्यास अंबरीष शुक शौनक भीष्म दाल्भ्य रुक्मांगद वसिष्ठ बिभीषणादीन् पुण्यान् इमान् परम भागवतान् स्मरामि'' I remember *Prahlada*, *Narada*, *Parashara*, *Pundarika*, *Vyasa*, *Ambarisha*, *Shuka*, *Shounaka*, *Bhishma*, *Dalbhya*, *Rukmangada*, *Vasishtha*, *Vibhishana* and other great devotees. Then he remembers the five *Pandavas*.

धर्मो विवर्धति युधिष्ठिरकीर्तनेन
पापं प्रणश्यति वृकोदरकीर्तनेन ।
शत्रु: विनश्यति वृकोदरकीर्तनेन
माद्रीसुतौ कथयतां न भवंति रोगा: ।।

The effect of remembering the *Pandavas* is described here. Remembering *Yudhishthira* inspires *Dharma*, memory of *Vrukodara* (*Bhima*) destroys sins and enemies. Diseases are removed by remembering the sons of *Madri* since they are the sons of *Ashwini*, the 'doctors' of gods.

Then he remembers the places of pilgrimage in our holy land. These places are capable of giving salvation.

"अयोध्या मथुरा माया काशी कांची अवंतिका
पुरी द्वारावती चैव सप्तैता: मोक्षदायका: ।।"

They are *Ayodhya, Mathura, Gaya, Kashi, Kanchi Avanti,*
Jagannath Puri and *Dwaraka* of Lord *Krushna.* Then before putting
his feet on the ground, he begs pardon of the Earth. She is a goddess
who supports life of human beings. She is the source of all the wealth
and food. She is the mother of all. He says,

समुद्रवसने देवि पर्वतस्तनमंडले ।

विष्णुपत्नि नमस्तुभ्यं पादस्पर्शं क्षमस्व मे ।।

"O goddess Earth, wife of Lord *Vishnu,* the oceans are your attire
and the mountains are your breasts. Forgive me for touching you
with my feet." Thus he creates holy feelings in the mind and life
before coming out of bed.

While taking his bath, he thinks of the sacred rivers.

गङ्गे च यमुने चैव गोदावरि सरस्वति ।

नर्मदे सिंधु कावेरि जले अस्मिन् संनिधिं कुरु ।।

He prays to the *Ganga, Yamuna, Godavari, Saraswati, Narmada,*
Sindhu and *Kaveri* to enter the water of his bath. So his daily bath
gets holiness because of the invocation of these seven rivers. Our
forefathers have taught us that eating is not a casual action of filling
the stomach with some stuff. It is like a *yajna* and accompanied with
mantra. The saints have said, "उदरभरण नोहे जाणिजे यज्ञकर्म."
Eating is not filling the stomach but it is a *yajna karma.*" He sprinkles
water around his plate with *mantra* 'सत्यंत्वर्तेन परिषिंचामि'. A morsel
is kept aside in the name of the ancestors. Ahutis are offered to the
five *pranas* of *Prana, Apana, Vyana, Samana, Udana. Mantra* is there
even while finishing the dinner. Before rising from the seat he says,

277

अमृतोपस्तरणमसि ।

अमृतोपिधानमसि ।

सत्यम् त्वर्तेन परिषिंचामि । ऋतं त्वा सत्येन परिषिंचामि ।

"I sprinkle water." He utters a *shloka* even for digesting the food.

अगस्त्यं कुंभकर्णम् च शनिं च वडवानलम्

आहारपरिपाकाय, संस्मरामि वृकोदरम् ।

आतापिभक्षणाय वातापिं च महाबलम्

समुद्र: शोषितो येन स मे अगस्त्य: प्रसीदतु ।।

"I remember *Agasti, Kumbhakarna, Shani, Bhima* and *Vadavaanala* for digesting the food. *Agasti* had digested the demons *Aataapi* and *Vaataapi*, and even the seas in his stomach. So he should help me."

After eating, the whole routine of the day also is accompanied with God's name. In the evening lamps are lit with *mantra* . He prays to lamps and the spirit of light.

दीपज्योति: परब्रह्म दीपज्योति: जनार्दन: ।

दीपो हरतु मे पापम् संध्यादीप नमोऽस्तुते ।।

or

शुभं करोति कल्याणम् आरोग्यं सुखसंपद:

मनोबुद्धिप्रकाशं च दीपज्योति: नम:अस्तु ते ।।

The flames of lamps are like *Brahma* and *Janardana*. I bow before the evening lamp and let it remove my sins. This lamp will bring in auspicious things, happiness, health and wealth. It will spread light in the mind and intellect."

अगस्ति: माधवश्चैव मुचकुन्दो महात्यल: ।
कपिलो मुनि: आस्तिक: पंच एते सुखशायिन: ।।

While going to sleep, he says,

शान्ताकारं भुजगशयनं पद्मनाभं सुरेशम्
विश्वाधारं गगनसदृशं मेघवर्णं शुभांगम् ।
लक्ष्मीकान्तं कमलनयनं योगिभि: ध्यानगम्यं
वन्दे विष्णुं भवभयहरं सर्वलोकैकनाथम् ।।

"I remember the sages and believers *Agasti*, *Madhava*, *Muchkunda*, *Mahatyala* and *Kapila* for helping me to get good sleep." Lying on the bed he thinks of Lord *Vishnu* who sleeps on the snake *Shesha*. This is a beautiful shloka about *Vishnu*.

"*Vishnu* has manifestation of bliss. He lies on a snake, there is a lotus in his navel. He is the Lord of gods and support of the Universe. His limbs are graceful, His complexion is bluish like the sky and clouds and His eyes are like lotus. He is Lord of Goddess *Lakshmi*. *Yogis* meditate upon Him. I bow before this God who removes fears in this world and who is the Lord of all the worlds in this Universe. He says the following *shloka* to be protected from bad dreams.

रामस्कंधं हनुमन्तं वैनतेयं वृकोदरम् ।
शयने य: स्मरेत् नित्यम् दु:स्वप्नं तस्य नश्यति ।।

I think of *Hanumant* who has Lord *Rama* on his shoulders. I remember *Vainateya*, the Eagle god, and *Bhima* while in bed, so that bad dreams are destroyed." Our tradition has given a hymn of *Gajendra* which helps to get good sleep. We have a *mantra* from *Dhanvantari yajna* for *Dhanvantari* who is a god of medicines and is regarded as incarnation of *Vishnu*.

नमो भगवते वासुदेवाय धन्वंतरये अमृतकलशहस्ताय ।
सर्वामयविनाशाय त्रैलोक्यनाथाय श्री महाविष्णवे नमः ॥

"I make obeisance to *Dhanvantari* who has a pitcher of nectar in his hands and can remove all ailments. He is the incarnation of *Vishnu* who is the Lord of the three worlds."

Thus, the *vaidic* always has some *mantra* on every occasion and in every ritual in life, whether it is regular or for some special purpose. Apparently it may seem confusing why even trivial matters of daily routine are accompanied and associated with *mantra*. But if we look deeply into this matter we will come to know that the small matters such as lack of good sleep or trouble of bad dreams or rising with bad mood from the bed can aggravate our health problems. A *vaidic* never forgets name and *mantra* of God. It is believed that *mantra* should be given by the *guru* to the disciple with proper ritual of initiation. But there are certain *mantras* that do not need initiation. They are sanctified by holy saints as stones become golden with the touch of philosopher's stone and so these protective mantras can be uttered without guru and the rituals. They are always powerful and efficacious. For example, ''हरे राम हरे राम राम राम हरे हरे, हरे कृष्ण हरे कृष्ण कृष्ण कृष्ण हरे हरे' is a favourite *mantra* of the Hindus and *vaidics* about *Rama* and *Krishna*. ''श्रीराम जय राम जय जय राम'' also is a *mantra* about Ram and ''अच्युतम् केशवम् रामनारायणम् कृष्ण–दामोदरम् वासुदेवम् हरिम्'' is a *mantra* with various names of Krushna. The hymn of *Ramaraksha* is a great *mantra* known to every Hindu. These *mantras* are part and parcel of Hindu life. The great *sadhanas* of *japa* or *naam* have developed from these *mantras*. The ways of worship of the deities have *mantra* at the core of them. *Bhavana* or devotion is the most important part of them. Yet it is also true that there are two kinds of *mantra* according to the science of *mantra*. One has prominence of *bhavana* and the other has prominence of sound. *Mantra* and *tantra* are used to make *mantra* successful. The *mantra* which has prominence of sound need proper oration with proper rituals and also proper application of them. These *mantras* succeed with the use of *tantra* and *yantra*.

According to Hindu and *Vedic* system of *upasana,* and in the context of *Vaishnavas,* the *Vishnu Sahasranama* is well known. It is in the *anushasana parva* of the *Mahabharata* and is popular among the *Shaivas,* too. This is recited with great devotion. But when it is used in the worship of *Vishnu,* it is used with *mantra, yantra* and *tantra.* Its ritual becomes important there. Same is the case with *Ramaraksha.* It is recited with devotion but when it is used as a ritual of worship or *sadhana,* the *tantra* becomes important.

When these hymns are used as a part of *upasana,* there is a ritual of it to be followed. The ritual of *upasana* starts with the *sankalpa* or objective. There is a ritual to sit for the *sankalpa;* how to sit? Where to sit and what to face? The *sadhaka* has to complete his regular worship, rituals of purification and *Sandhya* worship. The proper place and *asana* has to be chosen. Then *achamana* is done followed by *pranayama* to proceed further to *sankalpa.* While doing the *sankalpa,* the thought of the place, region and time also is important.

It is significant to note that *sankalpa* is done with *pranayama* and the *sadhaka* considers the questions-Where am I sitting? Why am I doing *sankalpa* and *upasana*? At what time and in which region am I doing this *sankalpa*? Of course, the answers of these questions are not related to political geography but to mystic or esoteric geography. It is not important in which district of which state of the country the *sadhaka* is sitting. This point is peculiar and interesting.

The purpose of reciting *Vishnu Sahasranama* may be to remove some ailment, to get rid of some evil or to achieve some goal. After doing *sankalpa* Lord *Ganesha* is worshipped.

Lord *Ganesha* is worshipped in the beginning of all functions and activities. Then there is a ritual of getting rid of curses. This kind of ritual is more important when it is the *upasana* of reciting *Vishnu Sahasranama* because it has the curse of *Rudra* and it has to be removed before *upasana*. Then there are hand gestures which are called *Kara Nyasa*. The five fingers are brought under spell and they are given a power. It is followed by *Anga Nyasa*.

The next step is ritual of *dhyana* with *dhyana shloka.* This *shloka* in the *Vishnu Sahasranama* is recited. Then the following *taantrika japa* is recited 108 times. It is

ॐ क्लीं ह्रां-ह्रीं भूम्-स्वाहा ।

Then water is sprinkled on the earth and a prayer is sung. It is

ॐ श्रीविष्णुसहस्रनामस्तवे रुद्रशापविमुक्ति: भवतु''

"In the *Vishnu Sahasranama* recitation I should be free from the curse of *Rudra.*" *Samputa* is performed after that. *Samputa* is performed before and after every *shloka* in the *Vishnu Sahasranama*. If *Vishnu Sahasranama* is recited along with this *Samputa,* 21 times every day, desires are fulfilled and success is achieved. What is the *Samputa*? There are six *Samputa* in *Vishnu Sahasranama*. The *sadhaka* should utter *Achyutanantagovinda* (*Samputa*) before every *shloka* and *Achyutanantagovinda* after every s*hloka*. Another *Samputa* is

ॐ कृष्णाय वासुदेवाय हरये परमात्मन ।

प्रणतक्लेशनाशाय गोविन्दाय नमो नम: ।।

"I bow before *Krishna Vasudeva* who is the great power and who removes afflictions of all who approach him." The third *Samputa* is

ॐ आपदामपहर्तारम् दातारम् सर्वसम्पदाम् ।
लोकाभिरामं श्रीरामं भूयो भूयो नमाम्यहम् ॥

"I again and again pay obeisance to *Rama* who is the most graceful in the world, removes calamities and gives glory and wealth. The fourth *Samputa* is

ॐ नम:शंभवे च मयोभवे च ।
नम: शंकराय च मयस्कराय च
नम: शिवाय च शिवतराय च

"I bow before *Shiva* and *Shivatara* who gives freedom from fear and does good things." The fifth *Samputa* is -

रामो विरामो विरजो मार्गो नेयो नय: ।
रक्षां कुरु श्रियं देहि त्राहि मा शरणागतम् ॥

"O *Rama*, you are the right path which should be followed. Please protect me and give me glory. I surrender to you." The sixth *Samputa* is the famous shloka with eight letters.

''ॐ नमो नारायणाय''

It is to pay obeisance to God *Narayana*.

So it is told in the rituals of *upasana* that this kind of *Samputa* is to be performed before and after every *shloka*. This gives fulfillment of wishes and success. *Sahasranama* is recited in this way. There are hymns like *Gajendrastotra* or *Adityarhridaya* used in *upasana* that helps to come out of difficulties. *Durgastotra* also is used in *upasana* and it gives freedom from penury and addiction of any kind. One can save himself from atrocities and injustice with this *stotra*.

The *Shantisukta* in the *Vedas* is well known. Recitation of this *sukta* removes evil thoughts and fear and sorrows. Regular recitation of this *sukta* is a remedy for worries, anger and lust. *Mitrasukta* is another *stotra* that is considered in the science of *mantras*.

Mantra enhances the power and influence of one's personality. Personality development is a key word in the modern world. Our ancient ancestors were very keenly aware of it and have suggested means for it. *Mantra upasana* in *mantra shastra* has this thought in detail. *Mitrasukta* is especially useful in this respect. Our tradition has also given some other *suktas* like *Ashma sukta*, *Ganapati sukta*, *Vijay* [victory] *sukta*, *Arishtanivarana* [removal of calamities] *sukta*, *Shatruvijaya* [conquering the enemy] *sukta*, *Agnidahashamana* [pacifying burning of fire] *sukta*. These *suktas* are useful in various incidents. *Mantra shastra* is not only for spiritual pursuits but it provides help in mundane and material matters of life. We need not only wealth but also health. Again, we need freedom from so many problems like fear, lust, enemies, and worries. There are measures for these problems in *mantra shastra*. *Nama* is the most important means in *mantra shastra*. *Nama sadhana* is advocated for *vaidics* and Hindus for both spiritual and material pursuits of life. We find a *Smarta shloka* in Shrimat Bhagavat, ''नामसंकीर्तनम् कलौ परमोपाय: ।'' In the modern age of *Kali, Nama* recitation is the greatest saviour of life. The 52nd shloka in the 3rd chapter of 12th Skandha of the same says,

कृते यत् ध्यायतो विष्णुम् त्रेतायाम् यजतो मखै: ।
द्वापरे परिचर्यायाम् कलौ तत् हरिकीर्तनात् ॥

"Whatever is achieved in the *Krita* age with *dhyana* of *Vishnu*, in the *Treta* age with *yajnas* and in *Dwapara* age with worship, all that can be achieved in the *Kali* age with the mere recitation of Hari or

284

God." Even Shri *Ramadasa* said that "मुखी राम विश्राम तेथेचि आहे, सदानंद आनंद सेवोनि राहे, तयावीण तो शीण संदेहकारी, निजधाम हे नाम शोक हारी," we get rest by reciting the name of *Rama*. It is not necessary to lie on the bed for that. God's name is the bliss in the heart. Weariness, doubts, grief can be removed by this recitation of God's name. Lord *Krishna* says in the 10th chapter of the *Gita* that "यज्ञानाम् जपयज्ञ: अस्मि" He is the *Japa yajna* among all kinds of *yajna*. So *japa sadhana*, *Nama sadhana* are significant in *mantra*, *mantra sadhana*, *mantra yog*. They are of the utmost importance particularly for the *yog sadhaka*. A spiritual *sadhaka* cannot do without *Nama sadhana*. It is like a wish fulfilling tree for him.

Nama Sadhana

Nama sadhana is important for any kind of *sadhana* in spirituality to make it effective, efficacious and successful. One important part of this *sadhana* is that it is convenient for all. There are no strict discipline, rules and regulations for doing this. You can do it at any time, at any place and in any way possible. There is no particular ritual for it. You can do it in any condition of body. The restrictions about holiness and purifications also are not there. *Nama sadhana* never denies help to the *sadhaka*. He sometimes feels that he is sick or troubled or entangled in some work, and then he wonders what he can do for *sadhana*. He can do *Nama sadhana* at any such moment. He can do it even when he is extremely busy in his work and affairs. It can be with him continuously and regularly with him. If you want to do *dhyana sadhana*, there is much thought of conditioning. You need proper atmosphere, appropriate surroundings, favourable internal and external factors. You need to have proper mindset for concentration and absorption in the object of *dhyana*. But *Nama sadhanaa* can be with you while eating, walking, talking

285

and so on. *Nama sadhana* is a great gift of *mantra shastra*. *Sadhakas* should be grateful to this science for it. Again, this *sadhana* makes no discrimination of the grade of the *sadhaka*. It is for a raw beginner as well as for an accomplished *sadhaka*. In no condition of life could you think of giving up *Nama sadhana*. You wouldn't. It can be done without a *guru,* too. If, unfortunately and unfairly, your *guru* abandons you, you can go on with your meek *Nama sadhana*. It is as desirable and useful in the beginning as in the next stages of *sadhana*. Its influence is always with the *sadhaka*, whether he is a simple *sadhaka* or a divine *sadhaka* like *Shuka Muni* or *Vyasa*.

The next part of *mantra shastra* deals with the question - which name of God is effective in which conditions and times? Let us turn our attention to that part.

Shri Krishnaarpanam astu

✛ ✛ ✛

Discourse - 23

Yogvidya – Mantra Yog-2

We have considered that recitation of God's name in any condition is *sadhana*. *Mantra shastra* is a science of vibrations. Different names of *Vishnu* are applied in different situations according to the theories of the science of vibrations. It is useful and effective. If you are suffering from illness, recite the name '*Vishnu*'. Remember '*Padmanabha*' while going to bed. The *Brahma* is created out of the lotus from the navel of *Vishnu* who is lying on the bed of the snake *Ananta* in the ocean, *Kshirsagara*. The name '*Prajapati*' is useful in the ceremony of marriage. The names *Chakradhara, Trivikrama, Narayana, Shridhara, Govinda, Madhusudana, Narasimha, Jalashayin, Varaaha, Raghunandana, Vamana, Madhava* are to be recited in the event of battle, journey, death, intercourse with one's own wife, evil dream, calamity, stay in a forest, contact with fire, that with water, climbing a mountain, travelling and for any work respectively. In this world of telecommunication today, we use codified and symbolic language. We have to use a particular code number to contact a particular place. Similarly, there are code words in the *mantra shastra* for contacting gods residing in other worlds. Our astrology makes use of *mantras* in *mantra shastra*. The *mantras* are freely used to remove troubles from some stars being at an unfavourable place or to avoid evil effects of an ominous constellation. The hymn of the nine planets (*Navagraha*) is well known. There are some *shlokas* for some planets that are in an unfavourable position. Recitation of these *shlokas* proves to be effective. There are symbols of the nine planets. Mercury is recognized by an arrow, a star represents Venus and the moon is shown with a square. A horizontal rectangle is the sign of Jupiter and the face of the sun is the sun.

Mars is shown by a triangle, a flag stands for *Ketu*, a bow for Saturn and a '*chatushfala*' for *Rahu*. These signs are used for *mantras*. *Mantras* are of many kinds.

There is a classification in the *shloka* 34 of chapter 53 of *Brahmanda Purana*. It tells us about nine kinds of *mantras* as *Murti*, *Ninda*, *Prashansa*, *Akrosha*, *Tosha*, *Prashna*, *Anujna*, *Akhyana* and *Asha*. Another classification is of 24 kinds. They are *Prashansa*, *Stuti*, *Akrosh*, *Ninda*, *Parivedana*, *Abhishapa*, *Vishapa*, *Prashna*, *Prativachana*, *Ashi*, *Yajna*, *Akshepa*, *Arthakhyana*, *Sankata*, *Viyog*, *Abhiyog*, *Katha*, *Sankhya*, *Varapradana*, *Pratibandha*, *Upadesh*, *Namaskar*, *Spruha* and *Vilap*. The Vedik mantras also are classified. It includes *Vidhatri Rucha*, *Yajna Vidhan mantra*, *Abhidhatri Rucha* and *Yajna kriya mantra*. There are some *mantras* that are called '*Pratyuhakarika*'. They can be used to overcome enemies and obstacles in the performance of the *yajna*. One more classification describes four *mantras* as *Siddha*, *Sadhya*, *susiddha* and *Ariari*. *Mantras* are also classified as having prominence of sound and that of meaning. The first kind is effective just by its pronunciation and the other works only if emotions are there. Some *vaidic mantras* as well as *shabar mantra* are useful for spirituality. One kind of *shabar* is *Daivi* and *Paishachi* and the other is *Preyas* for spirituality. *Mantra* is utterance. The classification in that respect is *vachic*, *manasic* and *dhyanaja*. The *vachic* also has three kinds. The first is *vaikhari* which is clear and audible utterance, the second *bhramara nada* is humming or whispering and the third has only movement of lips. *Manasic* and *dhyanaja mantras* are recited on mental and *dhyana* level respectively.

Another classification is *Bija mantra*, *Mula mantra* or *Pinda mantra* and *Mala mantra* or *Kartari mantra*. Generally *Bija mantra* has one letter but it never exceeds ten letters. *Mula* or *Pinda mantra* contains ten to twenty letters and *Mala* or *Kartari mantra* can have any number of letters more than twenty. *Datta mala mantra* must be the longest because it has as many as one hundred and eight letters. If it is recited for twelve hours every day for penance, it will take forty years to complete the *anushthana* or penance. श्रीं ह्रीं is for *Brahmins*, श्रीं for *Kshatriyas*, क्लीं for *Vaishyas* and ऐं for *Shudras*. When we recite *mantra* we use the organ of speech i. e. mouth. The mouth is a place of five elements. The element of earth is in the lips, water in the tongue, fire in the teeth, wind in the palate and ether in the throat. These five elements are considered in the pronunciation in the science of *mantra*. The science of mantra has thought of *mantra*, *tantra* and *yantra* comprehensively. This penance and *mantra*, *tantra* and *yantra* contains *hasta mudra*. *Hasta mudras* are used in the penance of *Gayatri mantra* and in *tantrik Sandhya* worship. There are *mudras* like *Sumukha, Samputa, Vitata, Vistruta, Dwimukha, Trimukha, Chaturmukha, Panchamukha, Shanmukha, Adhomukha, Vyapakanjali, Shakta, Yama, Pasha, Unmonmukha, Pralamba, Mushtika, Matsya, Kurma, Varaha, Simhankranta, Mahakranta, Mudgara, Pallava*. As a dancer uses his hands for *mudra*, so also the *saadhaka* uses the *mudraa* and movements of eyes in his penance. The science of *tantra* and of icons describe some more *mudras* like *Abhaya, Chit, Varada, Sakshatkara, Vidravani, Kaala, Siddhi, Yog, Rasa, Vaidhayasi, Samshobhana, Shatrukshayakari, Patala, Anjali, Parama, Aavahana, Jnana, Surabhi, Vairagya, Yoni, Shankha, Pankaja, Linga* and *Nirvana*. They also are used in *mantra* worship. *Purashcharana* of *Gayatri* is done. Twenty-four cycles of twenty-four lakh *Gayatri japa* is *purashcharana* involving five crore and seventy-six lakh cycles of mantra. The *mantra* is ॐ भूर्भुव: स्व: तत्सवितुर्वरेण्यं भर्गो देवस्य धीमहि धियो यो न: प्रचोदयात्. The penance is so great. The science of *mantra* tells us that if as many crore mantras as letters in the *mantra* are recited, it is a *japa* for salvation.

Swami Ramdasa did thirteen crore *japa* of the *mantra* श्री राम जय राम जय जय राम. He did thirty thousand *japa* every day for thirteen years. So he must not have taken any holiday of Sunday or festivals like *Dasara* or *Diwali*. If it is to be done with a proper speed one has to do *japa* for twenty hours a day.

We are dealing with *mantra yog*. It is obvious from the name that it is a kind of *yog* like *Jnana, Karma, Bhakti, Kundalini, Taraka* and so on. Apparently it is like other kinds of *yog* but it has unique significance. Because no kind of *yog*, even not excepting *karma yog*, can exist without *mantra*. No *yog* can be accomplished without *mantra*. No *yog sadhaka* can claim that he can be 'not concerned' with *mantra yog*. Naturally we have to think about it. *Yog* is *samaadhi*, *samadhi* is *dhyana* which cannot be without *japa*. *Japa* is not without *mantra*. *Japa sadhana* is the core of *yog sadhana*. This mutual relationship of *japa* and mantra must not be forgotten by the *sadhaka*. Our *dhyana* is not very much powerful but still *yog* has *dhyana*. It is told in the *Bhagavatam*, जपो ध्यानम्. *Japa* is *dhyana*. The concentration, absorption and enchantment in *yog* is *dhyana*. Our *yog* in the stage of beginning does not have *dhyana*. Our absorption is our *dhyana*.

Who can get initiation of *mantra yog*? What is the criterion of eligibility of the disciple? Any Tom, Dick or Harry cannot be worthy of this initiation because *mantra yog* cannot be accomplished before the *sadhaka* has become well versed in *ashtanga yog*. In a sense it is like a post-graduate course. A student is not eligible for admission to it unless he has completed the studies for graduation. A *sadhaka* going straight way to *mantra yog* without *ashtanga yog* has illusions

290

about himself. Only after achieving purification of emotions and strength of body and mind can the *sadhaka* get ability for *mantra yog*. There are two kinds of *mantra yog*—*Shakti upaya* and *Shamabhava upaya*.

Shakti upaya is a symbolic way in the context of *yantra*. While worshipping the personal deity, the *yantra* of the deities like *Laxmi*, *Ganesha, Dattatreya* is used. The particular *yantra* may not always be there but the devotion for the *yantra* or symbol should be there. The power of the deity is abstract and not expressed. *Yantra* is concrete. In *Shamabhava upaya* the object is abstract. The *sadhaka* does *anusandhana* or absorption in the power of the deity for worship. This is just primary information about the the two kinds. There are sixteen parts of these two kinds of *mantra yog*. They are *Bhakti, Shuddhi, Asana, Panchanga Sevana, Achara, dharana, Divya Desha Sevana, Prana kriya, mudra, Prana, Tarpana, Yajna, Bali, Yag, Japa, Dhyana, Samadhi* and so on. They should be borne in mind and then understood by the *sadhaka*. Now let us be acquainted well with each of these parts.

Bhakti – the first limb

Bhakti is the first part. Every deity has a *mantra* and *mantra yog* is accomplished with the support of *mantra*. If we want support of *mantra*, we must have *bhakti* for the *mantra* and for the deity. Even *bhakti* is needed because without it there cannot be absorption.

Bhakti cannot exist without accomplishing *ashtanga yog* and consequent increase of *sattva*. We cannot do *japa* without it. Our mind is worse than a monkey. This is a fact. We do not have vibration of *bhakti* as purity of mind is not there. *Mantra yog* is like a post-graduate course because it comes after *bhakti*. *Ashtanga yog* gives proper *dhyana* because it gives accomplishment of *bhakti* of many kinds like *vaidhi bhakti, ragatmika bhakti, para bhakti. Ashtanga yog sadhana* teaches the basics or alphabets of *bhakti*. It also makes the *sadhaka* learn *saguna* and *nirguna* worship. The concrete kind of *bhakti* is accomplished in *Ishvarapranidhana*. Let us avoid repetition and turn to the next part.

Purity in Mantra Yog

Purity is the second part of *Mantra yog*. Cleanliness and purity are not far away from holiness. So they are important in the worship in *mantra yog*. Even ordinary people are aware of these things while they worship idols and they are careful about it while performing daily worship and especially on *Rama Navami* or *Ganesha Chaturthi*. So the *sadhaka* has already developed this discretion. No *yog* can exist without holiness. Sometimes the *sadhaka* is so meticulous and scrupulous about purity that people take it to be mania or hypocrisy. His prudishness is considered as morbidity. But after all it is *mantra* worship which is a kind of penance. The wearer best knows how the shoe has to be used so as not to create pain. Impurity of any kind cannot have space in spirituality. It is rightly said in *Padma Purana*

मुखशुद्धिविहीनस्य न मंत्रा: फलदा: स्मृता: ।
दंतजिव्हाविशुद्धि: च तत: कुर्यात् प्रयत्नत: ।।

The *mantras* uttered with a dirty mouth are not fruitful. So teeth and tongue should be cleaned carefully. *Mantra* is to be uttered with mouth, so it is natural that it should be clean. After doing this physical cleanliness can the *sadhaka* proceed to reach purity of mind.

This purity is of many kinds. Three of them are the main ,and they are physical, mental and of speech. These are in order of their importance. If we talk about purity of food, we should not forget that food is not only for the body and stomach but for intellect, mind and

292

emotions. Two meals a day is not the idea here. This is a wide concept. Control and regulation are significant in this context. Just using clean material will not suffice and water, soap and powder are not the only means. *Japa* and *tapa* are the means for entire purity. Special attention has to be given to worshipping for purity. Of course, no cleansing agent is better or greater than knowledge, so the *yog sadhaka* should remember the importance of knowledge. We should think of what the *Gita* says about purity. The 38th *shloka* of the 4th chapter of the *Gita* says

न हि ज्ञानेन सदृशं पवित्रं इह विद्यते ।

There is nothing more sacred than knowledge.

We have to think of the relevance of knowledge in the context of purity. The thought of purity is comprehensive and profound. It comprises of knowledge, too. A *vaidic* knows that *yajna*, charity, penance, continence, purity of food and mind have to be observed. He will not forget that water, soap, cloth and powder are not enough for purity. Mind cannot be pure when the six enemies (*shadripus*) are playing pranks there. These are some facts about purity in general. But this thought of purity is still vaster in the context of *mantra yog*.

The thought of purity has four kinds in the context of *mantra yog*. They are purity of the surroundings, of the place, of body and, inward purity. These are technical points of information. The *vaidics* are acquainted with this in their rituals. The surroundings are purified by smearing with cow dung and sprinkling water. Purity of place gives nobility to the *sadhaka's* mind. Purity of place and body creates content and serenity. Purity of surroundings enhances strength of the *sadhaka* and his merit. The mind becomes cheerful as body gets cleanliness. Internal purity helps *dhyana* and all this pleases the deities. They give their blessings. These are the effects of the four kinds of purity.

Asana is the third limb

The importance of place is that a clean place creates cheer and merit. A temple is a holy place to give meritorious vibrations. Purity of surroundings gives physical and mental energy required for *dharana, dhyana* and concentration. Outward cleanliness removes inertia of body and mind. The electricity in water gives energy. Internal purity is a means of nobility and seriousness. This is the contribution of overall purity.

Asanas have particular and different meaning in *mantra yog* than in *ashtanga yog*. The place of *asana* is important in *siddhi* and use of *mantra. Japa* is at the core of *mantra yog* as *mantra* does not exist without *japa. Asana* has two meanings. One is the posture and the other is the seat to sit on. The *sadhaka* has to sit on a particular *asana* for *japa. Asanas* are of different kinds such as *Kushasana, Simhacharma, Mrugacharma, Vyaghracharma* i.e. the *asana* or seat made of *kusha* grass, lion skin, deer skin, tiger skin respectively. There is discipline for choosing *asana* for particular *sadhana*. It may be clean cloth, made of cotton or a wooden plank. A place smeared with cow dung is a kind of good *asana*.

There are restrictions also about particular postures for particular penance. Sitting in *virasana, vajrasana, padmasana, swastikasana* is necessary for *mantra upasana*. The *sadhana* requires strict observance of these rules. Wishful *mantra upasana* works if it is done sitting on a wooden plank, especially a red plank. It is a practice to use *Mrugacharma* for *japa*. It helps to achieve knowledge. *Vyaghracharma* is useful for *upasana* for salvation. Use *Kushasana* for longevity. Do *mantra upasana* sitting on cotton cloth and it expedites recovery from diseases. Sometimes many asanas together helps the *sadhana*. The tradition of *yog* tells that using cotton cloth on *Vyaghracharma* on *Kushasana* helps to get *yog siddhi*. The last instruction should be considered carefully in the context of *mantra yog*.

There are negative instructions about *asanas*, too. Sitting on plain floor is not good for *upasana*, as it brings sorrow and suffering. An *asana* of wood or reed is prohibited for *sadhana* because it gives poverty and penury. Stone *asana* for *upasana* is an invitation for ailments. Straw wood *asana* damages one's image instead of helping *sadhana*. The *asana* of tree leaves affects intelligence. Sitting only on cotton cloth for *japa* will ruin *japa* and penance, too. Skin of a lion should not be used unless the *sadhaka* has received initiation from his *guru*. Householders should not use tiger skin as *asana*. Only a confirmed and faithful celibate should use skin of black deer. He may or may not have received initiation. The only condition is that he should use *Pruthvi mantra*, purify the *asana* and also utter the '*sankalpa*', as it is said here. 'आसने विनियोग:'.

The other thought with respect to *asanas* is about sitting posture. *Padmasana* and *swastikasana* are the only two *asanas* useful for this *upasana*. Even those *asanas* cannot be used before purifying the place. *Hatha yog* and *mantra yog samhita* both mention how *asanas* should be taken and this is very important.

परमात्मदर्शिभि: पूर्वै: हठयोगविशारदै: ।
योगिनां श्रेयसे सिद्धि: आसनस्य प्रकीर्तिता ।।

It is said that the previous experts on *hatha yog* were able to see the great God. They have described the *siddhi* of *asanas* for the accomplishment of the *yogis*. This primary information must be obtained by the *sadhaka*. *Siddhi* of *asanas*, *ashtanga yog asanas* is a must for *mantra yog* He has to master the technique of *prana kriya, pancha prana kriya* and esoteric physiology in the context of spinal cord and other organs. He must be acquainted with the techniques of *hatha yog* that exist in *ashtanga yog*. He has to progress further from this primary information and should achieve the skill of esoterics of *asana* such as *bandha, mudraa, kriya.* The body has to be resonant for vibrations of *mantra.* It has to be made like that with proper *asanas.* The part of the technique of *prana, nada* and breathing are significant for this. It is necessary to apply *prithvi mantra* while using *asanas.*

Whatever *asana* the *sadhaka* is using for sitting on, he uses at least some *darbha* grass because it is important for *sadhana.* We can see the importance of *darbha* in the following *mantra.* This *mantra* is at 19.33.3 in *Atharva Veda* and is addressed to *Darbha* grass.

अत्येषि ओजसा
त्वं भूमिम् अत्येषि ओजसा त्वं वेद्यां
सीदसि चारुरध्वरे ।
त्वां पवित्रं ऋषय: अभरन्त त्वं पुनीहि
दुरितानि अस्मत् ॥

It says, O *Darbha*, you excel the knowable earth with your glory while dancing beautifully. You are so holy that rushis or sages set you on the altar of the *yajna.* Kindly remove our sins, too. Make us sinless.

The *mantra* has such powers as the *Darbha* possesses.

Shri Krishnaarpanam astu

✣ ✣ ✣

Discourse - 24

Yogvidya – Mantra Yog-3

In *mantra yog*, *Prithvi mantra* has to be recited with a ritual for taking an *asana*. This *mantra* is mentioned in 19:33:3 in the *Atharva Veda*. *Padmasana* and *Swastikasana* are recommended for *mantra yog*. *Siddhasana* and *Sukhasana* also are accepted. The thought of direction is important while thinking of *asanas*. Which direction out of east, west, north and south the *sadhaka* should face while doing an *aasana* is an important question. The *shruti* 1.7.1.12 in *Shatapatha Brahmana* says, 'प्राची हि देवानां दिक् ।' The east is the direction of gods. *Ishanya* or north-east also belongs to God and is sacred. The *vaidics* perform all their holy rituals like *yajna* and *yag* facing the east. *Mantra yog* also recommends *sadhana* facing the east. The morning rituals of *Sandhya* worshipping among the daily rituals are to be performed facing the east. Evening rituals are to be done facing the west. *Sandhya* worshipping is *sadhana* of the sun with the purpose of getting wealth, food, intelligence and knowledge. Naturally it is done facing the direction of the sun, the east. The south belongs to *Yama* and the dead forefathers. The forefathers are offered *arghya* in this direction. The north is for holy rituals, so spiritual *sadhana*, *svadhyaya* and studies of the *Vedas* are performed facing this direction. Training and studies of *yog, dharana, dhyana* and *japa* are more fruitful if the *sadhaka* faces the north. *Kandikas* 18.19 in '*Trishikhi Brahmana Upanishad*' say

तत: कालवशादेव हि आत्मज्ञानविवेकत: उत्तराभिमुखो भूत्वा स्थात्वा अनन्तरं क्रमात् मूर्ध्नी आधाय आत्मन: प्राणान् योगाभ्यासं स्थित: च ।

योगात् ज्ञानं संजायते ज्ञानात् योग: प्रवर्तते ।।

Then, at the right time and with the knowledge and thought of the self, the *sadhaka* should face the north and be stable there. Afterwards, he should pull his *prana* in the place between the brows and study *yog* faithfully. Then knowledge emerges from *yog* and knowledge develops *yog*. The north is good for the *karma* of the sages as well as for *yog* studies. The Himalayas stand in the north of India and this is significant in the context of knowledge and renunciation. Many *yogis*, sages and *siddha* persons live there, so we can say that the *sadhaka* obtains guidance from those holy persons when he faces the north.

Panchanga Sevana – The fourth limb

This is an introduction to the *asanas*. The next extensive part is *Panchanga Sevana*. We are going to consider this part which is five-fold. Any *mantra* is related to some deity, God and their power. So the *mantra* becomes the worship of that deity. It is necessary to have devotion for God, otherwise there can be no real worship. *Mantra* is a way of worshipping the deity or God.

Panchanga Sevana has great importance in the *Vedic* tradition. The *Gitaa* of the particular deity, *Sahasranama*, *Stavana*, *Kavacha* and *Hridaya* are the five parts of the worship of the deity. Naturally these five matters change according to the deity. The basic purpose of *Panchanga Sevana* is to create a great deal of *sattva guna*. *Panchanga Sevana* greatly increases the *sattvic* tendencies of the *sadhaka*.

Gita is the first part (limb)of the *Panchanga*. The well known the *Bhagavadgita* belongs to *Bhagavanta*, so all deities like *Shiva, Vishnu, Krishna, Narasimha, Datta, Devi* have their *Gitas*. What do these *Gitas* contain? They consist of morals and philosophy. It does not possess the knowledge and philosophy within the four walls of a university but that which is useful for living life properly and meaningfully. It contains important advice for the spiritual *sadhaka*. Any of these *Gitas* can give nobility, serenity and meaning to life, of course, only if it is followed properly. The study of this *Gita* moulds the life of the *sadhaka* because it gives nobility to his behaviour, thinking and habits of food and socialization.

The second part of *Panchanga* is *Sahasranama*. Every deity has *Sahasranama* as that of *Vishnu*, which is well known. The *Anushasana Parva* of the *Mahabharata* contains *Vishnu Sahasranama*. The *vaidic sadhaka* knows the *Sahasranama* of *Hanuman, Lakshmi, Rama, Sita, Shiva, Ganesha*, etc. The *Sahasranama* is in the form of *shlokas* and contains not only one thousand names of the deity but also innumerable qualities of God. This universe is like a playground of God and the happenings here are the sport of God. They are described in the *Sahasranama*. It contains the thinking and utterance about divine qualities of the Omnipotent that are beyond words. The recitation and memory of it enhance the *sattva guna* of the *sadhaka*. The vibrations of the utterance have an effect on the existence and emotions of the *saadhaka*. The praise of the deity increases nobility, humbleness, devotion and affection of the *sadhaka*. The *Purusha Sukta* in the *Vedas* describes the universe as the body of God. According to a mythological story, *Vamana* occupied the whole universe within three steps. A particle of God's body occupies the whole universe. The deity to be worshipped in the *Sahasranama* is given the place of *Brahman*. This is necessary for the particular mindset of the *sadhaka*. His devotion overflows with the recitation.

The third part of *Panchanga* is eulogy. The overflowing devotion of the *sadhaka* makes him praise the deity. His bliss overwhelms him and he gets the state of ecstasy. The poetry and melody of the praises heightens his bliss and makes him capable of union with God. While worshipping God with hymns the devotees experience eight kinds of *sattvic* emotions. The hymns composed by saints have become immortal with their devotion and love.

The fourth part of *Panchanga* is *Kavacha* or a shield. *Kavacha* is used for protection from evil forces of an enemy. The *sadhaka* uses it to protect his body and mind during his *sadhana*. There are evil, brutal and demonic forces inside and outside our mind. Spirits and ghosts are *Adhibhautic* and *Adhidaivic* afflictions and they as well as insects and germs can be kept at bay with this *Kavacha*. The *mantra Kavacha* gives a power to remove obstacles in the way of *sadhana*. It gives strength to fight difficulties and hostile forces. Favourable atmosphere for *sadhana* is created.

The fifth part of *Panchanga* is *Hridaya* or heart. Heart is as important in *sadhana* as it is in living beings. We will take an example instead of using technical language or terminology for understanding this concept. What is *Hridaya* when *Vishnu* is being worshipped? *Vishnu* is described as lying on the cobra called *Ananta* in the deep *Kshirsagara.* Now, the poisonous cobra is a symbol of anger, enmity, *tamas* and destructive forces. *Vishnu* lies quietly on such a terrible and destructive bed. Imagine our state of body and mind if a serpent just passes beside us. Then consider *Vishnu* lying on this kind of snake with thousands of mouths. The *sadhaka* should learn that in this world we are not in such a dangerous situation and we can remain quiet. The *Hridaya* description of *Vishnu* gives us this inspiration. We can see a rare example of balance of mind here. The *Bhrugu chinha* on the chest of *Vishnu* is like His ornament and another example of His quietness. A story in mythology tells us that sage *Bhrugu* kicked Him on the chest angrily but Lord *Vishnu* did not react angrily. Instead, he asked this devotee whether his feet were paining because of the kick. This height of tolerance can be an example to follow for the *sadhaka*.

The next part of *Hridaya* is that *Lakshmi* is at the feet of *Vishnu*. Actually she is the goddess of wealth and all kinds of riches, yet she is at his feet and still *Vishnu* is all humbleness and of sacrificing attitude. Think of our pride when we get some amount of wealth. So the devotee is overwhelmed while reciting the *Hridaya*. The approach of *Vedic* culture is

ईशावास्यमिदं सर्वं यत्किंच जगत्यां जगत् ।
तेन त्यक्तेन भुंजीथा: मा गृध: स्वित् कस्यचिद् धनम् ॥

Whatever there is in this world, belongs to that Omnipotent God. You should enjoy whatever he gives, even pleasures, with renounced mind and should not grab from anybody. This *Vedic* approach is found in the *Ishavasya Upanishad* and *Vishnu* shows the same. The lotus in His hand represents beauty, peace, content and neutrality. This quality of lotus is mentioned in the *Gitaa* as पद्मपत्रं इव अम्भसि - that means you should be like the lotus in the water. It is not affected by water. The four hands of *Vishnu* are symbolic of the four *Vedas* of *Rig Ved, Sama Ved, Yaajur Ved* and *Atharva Ved*. They may be taken as the four goals of life, namely, *Dharma, Artha, Kama* and *Moksha*. His qualities of unselfishness, humbleness, tolerance and love also are signified by them. Sometimes He is shown to have eight hands which stand for health, learning, wealth, order, success, organization, bravery and truth. These are supreme qualities of life.

There is *sudarshana chakra* in his hand. This is a symbol of mind because the mind has spokes like those of the *chakra*. Such a mind is controlled on a fingertip by Him. It makes us dance but He makes it dance on his fingertip. This is a symbol of his conquest of the mind. As said earlier, the lotus in His hands suggests detachment from the world. The lotus is born in the mud but its beauty is not at all affected by the dirty mud. The *sadhaka* should follow this example and be detached from this mundane life. It guides the *sadhaka* in this way. The conch in His hand makes a loud and deep sound which is like broadcasting of today. It advocates serious, noble and divine thoughts. The *kaustubha* jewel around His neck is a symbol of the soul. Both are detached and without gunas. The *Vyjayantimala* around His neck represents the five elements of the earth, wind, water, fire and ether. The sacred thread is a sign of *Omkara*. The sacred thread is made up of three threads and one knot as *Omkara* is made of three and half matras. This sacred thread is important in the context of *Brahma Vidya* or *Brahman*. It is not just a thread of cotton but can be borne only by a *Brahmana* with the glory of knowledge and holiness. It signifies *Omkara* which is all *sadhanas* concentrated. The eight sentries of *Vishnu* in the eight directions are the eight *siddhis*. His carrier is *Garuda* who is the enemy and destroyer of serpents that are signs of *tamas guna*. In this way this last part, *Hridaya* of *Panchanga* gives meaning to and shapes the core of *sadhana*. We have thought about the importance of *Panchanga Sevana* in *mantra yog*.

Aachara – the fifth limb

We thought about the four parts of *Bhakti, Shuddhi, Asana* and *Panchaang Sevana* among the sixteen. Now the next fifth one is *Achara* or behaviour as it is understood by the common man. *Achara* is very important in *mantra yog* and for *sadhana*. It is said in the *Mahabharata*, आचार: परमो धर्म: I *Achara* is the great *Dharma*. Whatever is understood in piety is *Achara*. But usually piety is taken to be moral ethical behaviour or values. Those who value only practical kind of life do not attach any importance to it. They accept only those values that count for mundane life and they forsake those values that are unfavourable for this life. In fact, it is not like this. Even following these values also is difficult. The the so-called practical minded materialist is ready for all kinds of compromises and to discard and flout values. He does not get any prick of conscience in doing this. Yet he is not at ease because life becomes more complicated. On the contrary, those who care for values ply smoothly. Normative sciences argue that those who follow values always stumble and gain less than what they lose. But if the *sadhaka* follows moral values in *yog* or spirituality, he may not be sure of developing his strength, still he does not see it degraded at least. This *Achara* should not be mistaken for the morals in ethics. *Sattva Achara* is development of strength and evil *Achara* is deterioration of strength and degradation of man. A spiritual *sadhaka* can easily be convinced of this. We have to be convinced that *Sattva Achara* develops strength. It can even give *siddhis*. That is why it is given an independent and high place.

When we start thinking about the question-what is *Sat Achara*? A very long list presents itself for the answer. It can go on with charity, penance, sacrifice, patience, mercy, tolerance and so on. The *sadhaka* can prepare a short list for himself, too. But there is a theorem in *mantra yog*. Truth in behaviour gives accomplishment of *mantra*. It is easy to understand the importance of mouth and speech in the expression of truth. The *sadhaka* should not forget it. He should remember the strength, *siddhi* and sacredness of speech. This purity of mouth cannot be achieved with mouth freshener. Only truth can give purity of speech. Only truth can give strength to speech that is needed for *mantra siddhi. Patanjali* says, 'सत्यप्रतिष्ठायां क्रियाफलाश्रयत्वं ।' If the principle of truth is accomplished actions will be fruitful. *Achara* in the context of mouth and speech is very important in *Achara*. The most important weapon in wars is

Brahmastra. Truth is as powerful as *Brahmastra*. This thought of truth is profound. We must wait a moment and think about it. Then we may be led to think that we must think for an hour about it. But in truth, it is as profound as to demand thinking for the whole life.

In order to get *siddhi* in *mantra yog* by observing this *Achara*, we need to get blessings or initiation. This blessing is of three kinds-the blessing of mother, father and of guru. This blessing enhances our *sattva* enormously. The importance of *guru* is explained in our tradition. *Mantra yog* explains the importance of this trio very clearly. To say it in brief, the *sadhaka* should have *Achara* in such a way that he gets the trio of blessings.

This thought has a background with manifold meaning. The *sadhaka* has to behave in such a way that he can collect qualities. These qualities can help to get the blessing of the trio of mother, father and guru. *Tantra* of *mantra yog* has three kinds of *Achara*. They are 1] *Divya Achara* 2] *Dakshina Achara* and 3] *Vama Achara*. We have to see the expected kind of *Achara* of the *sadhaka*. *Mantra yog* is accomplished only after *ashtanga yog* is mastered. The *sadhaka* of *mantra yog* has already become a *yogi*. We can comprehend his *Achara*. His qualities as a *yogi* give sublimity to all three of his *Achara*. All his *Achara* is *Divya* or divine in any sense. The words *Dakshina Achara* and *Vama Achar* can confuse our mind because *Vama Achar* has a vicious meaning in our language. But such a meaning is not logical and proper and it should not be taken in that way. The *Achara* of a *yogi* does not mean to be sinful. The concepts of these three *Achara* are *tantric*. The literal meaning would not be right. A *yogi* is a *mantra yogi* and renounced person, so his *Achara* is *Divya* or divine. It does not mean that he is permitted to behave or should behave in any way. The words *Dakshina* and *Vaama* are taken as contrasting in our language but they are not taken like that here. *Vama Achara* is not contrasting to *Divya Achara* but it belongs to the cult of *Shakti* worshippers which depends upon the worship of *Parvati*. This has the prominence of renunciation. *Parvati* is the goddess of supreme sacrifice. Also *Dakshina* in *Dakshina Achara* does not have the usual meaning. It is not contrary to *Vama Achara* even. It is a *tantrik* word here. The word is formed out of the name of the sage *Dakshinamurti*. This *Achara* of renunciation is promoted by this sage.

We have to look at the word renunciation very carefully. A person who has been unsuccessful in life also gets the feeling of renunciation. But it is created out of frustration and so it is temporary. It is not real renunciation. There is not an iota of knowledge in it. The renunciation that emerges out of knowledge is true renunciation. Again, if we open the books of *tantra shastra* the *Achara*s in it would sound ghastly. But it is their terminology and code language. There are many things in it which create a maze or labyrinth of words. For example, the five *'ma'kara*s in them can mean vicious things in our language but they have some different connotations. So *Vama Aachara* is not ugly and horrible behaviour but it is an extremely intricate and mystic *sadhana*. An ordinary man might take distorted meaning out of it and the confusion and wrong meaning might cause his downfall. He may not be able to come out of that abyss. So, never forget the complex and profound nature of this science.

We have considered the five parts of *Bhakti, Siddhi, Asana, Panchanga Sevana* and *Achara*. Now let us think about the sixth part of *dharana* among the sixteen parts.

Shri Krishnaarpanam astu

✤ ✤ ✤

305

Discourse - 25

Mantra Yog - 4

Dharanaa – the sixth limb

We have considered the five limbs of *Bhakti, Siddhi, Asana, Panchanga Sevana* and *Achara*. Now we turn to the sixth limb i. e. *Dharana*. There are two kinds of *Dharana* in *Mantra yog*. They are *Bahya* or external *Dharana* and *Antar* or internal *Dharana*. *Dharana* on some external and concrete object such as a lotus, some deity, an idol of some deity like *Rama* or *Krishna*, a sign like *Swastika*, *Shivalinga* is *Bahya Dharana*. This object is noble and suitable for *dhyana*. The *sadhaka* can concentrate on this object. *Antar* or internal *Dharana* has a subtle object. *Pranayama* has an important place in it. *Siddhi* of *japa* and blessings of deities are important in this *Dharana* or, rather, they are achieved by this *Dharana*. The spirit of *dhyana* of some goddess, the devotion and concentration are called *Dharana*. We can see here the importance of *dhyana* for *mantra siddhi*. The aid of *yantra* or *matruka* is taken for *Dharana*. Every deity has a *yantra* and *dhyana* in *mantra yoga* is directed on this *yantra*. *Matruka* [Appendix] supports *Dharana*. We have to understand the concepts of *yantra, tantra* and *mantra*.

If you have some acquaintance with *tantra*, you will know *Matruka yantra*. It has a particular shape and it may be called esoteric geometry. Any book on *tantra* can show us the pictures of *yantras* and *Matruka yantra*. *Matruka yantra* has squares and letters and *tantra sadhana* is performed through them. This is a kind of symbolism. *Dhyana* is directed to symbols in *mantra yog*. The object is suitable for *dhyana*. This is the way of spiritual *Dharana*.

Divya Desha Sevanam – the seventh limb

The next and seventh limb is *Divya Desha Sevanam*. Take the example of cow's milk. Actually this milk exists in the whole body of the cow and it is producing milk. All the systems of the cow are working for the making of the milk; but we get the milk through her udders. The Brahma pervades the whole universe. All the philosophies say that God is omnipresent. Even if this is true, it is also true that at some places the revelation of this all-pervading principle is prominent. It is so in some place of pilgrimage or some area. That is why we go for pilgrimage. So this part of *Divya Desha Sevanam* stands separately in *Mantra yog*.

The science of *tantra* tells us about sixteen *Divya Deshas*. They are *Agni, Ambu, Linga, Sthandil, Kandya, Pata, Mandala, Vishakha, Nitya Yantra, Bhava Yantra, Pitha, Vigraha, Vibhuti, Naibhi, Valaya* and *Mudra*. The *sadhaka* of *mantra yog* has to be ordained in this way. He has to do penance in this *Divya Desha* and through *Divya Desha Sevanam*. He chooses any one of these sixteen *Divya Deshas* and does the *sadhana*. This *Divya Desha* is to be chosen by the *guru* of the *sadhaka*. The *sadhaka* or disciple does *Dharana* in that *Divya Desha* and continues his *sadhana*. This is the tradition. In short, *Divya Desha* is very useful for *sadhana*.

Divya Desha means a place which is appropriate and suitable for *sadhana*, which fosters his mindset and encourages his desire for *sadhana* with proper atmosphere. *Divya Desha* is vitally favourable for *sadhana* and it gives inspiration and direction for expediting the *sadhana*. The *vaidic* tradition advises that the place should get *Prana Pratishtha* or get the place sanctified. The *sadhaka* cannot have compromises in the sanctification. This is quite understandable. When we install a computer, we have to take care about adequate place

307

and atmosphere. We prefer to have it in an air-conditioned room. We avoid dust and keep our shoes outside that room. If the computer needs so much care and discipline, we can see why, the place of abstract *sadhana* needs sanctity. The normal *sadhaka* compromises with the place but then it becomes a gym exercise of body and mind. We ordinary people do our so-called *yog sadhana* in this room today and that room tomorrow. We are not particular even about the town or city of our staying. We are not particular even about the timings. We do it in the morning or evening or night according to our materialistic convenience. Of course, it is another matter that it does not make a great difference for us. When the level of our *sadhana* is already so low, what difference can it make? But the high level *sadhaka* does need to take appropriate care about his place of *sadhana*.

अकथह चक्र

अकथह १	उङ्प २	आखद ३	उचफ ४
ओडब ५	लृक्षम ६	औढश ७	लृलय ८
ईधन ९	ऋजभ १०	इगध ११	ऋछव १२
अ:तस १३	ऐठल १४	अंणष १५	एटर १६

मीन अ: ठ भ कुम्भ अं ट व	मेष अ क ड म	वृष आ ख ढ य मिथुन इ ग ण र
कर्क औ त्र फ क्ष	अकडम चक्रम्	मकर ई ध त ल
धनु ओ झ प ह वृश्चिक ऐ ज न स	तुला ए छ ध ष	सिंह उ ङ थ ब कन्या ऊ च द श

Prana Kriya – the eighth limb

The next limb is called *Prana Kriya*. It is not necessary to tell the importance of *prana* to the *yog sadhaka*. *Prana* is significant in any kind of *yog sadhana*. So we can see the significance of *Prana Kriya*, the why and how of it. Perhaps we can understand the 'why' easily but not 'how' of it. As regards the significance of *prana*, we remember the *Brihadaranyaka Shruti*. It says, प्राणो वै बलं, प्राणो वै अमृतम्, प्राण आयुर्वै प्राण: राजा वै प्राण: This means that *prana* is strength, *prana* is nectar, *prana* is life and Lord of everything. There are many such statements in *Brihadaranyaka Shruti*. *Prana Kriya* is a kind of *pranayama*. This *pranayama* occurs in the context of *mantra yog*. The *yog* in *mantra yog* is with *prana*. The *japa* in *mantra yog* is not mental but is with *prana*. If the *japa* in *mantra yog* is taken to be important and really it is so, it is never mental but only *pranic*. Just the oral *japa* of *Omkara* cannot be mental *japa* or even *japa*. The

Mudras in Matra Yog

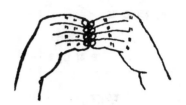

१ सुमुखम्

Sumukham

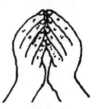

२ संपुटम्

Samputam

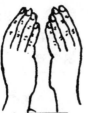

३ विततम्

Vitatam

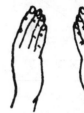

४ विस्तृतम्

Vistrutam

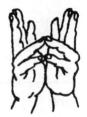

५ व्दिमुखम्

Dvimukham

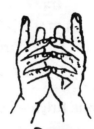

६ त्रिमुखम्

Trimukham

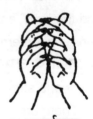

७ चतुर्मुखम्

Chaturmukham

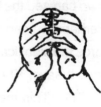

८ पंचमुखम्

Panchamukham

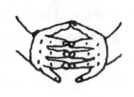

९ षण्मुखम्

Trimukham

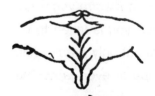

१०अधोमुखम्

Adhomukham

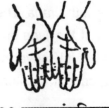

११ व्यापकांजलिकम्

Vyapakanjalim

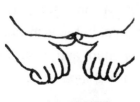

१२ शकटम्

Shakatam

310

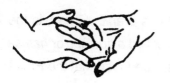
१३ यमपाशम्
Yamapasham

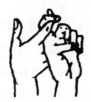
१४ ग्रंथितम्
Granthitam

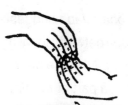
१५ उन्मुखोन्मुखम्
Unmukhonmukham

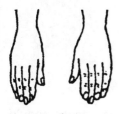
१६ प्रलंबम्
Pralambam

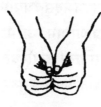
१७ मुष्टिकम्
Mushtikam

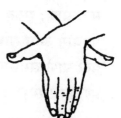
१८ मत्स्यः
Matsya

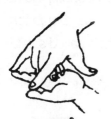
१९ कुर्मः
Kurma

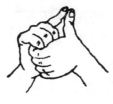
२० वराहकम्
Varahakam

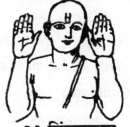
२१ सिंहाक्रान्तम्
Simhakrantam

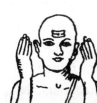
२२ महाक्रान्तम्
Mahakrantam

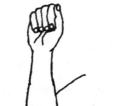
२३ मुद्गरम्
Mudgaram

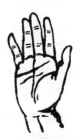
२४ पल्लवम्
Pallavam

311

soham japa suggests even in its title that it is *pranic*. *Soham* is the *japa* between inhaling and exhaling. This is called *ajapajapa* or *hamsa japa*. All these are *pranic*. So it can be easily deduced that the *Prana Kriya* part of *mantra yog* is very important in its *japa*. *Japa* is nothing if not *pranic*. Some quotations in *mantra yog* can tell us the importance of *pranic* element. The following *kandikas* can be considered.

मन: प्राण: मरुत् च एते अभेदसंबंधयोगिन:
मंत्रयोगे अपि सहित: प्राणायाम: अभिधीयते ।
यदा प्राणे समारोप्य पूरयित्वा उदरस्थितम्
प्रणवेन संसंयुक्त: व्याहृतिभिश्च संयुतम् ।।

Mind, *prana* and breath should be made one; then *apana* should be surrendered in *prana* while breathing. At the same time seven *vyahritis* should be recited. These seven *vyahritis* [Appendix] are as follows. *Om bhuh, Om bhuvah, Om svah, Om mahah, Om janah, Om tapah, Om satyam*. This knowledge of *pranayama* is called *sahita-pranayama* in *mantra yog*.

Kumbhaka – the ninth limb

Then follows *kumbhaka*. The *mantra* part of *kumbhaka* is ॐ तत्सवितु: वरेण्यं भर्गो देवस्य धीमहि धियो यो न: प्रचोदयात् and that of exhaling is अमृतं ब्रह्मा भू भुव: स्वरोम्. In this way *pranava* is with *prana*. Another point is that this is *prana kriya*. Those who have done *tantra* penance must be aware of this. This is *pranayama* in *mantra yog*. The important part of this is *anga nyasa, kara nyasa* and *pranayama* with *mantra*. *Pranayama* is not mere controlled inhaling and exhaling but it is accompanied with *mantra*. There is *pranayama* with *gayatri mantra* which is called *savyahriti gayatri pranayama*. So this is *mantra yogic pranayama*. It always has *mantra* and its *japa* is *pranic*. This is *prana kriya* in nutshell.

312

Mudra – the tenth limb

Now the next part is *mudra*. Those who are acquainted with the science of *yog* must be at least somewhat familiar with *mudra*. They must have at least heard the names of *mudras*. The *mudras* are part and parcel of *dhyana sadhana* of *mantra yog*. Books and treatises on *Hatha yog* tell us about them. I am mentioning some *mudras* here – *maha mudra, nabhi mudra, uddiyana mudra, jalandhara, mulabandha, maha bandha, maha vedha, khechari, viparita karani, yoni mudra, vajroli mudra, shaktichalana mudra, shambhavi mudra, ashwini mudra, pashini mudra, kaki mudra, matangini, bhujangini mudra*, etc. The books on *Hatha yog* can give us this knowledge and they are *Hatha yogic mudras*. *Mudras* of *mantra yog* are somewhat different. Those who are acquainted with the science of *yog* should not misunderstand those *mudras* with these *mudras*. *Hatha yogic mudras* are for *prana kriyas*.

It is important to note that *mudras* of *mantra yog* are different. The *mudras* in *mantra yog* are like hand gestures. They are used in the penance of *tantra* and *tantric* sun worship which is like *Vedic* Sun worship. The *mudras* in *Hatha yog* make use of body and particular poses of body. Indian classical art of dancing has various hand gestures and a variety of indications are given with them. The *mudras* in *mantra yog* are like them. They are *Unmonmukha, Sumukha, Samputa, Vitata, Dvimukha, Trimukha, Chaturmukha, Panchamukha, Vyapakanjali, Shanmukha, Adhomukha, Yamapasha, Shakata, Pallava, Pralamba, Matsya, Kurma, Varaha, Simhankranta, Mahakranta, Mudgara*. These hand gestures are used in *prana kriya*. They are used in *mantra yog* and in the worship of deities.

Eight *mudras* are used in *mantra yog* after *japa sadhana*. They are *Dhenu mudra, Jnana mudra, Vairagya mudra, yoni mudra,*

313

Shankha mudra, *Padma mudra* and *Nirvana mudra*. *Mantra yog* explains the benefits of these *mudras*. We are worshipping certain deity and reciting her *mantra*. The related *mudra* enhances the pleasure of that deity. *Japa* is divided as *ja* and *pa* and it is said जकारो जन्मविच्छेदक : पकारो पापनाशक : that *ja* means severing the thread of births and *pa* means destroying sins. *Mudras* are important in processes of *japa*. Their use in *mantra sadhana* or *mantra yog* destroys sins. The sciences talk about nineteen *mudras*. Each deity has love for particular *mudras*. *Vishnu* likes the *mudras* of *Shankha*, *Chakra*, *Gada*, *Padma*, *Venu*, *Kaustubha*, *Jnana*, *Shrivatsa*, *Vanamala*, *Bilva*, *Garuda* and so on. *Mahadeva* likes *Linga*, *Yoni*, *Trishula*, etc. There are different *mudras* for deities like *Shri Ganesh*, the Sun, *Shakti*, *Lakshmi*. These *mudras* are beneficially used while worshipping these deities.

Tarpana – the eleventh limb

The next part of *mantra yog* is *Tarpana*. The *Vedic* culture gives great importance to the debt of the forefathers. They look after us from the world beyond. The happiness we get is not only due to our efforts but also due to their blessings. Other cultures sever ties with dead people but the *Vedic* culture does not deny the existence of the dead in some form. So the dead forefathers are gratefully remembered. The rituals of *shraddha* are performed for their sake. Sacrifice is offered in the *yajna* for deities. In the same way it is offered to the dead forefathers which is called *Tarpana*. *Mantra yog* is *Vedic* and it is a *Vedic* belief that it is man's duty to do *Tarpana* for the forefathers. It is not waste of time because if he does *Tarpana* he need not do *Pitru yajna*. The *sadhaka* gets this concession, perhaps. He does it every day, so it is said that if he uses honey in it, his wishes are fulfilled. The *mantras* that he uses also become effective.

Destruction of sins is a part of it. If camphor or water with camphor is used in *Tarpana* the *sadhaka* is free from the ties of *karma*. Use of water with milk gives freedom from diseases. If *ghee* is mixed in water for *Tarpana*, the *sadhaka* gets longevity.

There are some factors in the process of *Tarpana* and some modifications are done so that it gives longevity, freedom from sins and fulfillment of desires. Mythologies tell us that Sage *Maricha* got freedom from sins because of *Tarpana*. *Tarpana* with coconut water has some special effect. *Tarpana* with milk, *ghee* and honey along with *mantra japa* and *rochana tilaka* can destroy enemies. This can tell us the efficacy of *Tarpana*. The nineteenth chapter of *Mantra Yog Samhita* describes this in detail.

We have considered the parts of *Mantra Yog* as *Bhakti, Shuddhi, Asana, Panchanga Sevana, Achar, Dharana, Divya Desha Sevana, Prana Kriya, Mudra* and *Tarpana*. The next or 11th part among the 16 is *Yajna*. The concept and institution of *Yajna* is at the core of the *Vedic* way of life. So because of its importance it is made a part of *mantra yog*. In our material life we have blessings of deities and gods. *Yajna* expresses our gratitude for them through the processes and rituals in it. The *Vedic* person knows that *yajna* means sacrifices to gods. Why are gods offered sacrifices? If we think of the *Adhidaivic* [Appendix] organization of this universe, we become aware that this universal revelation has its origin in their powers and blessings. As the *Vedic* person is grateful to the gods and forefathers, so also he is grateful to the society, culture and nature. The rituals of *yajna* are the *Vedic* expression of this gratitude. The *Vedic* person admits the debts of all of them and performs his duty towards them. This is a typical *Vedic* social and cultural system. In short, *yajna* is gratefully paying respects and offering sacrifices to nature, gods and our forefathers.

There is a concept in the *Gita* that this whole world is an altar of *yajna* and so it is holy. The concepts in the *Gita* belong to the science of the *Gita*. The human soul is spirituality and *adhiyajna* [Appendix] or divine presence is God. God resides at the centre of every proton, electron and neutron. So it is *adhiyajna*. Whomever you are worshipping and offering sacrifices in *yajna*, you are worshipping God only. So *yajna* is a different *Vedic* concept and it is a vast subject for studies with *adhiyajna*. Once again note that The concept and institution of *Yajna* is at the core of the *Vedic* way of life. So because of its importance it is made a part of *mantra yog*. We ordinary people can see one thing about *yajna*. It is that *yajna* is a great process of purification which is internal as well as external. Today the modern sciences also accept that the sacrifices in the *yajna*, whether *ghee* or any other substance, not only sanctify but also purify the atmosphere.

The sacrifices in the *yajna* are a part of the process of purification. They purify air, water, soil and the region. More importantly, *yajna* brings about the worship along with sacrifices for gods, goddesses and powers of the world. This is worship and penance. *Mantra yog* has accepted *yajna* as a part of it. It is described as *'havanam'* which means abandoning evil tendencies there. *Havanam* can be taken in a different ways. The *sadhaka* abandons his bad and selfish tendencies, evils and fluctuations of his mind. Abandoning all these evils, sins and bad omens is *yog*. The penance of *mantra* or *mantra yog* cannot succeed without *japa*. It is understandable that *mantra* worship cannot be done without *japa*. *Japa* is necessary for *mantra* worship. There is no *mantra* without *japa*. *Mantra* or *mantra yog* may be a kind of *siddhi* but *siddhi* cannot be obtained without *japa*. *Japa* or *mantra* can be successful only with *Havanam*. *Havanam* is a kind of sacrifice. Sacrifices are put in the fire accompanied with the *mantra* and observing the rites; and this is a part of the ritual. The *Havanam* also brings about worship and penance for the deity. The deity, especially the personal deity, is pleased with this and blesses the *sadhaka*. So   *Havanam* means the way or ritual for getting blessings of the deity. This suggests the importance of *Havanam*.

Blessings of the deity are important and *Havanam* is important for the blessings. After the worship and *Havanam*, there is sacrifice. *Homa* is offering particular substances to deities and *Tarpana* follows sacrifice. The order is *yajna*, *Havanam*, sacrifice *Homam* and *Tarpana*. Among the *Brahmanas*, there is one more ritual which is *Bali Vaishvadeva*. This ritual is among the regular ones and it is performed after the floor is sanctified. This is done through *Namana* and *Svaha mantra*. Sixteen offerings are made with *Mula mantra*. The *Vedic* code has *Pancha yajna* with *ahuti*. The *mantra yogi* should have faith for such *yajna* and *Havanam*. The spiritual part of the *Pancha yajna* is inherent in *mantra yog* and so it is a spiritual *Pancha yajna*.

Manusmriti has described *Pancha* or five *yajnas*. They are *Deva yajna, yajna* for gods, *Brahma yajna*, *yajna* for *Brahma*, *Pitru yajna*, *yajna* for forefathers, *Bhuta yajna, yajna* for all the beings and the fifth *Manushya yajna* for mankind. The spiritual kind is performed in *mantra yog*. This gives blessings of gods. *Tarpana* gives blessings of gods and forefathers. *Havanam* gives blessings of personal deity. The main thing is the temperament for *yajna*. The next part is *bali* or sacrifice. The world has immense misunderstanding about *bali*. The ordinary people and modern Hindus have a wrong idea about it. They think it is killing and sacrificing an animal like goat. We take it

317

as a stigma on our *Vedic* culture and feel inferiority complex about it. But this is an altogether different concept. The science of *yajna* tells- बलिदानात् विघ्नशांति: श्रेष्ठदेवस्यपूजनात् बलिदानेषु सर्वेभ्य: श्रेष्ठ: आत्मबली स्मृत: । बली श्रेष्ठ: । Sacrificing and worshipping of great gods removes all obstacles. The greatest sacrifice is of '*Aatma*' i. e. your own sacrifice. This is important and has a significant meaning. *Mantra Yog Samhita* says that sacrifice of animals is a sin. The book that accepts sacrifice as a part of *yajna* says that sacrifice of animals is a sin. This is significant. It suggests that this custom had not been there in the *Vedic* tradition originally but entered later from somewhere. The *Mantra Yog Samhita* clearly tells that sacrifice of animals is wrong, destructive and sinful. Sacrifice of animals is something born out of selfish and greedy tendencies of some people.

It has its origin in the cruel tendencies of people. They whitewashed and tried to justify it with the rituals of religion. This is not *Vedic*. There is a *tantra* concept of sacrifice of beasts. But who are beasts here? The inhuman cruelty and selfishness make beasts of human beings. We call cruel men as beasts. The *Upanishads* say, कामक्रोधलोभादिपशव : । The tendencies of extreme selfishness and cruelty are beasts. So the animal sacrifice is the sacrifice of anger, selfishness, greed, pride, lust and cruelty in us. The *Bhairava Tantra* has a *shloka* in it,

काम क्रोध सुलोभ मोह पशून् छित्वा विवेकासिना ।
मांसं निर्विषयं परात्मसुखदं भुञ्जन्ति तेषां बुधा: ॥

It means-The wise people kill the beasts of lust, anger, greed and infatuation with the sword of wisdom and enjoy the meat of these beasts which is devoid of sensuality and has great bliss. The five kinds of *Tantra* also say the same thing. The beasts of our sinister tendencies are to be eradicated with wisdom. *Yajna* is sacrifice and the sacrifice of these beasts of lust, anger, greed and infatuation is great *yajna*. Also it is admirable to kill our pride and audacity.

Extreme of pride, self-consciousness and the six mental enemies are beasts and their sacrifice pleases the deities. The science of devotion tells us that sacrifice of pride pleases gods more than their praise. The *Vedic* rituals have a custom of sacrifice to *Brahmadeva* which is called *Vaishvadeva*. Everybody should do this in his house. One *Tantra* in the *Vedic* rituals advocates sacrifice to *Dhanvantari* in the north, to *Indra* and the moon in the east, *Yama* in the south, *Varuna* in the west, *Dhata-Vidhata* at our door and demons in the direction of the sky. Sacrifice and *Tarpana* to the forefathers in the south is suggested in *mantra yog* and it starts with *achamana* [Appendix] of water. These sacrifices are offered to the nine *Grahas*. This ritual includes giving grain and food to birds, beasts, animals, insects and ants. So, right from animals to gods, all are pleased with appropriate sacrifices. This is the noble custom in the Vedic tradition. It is accepted specially on the spiritual level in mantra yog as sacrifice of the self and of evil tendencies.

The next part is *Yag*. We have to understand the *yag* on the earth. There are three *yagas* as *Antar* or internal *yag*, *Bahir* or external *yag* and *Upa yag*. *Antar* and *Bahir yagas* are known in the science of *yog* and they are performed to please gods. *Bahir yag* is a kind of worship included in mantra *yog* with sixteen, eight or five rituals. *Antar yag* is mental worship like *dhyana* and is superior to *Bahir yag*. The *sadhaka* has to observe purity of *Dik* or directions, of *Deha* or body and of *Desha* or the area. *Antar yag* does not need this. *Bahir yag* creates favourable atmosphere and situation for *japa*. The concentration needed for *japa* is given by this *yag*. Modern *vaidics* may not know the names of these rituals or their details.

Let us see the twenty-one rituals in it as there are sixteen in the *Mantra Yog*. They are *Avahanam, Svagatam, Asanam, Sthapanam, Padyam, Snanam, Vasanam, Upatilakam, Bhushanam, Gandhapushpam, Naivedyam, Achamanam, Tambulam, Malyam, Niranjanam, Namaskaram and Visarjanam*. The well known sixteen religious rituals are *Avahanam, Sthapanam, Padyam, Arghyam, Snanam, Vastram, Bhushanam, Gandham, Pushpam, Dhupam, Dipam, Naivedyam, Achamanam, Niraanjanam, Tambulam and Pranamam*. There is a set of ten rituals, too. They are - *Padyam, Arghyam, Snanam, Madhuparkam, Achamanam, Gandham, Pushpam, Dhupam, Dipam*, and *Naivedyam*. There are also five short cuts. They are *Gandham, Dhupam, Pushpam, Dipam, Naivedyam*. These are included in *Bahir yaga*. *Antar yag* does not need these but it has *dhya*na and *japa*. The third *Upa yag* includes studies of the *Vedas* and the *shastras* and *mantras* for personal deities. There are *Tantras* and *Gitas* of *Vaishnava, Shaiva, Shakta* and *Saur* sects and of the deities. We have referred to them in *Panchanga Sevanam*. *Upa yag* means studies, thinking and consideration of these. Following the discipline of these three *yagas* is a part of *mantra yoga*.

Japa

The next part or rather the core of *yog* is *japa. Japa* is a part of *yog* of any kind and especially of *mantra yog* and *dhyana. Japa* is very important in our spiritual *sadhana* and worship.

This is a special characteristic of our culture and *Vedic sadhana*. The *Bhagavatam* even calls *japa* as *dhyana*. जपो ध्यानम् Everybody has a right to do *japa* and *dhyana*, because *japa* and *dhyana* are taken to be equal. It is not the sole privilege of a *yog sadhaka*. The *Vedic* culture and code allow everybody to do *japa* or *dhyana*. There cannot be worship or *sadhana* spirituality without *japa. Japa* exists at every stage of spirituality. As it is there in the stage of raw beginning, it is there at the highest spiritual level. Right from the beginners like us to *Jnaneshvar* and *Chaitanya Mahaprabhu* every sadhaka tries to get concentration through *japa*. The great devotees *Tyagaraja, Mirabai, Pralhada* used *japa* for *sadhana*. It is like their heart. It is an unfailing companion of the *sadhaka* in all the stages. *Japa* is at the centre of any kind of *yog* whether it is *Karma yog* or *Jnana yog* or *Hatha yog* or *Raja yog* or *Bhakti yog*. Its importance in the science of *mantra* and in *mantra yog* goes without saying.

Japa is there in the material and spiritual aspects of *Vedic* code. *Japa* is used for attaining material success also. Any *mantra* is *japa* ultimately. The *Vedas* are in the form of *mantra* only. *Yog* is important in *mantra* and the state of *yog* is not without *japa*. In the 25th *shloka* of the 10th chapter of the *Gita*, Lord *Krishna* says, यज्ञानां जपयज्ञः अस्मि I I am *japa yajna* among all kinds of *yajna*. We are thinking of *japa* in the context of *yoga*. Our spiritual sciences and those of *yog* give a central place to *japa*. We are going to think of it in detail.

We will consider the kinds, rituals and instruments of *japa*. Since *japa* is done in various stages of *sadhana*, there are different kinds of *japa*. It is done in the stage of the beginning and in that of ultimate *siddhi*. Since purposes of *japa* are various, it is done in different ways.

The first kind of *japa* is *Nitya* or regular *japa*. As our body needs bath, food, air and water every day, so also our subtle or esoteric body needs many things such as rest, sleep, food, bath, water. But they are needed in different forms. All this is provided to it by *japa*. *Japa* is bath, food, air and water for our subtle or esoteric body.

It is also an exercise for this body. This *Nitya japa* may be *japa* of the personal deity. Sometimes it is given by the *guru* or by the saints.

Some are traditional. This *japa* develops our strength and powers of the *sukshma sharira*.

A simple ritual is prescribed for this *japa*. Anybody and everybody can follow this ritual and some rules. One has to take care of purity, cleanliness and nobility and discipline of mind.

The other kind is *Naimittic* or contingent *japa*. This *japa* is done for certain occasions like *shraddha karma*, the fourth or eleventh date of the lunar calendar, full-moon or no-moon night, *Shivaratri, Shrikrishna ashtami, Shrirama Navami,* etc. In short the *japa* is done on the day of our personal deity. It is performed also for making planetary condition favourable or reducing evil influences. We will consider this subject again later.

The third kind is *Kamya* or wishful *japa*. As the name suggests, it is done with some specific purpose, for achieving something or for removing some evil influence. One more kind is *Nishiddha japa* or *japa* with some prohibitions or restrictions, which has restrictions about rituals and rules. He has to abide by them and has to avoid all the conditions, situations and places that are bad for *japa*. A particular *japa* has to be done at particular place with full care about cleanliness and purity.

Another kind of *japa* is *Prayaschitta japa*. The religious treatises tell us that this *japa* helps to expiate the sins that are committed by us unknowingly. This sin might have been committed before some *karma*. It might have been done during childhood or youth or old age. So the *japa* is for expiation of sin or for the beginning of some *karma*.

The next *Chala japa* can be called 'mobile' *japa*. The *sadhaka* can do this while walking, talking, eating or travelling. This weapon of spiritual *sadhana* can be used in a difficult situation also. The *japa* can be done with its holiness and purity even when the rules and discipline is kept aside. So this is a convenient kind of *japa*.

This classification of Regular, Contingent, *Nishiddha*, *Kamya*, *Prayaschitta* and *Chala japa* is based on the particular kinds of *sadhana*. We can classify *japa* on the basis of the media of *japa* i. e. speech and mind. The first *Vachic* or *Vangmaya japa* is done with the vocal organs and all the ingredients of oration are used in it. So this gives *siddhi* of speech on account of the regulated use of teeth, lips, palate and tongue. Speech becomes clear, effective and resonant. Proper utterance of *beeja mantra* with such speech gives the *sadhaka* the powers of the *mantra* and the six plexi. An ordinary person may not be able to understand this but he can at least experience that the long pronunciation of the *mantra* gives exercise to body, mind and brain. We always see that those who practise Sanskrit reading have clear and pure speech.

Another kind of *japa* is *Upanshu japa*. This *japa* cannot be heard by others but it gives internalization to the mind. The mind is diverged from outside objects and starts a journey towards concentration. Naturally this *japa* can be kept secret.

The third *japa* is *Bhramara*. It is like humming of bees where the sound of the *mantra* is heard but not understood. It is like hypnotism and gives happiness and peace of mind. Even though lips do not pronounce loudly the sound of the *mantra* creates an effect on the brain.

Bhramara japa leads to the fourth kind of *Anahata japa*. It is mental and soundless as the title suggests. Sound is always necessarily created out of some stroke but *Anahata japa* emerges without any striking and without any movement of muscles of the mouth and without pronouncing the vowels and consonants.

The title of the fifth *japa*, *Akhanda* or continuous, suggests that it is going on incessantly. It is constantly going on, sometimes loudly, sometimes on the mental level, sometimes whispering or with speech or *pranic* or with *dhyana*.

The *dhyana japa* is of and for an accomplished *yogi*. His meditation and mental *Svadhyaya* is continuously going on. The *japa* out of this *dhyana* is *dhyana japa*. If it is done for twelve years it is called *Tapa* which means penance. *Tapa* also means twelve years but if the penance is done for the entire twelve years, then only it is real *Tapa* or penance.

The next *japa* is *ajapajapa*. We have twenty-one thousand six hundred breaths every day. In each of these breaths *soham* is going on. *Shloka* 30 of the 4th chapter of the *Gita* describes this *japa*. अपरे नियताहारा: प्राणान् प्राणेषु जुह्वति। These *sadhakas* regulate their food habits and offer sacrifice of *prana* into *prana* while doing *japa*.

The last *Pradakshina japa* is done while moving around the idol in the temple or around the sacred trees of banyan or fig.

So this is the classification of *japa* as *Vachic, Upanshu, Bhramara, Manasic, Akhanda, Ajapajapa, dhyana japa* and *Pradakshina* based on the medium.

Some elements are necessary in whatever kind of *japa* it is. The main element is faith. The *japa* of *yog sadhana* is devotion oriented. Devotion enhances faith, so it is important in *yog* and *japa sadhana*. It is not only sensitivity but it is faith in God that creates concentration needed in spirituality.

नास्ति बुद्धि: अयुक्तस्य न च अयुक्तस्य भावना ।
न च अभावयत: शान्ति: अशान्तस्य कुत: सुखम् ।।

A person who is not fit for *sadhana* has no intelligence and no faith or devotion. Such a person is never calm. An agitated person can never be happy. The real *sadhaka* has these qualities. He has purified his heart with *pranayama*. He should have pure food and good habits of socialization. Food is not only for the stomach but also for the eyes, ears and touch. The purity of all these gives a good background and power to the *sadhaka*.

Meaning is important in *japa*. *Patanjali* says, **तज्जपस्तदर्थभावनम्।** While thinking of the explicit and implicit meanings of the *japa* faith for God is created. *Rama* is not only the son of *Dasharatha* but the word has a spiritual meaning. The sound of *japa* is important. The vibrations of the sound create an effect on the heart and body. Thought must be given to it. The body should be sensitive for the vibrations. The rituals of *japa* have to be observed carefully. *Japa* should be done at a proper and favourable place. Observing the discipline and rules of bath, worship, fasting, etc. is imperative. The *sadhaka* should take care of his speech in the sense that he should practise *mouna* or silence and increase his mental energy with truth and by being quiet.

The *sadhaka* should also be well versed in the sciences of *mantra*, *japa, yog, prana*, spirituality, *tantra* and gods. He should know at least the primary things about these. Knowledge and faith of *Adhibhautic* and *Adhidaivic* constitution of the universe must be there. He should possess spiritual calm and content. All this can give us the idea of the required equipment of the *sadhaka* for his *sadhana*. He should think of the questions-What is *japa*? What is *mantra* ?

मननात् त्रायते यस्मात् तस्मात् मंत्र: प्रकीर्तित: ।

जपात् सिध्दि: जपात् सिध्दि: जपात् सिध्दि: न संशय:

The sciences tell us that *mantra* helps us with the meditation. It is assured that *japa* can give *siddhi*. *Mantra* is a set of letters or words, utterance of which and contemplation of meaning of which lifts man from mundane mire, therefore, *mantra* is always a saviour. You should not doubt it. Of course, the *japa* should be for God and not for money. What is the meaning of *japa*? जकारो जन्मविच्छेदक: पकारो पापनाशक: । The letter *ja* in it suggests freedom from being born again and again. The letter *pa* in it signifies redemption of sins. The *japa* for money destroys life. People running after money die early. *Japa* of the *mantra* of gods gives salvation. *Mantras* like *Shri Rama Jai Rama Jai Jai Rama, Shri Krishna Govinda Hare Murare, He Nath Narayana Vasudeva, Om Namah Shivaya, Om Namo Narayanaya, Om Namo Bhagavate Vasudevaya* give salvation and destroy sins.

When we think of *japa* from the angle of *mantra yog*, we have to think of *tantric* aspects of *japa*. *Tantric japa* has to use *mudra*. There is a *shloka* in *Mantra Yog Samhita*

मंत्रयोगस्य माहात्म्यं इदं अत्र अपरं मतम् ।
हठे लये तथा राजयोगे सहकरोति अत: । (७० – ४७)

This means that the greatness of *mantra yog* is accepted by all. *Mantra* is essential in any *yog*, *Hath yog* or *Raja yog* or *Laya yog*. *Dhyana* cannot be there without *japa* and *japa* is impossible without *mantra*. *Japa sadhana* has *Beeja mantra* in it. The sciences tell us that the greatest *mantra* is ॐ प्रणव:

Beeja Mantra

Now let us think about *Beeja mantra*. *Mantra* is important in any *yoga* and *Beeja mantra* is specially important in *mantra yoga* and *Tantra*. It is important in the context of the six plexi. *Japa* has to be done with *mala* or rosary, so the spiritual sciences have explained everything about rosaries. They explain the purpose behind every rosary, how to hold it in the hands, which hand should be used for holding it, how to tell the beads and how to do japa. They have given the hierarchy of rosaries. The lowest one is *Arishtapatra Mala*, better than that are *Beeja mala, Shankha Mala, Padma mala, Mani mala, Kushak Granthi* and the greatest is *Rudraksha mala*. Another classification of rosaries is based on the beads, such as *Pravala* or coral *Mala, Mukta* or pearl *Mala, Sphatika* or crystal *Mala, Hiranyagarbha Mala, Indraksha Mala, Rajat* or silver *Mala* and *Suvarna* or gold *Mala*. The best among these are *Tulasi*-basil and *Mani mala*.

Mantras are of two kinds. The first is sound oriented which gives greater importance to clear and flawless pronunciation. Utterance of *mantra* like this is powerful. This *mantra* is not very important in *yog sadhana. Vedic mantra* is important for spiritual progress. *Sabar mantra* is useful for material progress. *Mantra yog* does not contain *Daivi* and *Paishach mantra* because they are used in black arts or magic. Those interested can look for its subtle explanation in *Mantra Shastra*. We are concerned here only with *Mantra yog*. The other kind is *Bhavapradhana* where the emotions and feelings for the meaning of the *mantra* are of paramount importance.

Dhyana – the fifteenth limb

We have so far considered the 14 out of 16 parts of *sadhana* that are *Bhakti, Shuddhi, Asana, Panchanga Sevana, Achar, Dharana, Divyadesha Sevana, Prana kriya, Mudra, Tarpana, Yajna, Bali, Yaga and Japa*. Now we can go to the 15th part of *Dhyana. Samadhi* is the 16th part. Obviously the *dhyana* in *Mantra yog* depends on *mantra*. We cannot have *dhyana* on lotus and *Samadhi* on *mantra*. It cannot be centred on an object or an element like the earth or sky. It is clear that *dhyana* is where *Dharana* is and *Samadhi* is where *dhyana* is. *Mantra* may have one or more letters. *Bija mantra* has one letter. *Dhyaana* in *mantra yoga* develops with *Bija mantra*. *Mala mantra* can be very long or vast even. *Datta Mala Mantra* has as many as one hundred and eight letters. We do *dhyana* while worshipping the idols. *Dhyana* is of many kinds. *Mantra yog* and *Tantra yog* state that *Vishnu dhyana* is of seven kinds. *Dhyana* of goddesses like *Laxmi, Saraswati or Kaali* has 24 kinds. *Dhyana* of *Mahadeva* is of five kinds. *Dhyana* of *Surya* or sun and *Ganesh* is of two kinds.

We can do *dhyana* of the image of our personal deity. We raise an image of the deity in the mind for *dhyana* or do it with mental imaging. According to *mantra yog*, *mantra* makes the soul to be one with God as salt dissolves in water. Soul or salt is dissolvent and God or water is dissolver. *Mantra* helps the process of dissolving.

Dhyana has many kinds such as *Vishnu dhyana, Shiva dhyana, Saura dhyana, Ganesha dhyana*. We have to turn to *Agama Shastra* if we want to think and know more about it. *Aagama Shastra* is a very vast subject and it gives minute description of kinds of *dhyana*. For example, *Vaishnava Agama* gives all information about *Vishnu dhyana*. *Mantra* is the centric force in the *dhyana* in *mantra yog*. The meaning of the *mantra* portrays the deity in our heart. *Dhyana* gives us the experience of it. With the *mantra* of *Narayana* the image of *Narayana* emerges in the mind and *dhyana* gives us experience of *Narayana*. *Dhyana* shows us the glory of *Vishnu*. This is the mysticism of it.

The *japa* that leads to *yog* is not *manasic* but *pranic*. The concept of *pranic japa* has been created out of *mantra yog*. It has entered the other kinds of *yog* later. The *pranava japa* in the *Yog Sutras* of *Patanjali* or the *pranava japa* in *Jnana yog* is according to the science of *mantra yoga* only.

Samadhi – the sixteenth limb

It is said in *Mantra Yog* that the *Samadhi* in *Laya yog* is *Mahalaya*. The *Samadhi* of *Hatha yog* is *Mahabodha* and that of *Mantra yog* is *Mahabhava*. *Bhava* is important in the *Samadhi* of *Mantra yog*. *Patanjali* says with regard to the process of *japa* तत् जप: तदर्थभावनम् । So he gives importance to *bhava*. The *Mantra Yog Samhita* says that as long as the trio of *Dhyata*, *Dhyana* and *Dhyeya* i. e. one who does *dhyana*, the actual act of *dhyana* and the object of *dhyana* remain, the importance of *dhyana* is there. The trio ceases to exist when *Mahabhava* or *Samadhi* emerges. *Mahabhava* is the supreme state of mind. Mind has completely submerged in the deity. As salt dissolves totally in water, so mind dissolves in the deity. The trio vanishes. At that time the eight *Sattvic Bhavas* come out. The journey towards *Samadhi* begins. When *Mahabhava* is achieved, the conclusion of *Mantra yog* is the beginning of *Hatha yog*. The ultimate *Samadhi* of *Hatha yog* is *Raja yog*. The *shloka* 2/76 in *Hatha yog Pradipika* is

हठं विना राजयोग: राजयोगं विना हठ: ।
न सिध्यति ततो युग्म आनिष्पते: समभ्यसेत् ।।

Hatha yog is not fruitful without *Raja yog* and also *Raja yog* is not fruitful without *Hatha yog*. The *sadhaka* should study both of them from the beginning. *Raja yog* reaches its culmination in *Rajadhiraja yog* or *Kundalini yog*.

Today so-called *yogis* claim to be teaching *Hatha yog* in the very beginning of *sadhana*. The supposed *Kundalini yog* is sold like hot cakes in the market. Ten or fifteen thousand people get initiation of *Kundalini yog* simultaneously. All of them get their *Kundalini* raised at the same moment. Actually mere *dhyana* cannot raise *Kundalini* without using *Bija mantra* and the process of *mantra*. The ritual of

329

Shaktichalan even cannot do this difficult task. *Kundalini* is not a sleeping person who could be woken up by giving him jerks. The subtle processes of *Hatha, Raja* and *laya yog* all stand on the use of *mantra*. *Mantra yog* cannot exist without *mantra* and it has *mantra* in its title itself. Similarly *Hatha yog* does not exist without *mantra*. *Hatha yog* is not accomplished by knotting different limbs and assuming contortions of the body. If these *yogis* are talking of *yog* without *mantra*, then they are talking of a lake without water.

No *yog* exists without *mantra*. The claims of these fake *yogis* are preposterous. The theory can be stated briefly- *Yog* cannot be there without *mantra*, whether it is *mantra yog* or *raja yog* or *Hatha yog*. There is no exception for this rule. The *dhyana* of *mantra yog* culminates in the dissolution of '*triputi*'. This *mantra yog Samadhi* is the subtle process in intuitive mysticism. So these are the sixteen parts of *Mantra Yog*.

Guru

The tradition tells us that the *mantra* should be given by the *Guru*. It is not proper to set out for *sadhana* by taking *mantra* from somewhere at random. Our tradition has talked about the importance of *Guru* and his advice and initiation. The thought about *Guru* in *Mantra yog* is very interesting. We have to understand it.

The book '*Pandava Pratapa*' talks about twelve types of *gurus*. Their source is the science of *Mantra yog*. The first type is *Dhaturvadi guru*. He asks the disciple to do pilgrimage and gives initiation after the pilgrimage. The second is *chandana guru*. Like *chandana* or sandalwood which makes fragrant anything that is around, this *guru* influences everybody. Of course, *chandana* has no effect on banana and a plant called *hingul*. There are some profane people who remain untouched by his influence. The third *Vichara guru* works on the disciple only with his *vichara* or thought. He transfers his thoughts to his disciple and redeems him. Naturally this path is very slow and has a speed of a snail. But, of course, spirituality, like success has no short cuts. The fourth *Anugraha guru* redeems his disciple just with his *Anugraha* or gracious glance, even in their absence from each other or blessings. The disciple is fortunate to be blessed without any hardships.

The fifth *guru* redeems only with the touch. This is like the touch of the philosopher's stone that turns iron into gold. This is a channel of the privileged disciples. The sixth *Kachhapa guru* redeems his disciple just by looking at him lovingly. It is believed that *Kachhapa* or tortoise feeds her young ones with her looks at them with love. This poetic idea is elaborated beautifully by *Jnaneshvar* in '*Jnaaneshvari*'. The seventh *Chandra guru* redeems his disciple from a distance even. He works like *Chandra* or the moon who makes the stone *Chandrakanta* melt with her cool rays. He gives knowledge to his disciple in this way. The next *Darpana guru* is like a mirror who redeems his disciple when the disciple is before him. There is a bird named *Chhayanidhi*. If a person comes in its shadow, he becomes a king. Similarly, *Chhayanidhi guru* redeems his disciple with his shadow. The tenth *Nadanidhi guru* helps his disciple just with his *nada* or voice. The bird *Krouncha* or heron fosters his young ones by remembering them. So also *Krouncha guru* redeems the disciple by remembering him. The twelfth *guru* is *Suryakanta guru*. The *Suryakanta* stone creates fire without efforts. In the same way *Suryakanta guru* blesses his disciple with his blessings when they are in the proximity. So the relationship of *guru* and disciple is important. *Mantra yog* cannot start without initiation from the *guru*. The students start their education by getting admission in an educational institute. This does not take place in spirituality.

Dikshaa

Initiation or *diksha* is explained in the science of *Mantra yog* as follows,

दीयते दानं सद्भावनात् क्षीयते पशुवासना ।
दीनक्षपणसंयुक्ता दीक्षा तेन इह कीर्तिता ।।

The offering of *diksha* is done with good feeling and brutal feelings are reduced. In this way *diksha* consists of both offering and destruction. *Kumardiksha* is advised in *yog* tradition. *Sanatkumara*, *Sanandan*, *Sanatsujata*, *Sanatsanatana* belonged to the path of renunciation and were given *Kumardiksha*. The seven *rishis* are for the seven celestial plains. Tradition says that *Sanatkumara* is our *guru* for this earth. This *guru* directly gives *mantra yog* in the *Manomaya kosha*. There are many kinds of this *diksha*. The first is *nada diksha* which has almost 262 kinds. *Nada* means sound or the ether. This *diksha* brings about reorganization of the atoms of the element of ether or *akasha* in the body. The second *mantra* or *vidya diksha* is given with *mantra* and rituals. As *Gayatri mantra* is given in the thread ceremony, similarly *mantra* is transmitted on the *akash* element of our body. The third *vidyadi devta diksha* makes the *sadhaka* see the particular deity of the respective *mantra*. The fourth *Narayana diksha* is given by *Narayana rishi* and is described in a book of *Tantra*, 'Vasudeva Rahasya'. *Samaya diksha* is given with respect to the deities of the six plexii. The deities *Brahma, Vishnu, Rudra, Ishvara, Parabrahma* and *Sadashiva* belong to heart, throat, palate, central spot between the eyebrows, *Brahmarandhra* and forehead. These kinds of *diksha* have further kinds like *Kriyavati, Varnamayi, Kalavati* in the form of touch and speech, *Vedhapadi* and *Sampradayiki*. Those who give these *diksha* are *sadgurus*.

Vidhi diksha and *yog diksha* remove the impurities and afflictions in us. Our *karma* is eradicated and the feeling of renunciation starts pervading. The key word of all these *dhyana yogas* is *mantra*. *Laya yog, Hatha yog, raja* or *dhyana yog Samadhi, Kundalini* do not exist without *mantra*. What is the *maha mantra* about *mantra*?

ओम् इति एकाक्षरं ब्रह्म व्याहरन् मां अनुस्मरन् ।

य : प्रयाति त्यजन् देहं स: याति परमां गतिम् ।।

As it is said in the *Gita* "the *sadhaka* who leaves the body while reciting the *mantra* of *Omkara* and thinking of Me, goes to the spiritually highest place". *Pranava* is the crown of *mantra yog*. We have thought about the sixteen parts of *mantra yog* here. This concludes the explanation of *Mantra yog*.

नादरूपो स्मृतो ब्रह्मा नादरुपो जनार्दन: ।

नादरूपा पराशक्ति: तस्मात् नादात्मकं जगत् ।।

Brahma, Janardana and the highest power of the universe exists in the form of sound. So the universe is sound itself.

Shri Krishnaarpanam astu

✢ ✢ ✢

Discourse - 26

Japa Yog

We have seen that *Japa* is like a divine tree that grants wishes. The purpose behind *japa* may be spiritual or worldly, the purpose is served by *japa*. It is inherent in the *sadhana*. The kinds and methods of *japa* depend upon the purpose of the *japa*. It is also true that there may be different categories and hierarchy of *japa* even for one purpose. The important point is-the purpose may be one but on what level the *japa* is being performed. If *japa* is to be done as a *yog sadhaka*, it becomes *svadhyaya*, a component of *Niyama* which is a component of *yog*. Even the kinds of *japa* for *svadhyaya* may be different depending upon the level of the *sadhaka*, whether he is *adhamadhikari, arambhadhikari uttamadhikari* or *madhyamadhikari*. Observance of *Niyama* on our level, on the level of an accomplished *yogi* and of some *Jnaneshwar* differs vastly. Naturally the method of *japa* differs according to the hierarchy of the *sadhaka*. Suppose, the purpose is to achieve merit, but there is no specific kind of *japa* for achieving merit. The kind of *japa* depends upon the level of *sadhaka* and also the kind of merit the *sadhaka* wants to achieve. So the rites and rituals of *japa* mainly are decided by the hierarchy of the *sadhaka*.

The spiritual sciences mention and accept *japa* for different purposes like exoneration of sins, retribution and achieving merit. Many kinds of *japa* are described in the sciences of *karma* and *Dharma*. It is among the kinds of penance and observances for these purposes. It is included among the rituals for the sake of gods and ancestors. The various *yajnas* in the *Vedic* culture have various *japa* in them. Health sciences have *japa* in them. There are *mantras* as remedies as well as medicines and these *mantras* are *japa* only.

Japa is a vital part in all these places. It is found to be important in all these sciences. So *japa* itself is a vast science and it needs several births to study all these kinds of *japa*.

Japa is applied for many purposes and on many levels. We do *japa*. *Mirabai* also did *japa*. *Surdas, Ramdasa, Vashishtha* and *Vishwamitra* also did *japa*. It is difficult to classify *japa* and it is unwieldy. The kinds of *japa* are almost innumerable. The *sadhana* of *Nama yog* is *japa sadhana*. *Nama* means nomenclature or name. Kinds of *japa* are important in *Nama yog*. We can consider a broad classification here.

Eighteen kinds of Japa

We are going to consider eighteen kinds of *japa* and almost all kinds of *yog* are included in them. The context here is *yoga sadhana* only. We are not thinking of *japa* of any other kind of *sadhana*. We are thinking of *Nam yog*. We can only imagine what must be the number of kinds of *japa* in the sciences of *karma* and *Dharma*. The eighteen kinds of *japa* in the context of *yog sadhana* are vast. The first kind is *Nitya* or regular. As the name suggests, it is done at a particular time, in a particular condition and is performed as *sadhana*. So it is important from the point of view of discipline for the mind, *chitta* and mentality. This creates overall discipline while taking care of other rituals. The restriction of regularity is important for the *yog sadhaka*. The second kind is *Naimittic* or ad hoc. It depends upon particular occasions, such as festivals or holy days. Time of *Parva*, of eclipse of the moon or sun, the day of the birth of Lord *Shri Rama* or *Shri Krishna, Ekadashi* or *Shiva* festival are some of the occasions when they do *japa* of the personal deity. This kind of *japa* is done also in adverse times, when the stars are not favourable. They do this kind of *japa* when the stars like Saturn, Jupiter or Sun are not favourable. The third *japa* is called *Kamya japa* which is done for wish fulfillment. This is done to get the guidance and blessings of *Guru* or Master. The fourth kind is called *Prayashchitta*, exoneration or exculpation. Sins are committed by us knowingly or unknowingly, while in dreams or in wakeful or half wakeful state. They are committed in young or old age, in childhood or adulthood. *Prayashchitta japa* is done for exoneration of these sins. The fifth one is *Achala japa*. This is also *Nitya japa* but it is *Nitya japa* of a *yogi* who need not do any compromises for the regularity of *japa*. The ordinary persons have to make compromises because of their worldly engagements. This makes their *japa* hardly *Achala*. The *yogi's* frame of mind has *Achalata* of mind. This is done while following *Yama* and *Niyama*. The next one is *Chala japa*. This may be called mobile *japa* because it can be done at any time, in any way and at any place, while eating and drinking, while walking and talking. It is useful for controlling the wandering mind and stopping the waves of whims. The religious texts allow these actions and movements while doing *japa*. There are no restrictions for this *japa*. This *japa* helps to retain the good habits and guards from slips. The next *japa* is vocal which is done using all the organs of speech such as lips, teeth, tongue and palate. Naturally this is articulate but the next one is *Upanshu* or speechless. There is no utterance of words but lips are moving. *Bhramara japa* is like the sound of *bhramara* or humming of a bee. The humming is heard but the words of the *japa* are not understood. *Manasic japa*, as the title suggests, is done with the mind only. *Nishiddha japa* is a kind which has many restrictions and rules. It is probihited to be done at specific place, time, occasion and so on.

One more kind of *japa* is *Akhanda japa*. This *japa* goes on as long as breathing goes on. Whenever the person is waking, he starts doing *japa*. Whatever he is doing with his hands, mouth and feet, the *japa* continues. One similar japa is *Ajapajapa*. This goes on along with inhalation and exhalation. *Pradakshina* japa is performed while the *sadhaka* is moving circularly around an idol or around himself. *Pradakshina* is circumambulation around the sanctum sanctorum. Patanjali tells us a sutra- 'यथाभिमतध्यानात् वा'. The *Japa* for peace of mind suggested in this *sutra* is *Chitta pari karma*. Naturally this is important for *yog sadhaka*. *Dhyanaja japa* is for *dhyana* and has the nature of *dhyana*. *Patanjali* tells us a sutra- 'यथाभिमतध्यानात् वा'. Proper *dhyana* helps purification of mind. *Pranic japa* is done with *pranayama* which is called *samantraka pranayama*. The *sadhaka* takes support of *Omkara* in *Samadhi sadhana*. This *japa* is *Samadhi japa*. It is related to *Samadhi*, born/emerging out of *Samadhi* and also giving *Samadhi*. So these are different kinds of *japa* as *Nitya*, *Naimittic*, *Kamya*, *Prayashchitta*, *Chala*, *Achala*, *Vachic*, *Upanshu*, *Bhramara*, *Manasic*, *Nishiddha*, *Akhanda*, *Ajapa*, *Pradakshina*, *Chittaparikarma*, *Dhyanaja*, *Pranic*, *Samadhija*. This is a big classification.The *yog sadhaka* does all these kinds of *japa*.

Bhavana or dedication is extremely important in the *japa* in *Nama yog*. So now we shall think about *Bhavana* which is the heart, soul and *prana* of *Nama yog*. *Bhava* is emotional response to the act of *japa*. *Japa* is done with emotionality which is given by the meaning of *japa*. The psyche has a sympathetic resonance to the profile of emotions. Like in music or in our nervous system, there is a sympathetic body. Here the psyche is sympathetic to emotional profile of *mantra* or *nama*. Thus the mind has resonance to the emotions of *nama*. *Japa* is meaningless without *Bhavana*. Some technical kinds of *japa* give importance to sound or utterance. *Bhavanaa* is not so important here, because only the pronunciation activates the *japa*. If the pronunciation is correct, then only the *japa* is effective. In another kind of *japa* the meaning is significant. The meaning creates the *Bhavana* in the mind. *Patanjali* says in the topic of *Pranava japa* in his *yog sutras*, 'तस्य वाचक: प्रणव: तत् जप: तदर्थभावनम्' I So the japa should be done with the feeling of the meaning. *Nama yog* gives importance to meaning in the heart. It is the *yog* which requires *dhyana* which requires *Bhavana* and it should be intense.

Meanings of mantra

Nama yog has *mantra* in it. In the context of *mantra*, it should be noted that mantra has many meanings. They are mainly six. The first *Bhavartha* can be obtained from a dictionary because each and every word has been given a meaning by the tradition of that particular language speaking community. The second meaning is *Sampradayika* and it depends upon the *Sampradaya* or sect. The tradition of the *Sampradaya*, of the *Guru* or of the race decides the meaning. The third meaning is mystic, spiritual and ethereal. It is based in intuition and its nature is extra-terrestrial or celestial. Its source is *Samadhi* which is not meant for ordinary people. It belongs to epiphany in *yog* and accomplished sages, saints and *rishis* are the chosen ones to possess this kind of meaning. Naturally, no words in any language can be the carriers of this meaning. It is trans-verbal and trans-auditory. It is just to be felt. It is lost if it is brought to the level of articulation. It is beyond the reach of the *jnanendriyas*, the senses or the organs that receive knowledge. None can claim to have heard or seen it. This speechless meaning would get sullied if words would touch it. It just emerges without words. It may be called the '*para*' stage, or the first stage of speech out of the four stages. The difference is that it never reaches the 'second '*pashyanti*' stage, so there is no question of its reaching '*vaikhari*' or the fourth articulation stage. It can be rightly described as 'यतो वाचो निवर्तन्ते अप्राप्य मनसा सह I'. But this meaning creates *Bhavana* effectively which is vital for japa or *Nama yog*. Meaning is not the prerogative of grammarians only. That is why *Patanjali* has used the concept '*artha Bhavana*' in the topic of *japa*.

Nama is the core of *Nama yog* and *Nama* is nothing if we do not know the meaning of it. The *Nama* with its meaning arouses dedication and emotionality. This meaning depends upon the particular entity that we denote by it. Suppose that somebody's name is *Naaraayana*. In this case the word *Naaraayana* has no great meaning. Also the name of God is *Naaraayana*. Our mind is different when we call that somebody and when we address and pray to God. So the connection and relation between the meaning and the *Bhavana* that is aroused is important. When the devotee utters *Narayan* as the name of God his body and mind are overwhelmed. This is the impact of *Bhavana*. When *Sant Tukaram* says '*Ramkrishna Hari*' he experiences a total transformation. True *Bhavana* does not remain limited to certain parts of the heart but occupies the whole being. This is the tremendous range of the influence of *Bhavana*. That is why eight *Sattvic bhavas* are expounded in the context of *Bhavana* in *Bhakti yog* or *Nama yog*. What are they?

They are *Romancha* or hair standing on the ends, *Sveda* or sweat, *Ashru* or tears, *Kampa* or tremours because of emotional outpour, *Stambhana* or spellbound condition, *Svarabhanga* or tremours in the voice, *Vaivarna* or losing the identity, *Pralaya* or submerging. All these emerge because of the influx of *Sattva guna*. A flood of *Sattva guna* is created in the heart and it is so vast that it permeates and overflows the inner and outer being. The first *bhava* is *Romancha*. The hair on the body stands on the ends. Usually this happens because of fear but here the cause is remembering the deity or reciting his or her name. The next step is sweat on the whole body. This is the overflow of love. It brings tears in the eyes and makes the body tremble, but very soon it gives way to stunning. The devotee stands still like a statue. This is a kind of ecstasy. The face has no expression. Then his voice gets tremours. The next stage is losing identity because of transcendent condition of mind. He crosses his body and also his I-ness. This is followed by the flood or deluge of emotions of devotion. These are eight *Sattvic bhava*. *Japa* is the core of *Nama yog* because *japa* of *Nama* is continuously going on. So let us think about *japa* and its theory.

Japa is the heart and soul of *Nama yog*, rather of any *yog*, because it has *dhyana* process and *japa* is at the core of *dhyana*. Remember one important equation very carefully. No *dhyana* exists without *japa* and no *yog* exists without *dhyana*. Moreover, *japa* has extraordinary importance in *Nama yog* as the *Nama sadhana* of *Nama yog* is performed through *japa*. *Japa* fulfills many purposes. We have considered many purposes in the previous chapter. Since we are thinking of the theories and secrets of *japa*, let us once more think of the various causes and purposes of *japa*.

The short list that we made there is going to be long here. *Japa* can be *sadhana* of penance. It can also be the ritual of worship of God or the deities. It is there in the process of *yajna* or sacrifice. There can be *japa* for exoneration or expiation of sins. It can be for obtaining and increasing merit. *Japa* can give exercise to the mind and it can create discipline in the mind. *Japa* can refine and culture the mind. The mind comes out of fluctuations and becomes stable with *japa*. It is a process of *chitta pari karma* because it is a mental *sadhana*. It can make the mind noble, serene and peaceful. It can be done as *mantra sadhana, tantra sadhana* and also *yantra sadhana*. The worship of an idol consists of *japa*. When the devotee worships the idol with sixteen kinds of rituals he uses *japa*. It can purify the speech and make it clear. One important fruit of *japa* is obtaining knowledge. It is an important part of *Gayatri* recitation. Twenty-four cycles of twenty-four lakh *Gayatri japa* is *purashcharana* involving five crore and seventy-six lakh cycles of *mantra* and it gives knowledge. There are historical evidences of this.

Again, *japa* is for *dhyana* and *Samadhi*. Twenty-four kinds of *japa* are used in *yog*. So we can see what *japa* can achieve. When we consider the number of kinds of *japa* and purposes of *japa* we are enabled to know the theories of *japa*. The external form of *japa* is for making our speech clear and pure. It is also a mental exercise. When *japa* is done in a noble way, the mind also becomes noble. Nobility of mind is achieved by doing *japa* in *dhyaana*, for *dhyana* and for *sadhanaa*. *Japa* is important for *Tantrik sadhana* and *siddhi*. It is in *karma yog*, too. *Karma yog* has *japa, nama* and *nama sadhana* in it. As the musical instruments like *tanpura* are working while the singer is singing, so *japa* works when his *karma* is going on. This is a true *karma yogi*. This *karma yogi* is different from the *karma yogi* who does social service, digs wells, builds temples or hospitals or free inns. That *karma yogi* is no less important than this *yogi*. *Karma yoga* has devotion for God. In *dhyana yog japa* is at the core. We have already seen that no *dhyana* is there without *japa*. The breath of the *sadhaka* is accompanied with *japa* in *dhyana yog*. *Bhakti yog* has its soul in *naama sadhana*. So it is repeatedly told that japa is there in *Jnana yog, dhyana yog, karma yog, Bhakti yog*, worshipping, *sadhana* and also in prayers. It is in *Tantra sadhana* and *mantra sadhana*. This *sadhana* with *japa* can give the *sadhaka* superhuman or supernatural powers. *Japa* is in religious conduct, religious attitude and religious sadhana. *Japa* can awaken and increase physical, mental, intellectual and psychic powers.

Japa is there in jurisprudence. Japa is used for deliverance from sinning tendency. It is for expiation, as punishment and also for improving and converting the person. Jurisprudence also included *japa* and such *japa* can work as atonement.

Three parts of Japa

After taking into consideration the background of *japa*, let us turn to the core part of *japa*. We come to know three parts of it. The first one is sound. This sound might be heard, audible or unheard or inaudible but it does exist. We know the subtle sounds described by the Victorian poet, Lord Tennyson. They are the sounds of rose petals falling on the ground, of dew drops falling on the grass and of eyelids of a tired worker dropping down when he goes to sleep. This sound in the spiritual field is naturally subtler and holier than those sounds. *Japa* has a sound effect, whether the sound is made by *vaikhari* or the physical and audible speech or by mental speech. Sound effect can be broad and subtle depending upon whether it is mental or oral. If *japa* is in *dhyana*, is not an object of ears. The sound effect may not always be the object of the ears. Sometimes we are thinking and we think that there is no sound but this is not correct. Even mental thinking has a sound effect. The second part of *japa* is the number. One utterance is not *japa*; there are many cycles of it. Some *japa* have specific number like eleven, twenty-four or one hundred and eight, etc. So the number is important. The third part is emotions and meaning. They are important even in the *japa* where sound is important. *Artha Bhava* is related to mind. So we have to think about *japa* with these three elements.

Three kinds of Japa

One more point about *japa* theories is that it is of three kinds— *vachic* or of speech, *manasic* or related to mind and *praanic* or related to *prana*. Naturally sound effect is important when *japa* is *vachic*. Number is countable in *nama yog* and *japa yog* in the context of *pranic japa*. The number of inhalations and exhalations with the utterance of *nama* is significant here.

The three factors of *japa* i. e. speech, mind and *prana* are related to three gods. The speech is governed by *Agni* or fire. It is believed and *Adhidaivic* constitution of body says that fire resides in the mouth and on the tongue. *Prana* is related to *Aditya* or the sun. The mind is under governance of the moon. In the western tradition also the moon or lunar is related to mind. The psychologists observe that fluctuations of the mental patients have a connection with waxing and waning phases of the moon. So the ultimate classification is-

Speech	Mind	Prana
Sound	Artha bhava	Number/Quantity
God of Fire	God of Moon	God of Sun

The organization of the *japa* of mind is vibration + rhythm + harmony. The second part of *japa* is number. The number 108 has some significance in this part, according to our tradition. What is the reasoning of this significance? Perhaps the 4 kinds of speech- *vaikhari, madhyama, pashyanti, para*-x 3 factors of speech, mind and *prana* x 3 factors of Sound, *Artha bhava*, and Number/Quantity = 4x3x3x3=108 is the explanation. *Nama* is the core of japa or *nama yog*. The science of *bhakti yog* tells us that God is omnipotent, omnipresent and omniscient; He possesses the Spirit of Glory itself. Yet he has a need and fascination for *bhava*. The saints tell us that He is thirsty for *bhava*. He is a slave of the devotees, of their *bhava*.

343

God helps the devotees, rather does their work. As the stories of *Janabai, Sena* and *Gora* go, God performed the duties of a maid servant, a barber and potter, respectively. He is ready to do anything for the devotees. It is the devotion of the devotees that makes Him do this. What is the medium of the devotees for doing this? It is *nama* of God. Recitation of the *nama* of God makes Him a slave of the devotee. This is not exaggeration but a fact. *Namdeva* made a dead cow live with the power of *nama* and *Ramdas* made a dead man stand on his feet with the same power. So *nama* has a miraculous power. The temporal and rationalist people will not agree with this and say that this will make people inert and weak. The modern culture does not accept the power of *nama* but history gives evidence for it. The biographies of saints tell us the same thing. Atheists do not respect *nama* because they do not know the mystery of *nama. Kabir, Chaitanya. Tyagaraja, Tukaram* became what they were only because of *nama. Nama* has helped people come out of their afflictions. So the *sadhana* of *nama* is very important in the present age of *Kali.* The power of *nama* can give everything in the world. Some lines from *Vishnu Sahasra Nama* say this clearly.

रोगार्तो मुच्यते रोगात् बद्धो मुञ्चेत बंधनात्, न अशुभं प्राप्नोति मानव:।
यशो प्राप्नोति विपुलं भवति अरोगो द्युतिमान् ।

A sick man will be cured and a bonded person will be free from his chains with the power of *nama. Nama* can save a person from evils, can give great success and make him healthy and full of glow. स्तुवन्सहस्रेण पुरुष : सततोत्थित : । A person who praises God with *naama* is always on the path of progress. Also, 'न क्रोधो न च मात्सर्यं, न लोभो नाशुभा मति: । *nama* saves a person from anger, jealousy, greed and evil thoughts. We can see the importance of this in the context of a *yog sadhaka.*

Patanjali has said that *japa* of *Omkar* removes obstacles in the way of *yog sadhana*. He gives a long list of the benefits of *japa*. *Omkar* can give freedom from illness, inertia, guilt, doubts, laziness, dwindling of dispassion, delusions, lack of firm decision, lack of stability which is attained, sorrows, unhealthy mindset, infirmity of body and from faults in breathing. In this way *nama* is a great boon to the *yog sadhaka* for his *sadhana* to be free from hindrances. Internal and external obstacles in the *sadhana* will be removed with nama lest he should be discouraged and careless. He goes on trying to remove the thorns and boulders in his path of sadhana so as to make the way smooth but in this material world it will be in vain. The only effective way is *nama sadhana*. Actually *Patanjali's Yog Darshana* gives importance to reason; yet he prescribes *nama* and *japa* for removing obstacles and making the way smooth. How many *sadhakas* have taken note of this point? Let us consider the *nama sadhaka*.

It is already told that *nama* has a great power. It makes God the slave of the devotee. Of course, our *nama sadhana* cannot be like that of *Tukaram, Ramdas* and such devotees. It is also told that nama can remove afflictions and it is a panacea for all problems. One can ask what logic there is behind it. Then we should remember that there are different categories of *naama saadhaka*. It is important to note that *nama sadhana* or *japa sadhana* can do this work at a particular stage and so the stages in *nama sadhana* should be remembered. *Nama sadhana* is there in the beginning stage at our level but it is there as a part of *ashtanga yog*. The *Ishvara Pranidhaana* part of *ashtanga yog* has its starting point in *nama sadhana*. So at this stage we cannot expect the proficiency or fruits of *nama sadhana* as *Tukaram* obtained it. We cannot get his experience at our primary

345

level. This would be as contradictory as if a learner is learning a b c of English and wants to get mastery over Shakespeare. And even then it is necessary and it has its own importance.

Patanjali has brought it in as a part of *Niyama*. In the first *Pada* he has explained the importance of *japa* which can destroy the enemies of the mind. So this *sadhanaa* starts in the *Ishvara Pranidhana* part of *Niyama*. The *yog sadhaka* should remember this and give an appropriate place to *nama japa* in their *sadhana*. In the beginning it might be mechanical; that does not matter. After all, it is a part of the penance and so he should obtain the prerequisites such as faith, devotion, theism, piety, purity, steadfastness and so on. He should think of all the ways of sublimating the mind. Oblation, worshipping, *pranayama* are some of the ways. If the mind is first made noble, serene and magnanimous through these and then *japa* is performed, it certainly proves to be effective.

Yoga tells of many techniques to make the mind noble, serene and peaceful. *Nama japa* can be used along with these techniques. *Satsanga, Sadhanasanga and Shastrasanga* are also ways of enhancing nobility among ourselves. This nobility sharpens the weapon of *nama* and it gets efficacy. *Satsanga, Sadhanasanga and Shastrasanga* increase *sattva guna* and these three *sangas* are the regulators of our habits about food, movements, behaviour, thinking, studying and so on. They bring among ourselves intensity and profoundness of feelings. It also creates the power capacity needed for *nama sadhana*.

Yog sadhana gives the techniques of doing *nama sadhana* through *prana*. The *Chhandogya Upanishad* consists of *Udgeetha Vidya*. This *Vidya* tells about *Omkar* penance. It is told there that this *Omkar* penance proved fruitless when it was done with other organs

346

but it became successful when it was done with the main *Prana*. The *yoga sadhaka* handles this important technique. He uses *sadhana* with different aspects such as *Satsanga, Sadhanasanga and Shastrasanga,* good habits about food, movements, behaviour, thinking, studying *yama, niyama, asana, pranayama, bandhas, mudras.* The *nama sadhana* of the *yog sadhaka* is not done only with the rosary in the hand and it has many such aspects. That is why he can climb the great mountain of the *sadhana.*

The spiritual *sadhaka* or *yog sadhaka* has to give some time to *japa sadhana* during his regular *sadhana.* He needs this particular and regular *japa sadhana.* The *ashtanga yog sadhaka* does not forget that *japa* is a part of *ashtanga yog sadhana. Shaucha* is a part of *Niyama* which is related to *japa* and it is important for internal purification. Every devotee knows that *japa* gives purification of mind and *chitta.* यः स्मरेत् पुण्डरीकाक्षं स बाह्याभ्यंतरशुचिः । You may be in an impure or pure state of mind, You may be in any state of mind and body. If you think of the Lord with lotus eyes, you are bound to get internal and external purity. So *japa* gives purity and *japa* also gives *Santosha,* another part of *Niyama.* Mythologies, biographies of saints and their literature give us plenty of examples to prove that *nama* gives peace and purity of mind.

One more element of *Niyama* is *Tapas* or penance. *Japa* is a kind or way of penance. The *yog sadhaka* has to get his organs-*indriyas,* senses purified, which is almost a *siddhi* for him. *Yog sadhana* may be in the form of *dhyana, pranayama, pratyahara* or *asana,* and the contribution of organs is exemplary. *Japa* helps him to accomplish strength for these organs. *Japa* is important also for getting freedom from the natural tendencies of these organs. As *Kalidasa* has mentioned, just like water, these natural tendencies are prone to flow downwards. They are susceptible to fall in the trap of pleasures easily. We have to try hard to pull them upwards and towards sublimation. *Japa* helps to dissuade them from pleasures. *Japa* gives the mind discipline, control, balance and governance. Even the *Svadhyaaya* part has *japa* in it. *Vyasa Bhashya*, the treatise on the *Patanjali Sutras*, also mentions the importance of *japa* in the explanation of *Svadhyaya*. *Svadhyaya* includes the study of the spiritual sciences of religions, of *karma*, of the *Gita* and so on. Along with it, *Svadhyaya* has *japa* of deities and of *Omkar*. Even the part of *Ishvara Pranidhana* contains worshipping which has prayers. Prayers cannot be done without *japa*. In this way all the five factors of *Niyama* contain *japa* in them. *Japa* exists for the *sadhaka* in so many ways, for so many purposes and he has to use it in many ways.

Generally, the *sadhaka* is not aware of the importance of *japa* as it comes in different forms in his *yog sadhana*. He may not be doing it every day as a rule but it comes in many forms. As we have seen, it may be for *Shaucha, Santosha, Tapas Svadhyaya, Ishwara Pranidhana* or for purification or sublimation of mind. He has to do it at a particular or specific time. He does *japa* of *Gayatri* which is very beneficial for him. He does *Aghamarshana japa, Ajapajapa,* pre-*dhyana japa* and other kinds of *japa*. He cannot do without *Gayatri japa* if he is ordained in the *Gayatri mantra*.

The *Aghamarshana japa* mentioned above has a specific purpose. Man is bound naturally to be a prey to deviation from sacred frame of mind. This may be avoided by him when he is waking but he has little control over it when in sleep. Even a strict disciplinarian and *sattvic* person loses control of himself in his dreams. This was recognized by our wise and practical ancestors. They called it *Svapna Dosha*. Manu has mentioned a *Sutra* about this in his *Manusmriti*.

This is a *Sutra* for expiation of sins. So the *vaidic*, the *Brahmana* has to recite it every day. It occurs in the first part of *Taittiriya Aranyaka* in the 31st *Kandika*. 'पुन: मां एतु इंद्रियम् । पुन: आयु: पुनर्भग: । पुनर्ब्राह्मणमैतु मा । पुनर्द्रविणमैतु मा ।' The *Aghamarshana* mantra is 25th *mantra* occurring in tenth part in *Taittiriya Aranyaka*. This is a part of the *Sandhya Vandana*, too. सूर्य: च मा मन्यु: च मन्युपतय: च मन्युकृतेभ्य: पापेभ्यो रक्षन्ताम् । यत् रात्रो पापं अकार्षम् । मनसा वाचा हस्ताभ्याम् । पद्भ्यां उदरेण शिश्नेन । रात्रि: तत् अवलुम्पतु । यत्किंच दुरितं मयि । इदं अहं अमृतयोनौ । सूर्ये ज्योतिषि जुहोमि स्वाहा । The sun god is prayed and worshipped with this *mantra*. The worshipper says, "O sun god, whatever sin is committed by me in sleep or in the waking state, all that should be removed. Please guard me. Whatever sins are accumulated in me, make me free from them. Make me free from all those sins that are committed by my hands, feet, stomach, penis or any other organ. I am praying you for this." The tradition tells that every person twice-born i. e. *Brahmana, Kshatriya, Vaishya* should do *japa* of this *Aghamarshana* mantra. The *pranayama mantra* or *mantra* of *soham sadhana* helps to give a *yogic* mindset and makes the *chitta* eligible for *dhyana*. *Pranayama* with *mantra* is important in *yog sadhana*. A *shloka* in the *Garuda Purana* is very important for the *yog sadhaka*. It says, 'करिष्यसि सांख्येन, किं योगेन नरनायक, मुक्तिमिच्छसि, राजेन्द्र, कुरु गोविंद कीर्तनं' O King, you may be a *sadhaka* of *yog* or *samkhya*. But if you want salvation, do *japa* of *Govinda*." In *Purana Tantra* it is said, 'जपयज्ञात् पर: यज्ञ: अपर: न अस्ति इह कश्चन, तस्मात् जपेन धर्मान् काममोक्षार्थ साधयेत्' The *yajna* of *japa* is the most important *yajna*. You can achieve *Dharma, kama* and *moksha* also with *japa*. A shloka in *Bruhan Naradiya Purana* also tells, 'हरेर्नाम हरेर्नाम हरेर्नाम एकं केवलं कलौ न अस्ति एव न अस्ति एव न अस्ति एव नास्त्यैव नास्त्यैव नास्त्यैव गतिरन्यथा ।' In this age of *Kali*, the only way out of afflictions is *nama japa* of *Hari*. There is no other way out.

Vedavyasa who wrote the commentary on *Yog Sutras*, has said, 'स्वाध्यायात् योग आसीत् योगात् स्वाध्याय: स्वाध्याययोगसंपत्त्या परमात्मा प्रकाशते ।' We should accomplish *Svadhyaya* with *yog*, we should accomplish *yog* with *Svadhyaya* and with both of them, we should accomplish light for our soul. *Svadhyaya* is *japa* or *Omkar japa* here. A *shloka* in *Pandava Gita*, tells us that we should recite *nama* of God while eating or drinking or talking or walking. This helps us immensely. It is as follows- 'गोविंदेति सदा स्नानं गोविंदेति सदा जप:, गोविंदेति सदा ध्यानं सदा गोविंदकीर्तनम् ।।' So *nama* is a panacea, it is a great religion, a penance. Saints have talked about it at length with great meaning.

Place of Japa

Nama japa will be effective if the discipline about its utterance is followed faithfully. The place of *japa* should be holy and full of noble vibrations. Fruition of *japa* depends upon the quality of the place. A *shloka* in *Linga Purana* says, 'गृहे जप: समं विद्यात् गोष्ठे शतगुणो भवेत्'. The *japa* in the cowshed is more effective than in the house.The *Devi Bhagavata* says, पर्वताग्रे नदीतीरे बिल्वमूले जलाशये गोष्ठे देवालये अश्वत्थे उद्याने तुलसीवने 'पुण्यक्षेत्रे गुरो: पार्श्वे चित्तैकाग्रस्थलेऽपि च । पुरश्चरणकृत् मंत्र: सिध्यति इति न संशय: । *Japa* is more effective at the top of the mountain, on the bank of the river, at the bottom of a *bilva* tree, near a lake, in a cowshed or a temple, in a garden of *ashwattha* or basil, near a Master. This kind of *japa* gives concentration and so can give great fruits. The place of *japa* should be clean and without insects, ants and dust. It should not be brightly lighted or windy. It should be slightly lighted, peaceful and without fear. It should have a divine touch about it.

350

Rosary for Japa

The next point is - how should be the rosary? Usually it has one hundred and eight beads. Famous sacred rosaries are *Rudramala*, *Tulsimala* (basil), *Chandanamala* (sandalwood), *Sphatik* (crystal) *mala* etc. The *Tantra* describes two kinds of *malas* - *Jayamala* and *Vanamala*. *Vyjayantimala* or *manimala* is *Jayamala* and *mala* of pearls is *Vanamala*. *Garudimala* is made of bones of animals like snakes. It is a part of *Tantra* and it is used for effective treatment of certain diseases. *Malas* of Hindus have 108 beads and those of Jains have 111 beads, those of Buddhists have 108 or 112, *Yavana* sects have 99 or 101, Christians use 100 or 150 and Jews use 32 or 99 beads. So, all the religions use *japa sadhana*. *Tulsimala* (basil) is sacred for the *Vaishnavas*, ivory for devotees of *Ganesha*, red sandalwood for Goddesses and *tripura sundara Rudraksha* for *Shiva* and for Goddesses.

Purposes of Japa

We have seen that *japa* is performed for different purposes. *Japa* is capable of giving various fruits. Though it is important for the *yog sadhaka* its importance varies according to the grade of the *sadhaka*. The basic importance of *japa* remains right from the beginning to the condition of *siddha*. The central place of *japa* in the *yog* or spiritual *sadhana* does not change. Proficiency in *japa sadhana* enhances the effectiveness of *japa*. *Japa* gives a ladder for the evolution and progressing of man. He gets penance, knowledge, sublimity gradually with the help of *japa*. He gets devotion and *mantra* with this instrument of *japa*. If we make a list of what all *japa* can give, it will be long. *Japa* can give the desirable, can remove what is undesirable, give wealth, health, removal of troubles, strength, power to fight evil tendencies and so on. *Japa* is a *sadhana* of so many things. It is *sadhana* of *karma, dharma, mantra, tantra, yantra*, mind, *chitta*, speech, intelligence, memory, *yoga*, worshipping, spirituality, *dhyana* and so on. *Japa* of *Gayatri* can give great knowledge which is proved in history. Recitation or memorizing is a kind of *japa* only. The power of giving attention is important. We find the mention of *avadhani*, *ashtavadhani* and *shatavadhani* which means ability of memory and of giving attention to many things at the same time. *Japa* can give the capacity to master all these.

Japa is mentioned in the sciences of religions as regular, contingent and *kamya* or desire-based. We do *karma* but *japa* is needed to make *karma yog* of the *karma*. The *vaidic* man recites the *mantra* before doing *karma* – 'श्रीमत् भगवदाज्ञया भगवत् कर्म रूपं करोमि' I am doing *karma* because of the order of God. A successful and accomplished *karma yogi* has *japa* of God attached to his *karma*. The idol of God is established with some ceremony for making it sacred. In the same way the *karma* becomes sacred when it is accompanied with the *japa* of God. *Japa* gives strength and purity to mind. *Japa* helps our health and proves to be a medicine. A certain *japa* described in *Soundarya Lahari* "ॐ ह ॐ" performed for 45 days can give great power.

Every language has certain *mantras* for different purposes. In Marathi, there are some *mantras* for removing migraine and headache. The *Sudarshana mantra* in Sanskrit 'ॐ ह्रीं सुदर्शनाय विद्महे, महाज्वाल्याय धीमहि तन्नाचक्र, महोदयात्' is useful for health. Some *mantras* are powerful medicines or antidotes for poison, snakebite and so on. The *mantras* of *Hanuman* and *Kalabhairava* are useful if one is possessed by evil spirits. Our tradition advises recitation of the *nama* of *Rama* for removing fear, confusion and weakness of mind.

Sadhana of *mantra* can give salvation. The science of *mantra* tells that *japa* of as many crores as the letters in the *mantra* can give us salvation. For instance, the *mantra* 'ॐ नम: शिवाय' has six letters in it. If we do *japa* of this *mantra* six crore times, it gives salvation. 'ॐ नमो नारायणाय' is a mantra with eight letters. If we do *japa* of this mantra eight crore times, it gives salvation. Similarly, 'ॐ नमो भगवते वासुदेवाय' and 'श्रीराम जय राम जय जय राम' have twelve and thirteen letters respectively. They also can prove fruitful in this way.

In conclusion, we have to say that *japa* is so important that it is almost like a *yajna*. We know the importance of *yajna* in the *Vedic* tradition and *japa* is equalled to *yajna*. Lord *Krishna* says in the 25th *shloka* of the 10th chapter of the *Gita* 'यज्ञानां जपयज्ञ: अस्मि. I am *japa yajna* among all the *yajnas*. So this is the greatest *yajna*. Again, this *yajna* needs no material like money or man power. This *yajna* has no kind of violence which had entered in the *yajnas* in the Middle Ages. Rather it is a counter to violence. There is no sense of pride in it. It is needless to explain how important it is for *yoga*. *Japa* is another name for God. This concludes the thinking regarding *Nam yog* and *japa yog*. Both these are higher kinds of yog. They are post-graduate courses in the spiritual sciences. The *sadhaka* can go to them only after the graduation of *ashtanga yog* is qualified. Of course, this is needed for any kind of *yog* such as *dhyana yog* or *jnana yog*. Any *yog* starts only after *ashtanga yog* is accomplished. *Nama sadhana* is so precious that it is at the core of the Hindu tradition. The factors of *ashtanga yog* included in *Niyama* naturally make us do *japa* of some kind. *Ashtanga yog sadhana* makes us gain the culture of *chitta* that is necessary for *japa* and *nama yog*. In this way we have thought of *nama* or *japa yog* as a kind of *dhyana yog*.

Shri Krishnaarpanam astu

✣ ✣ ✣

Discourse - 27

Laya Yog - 1

While doing the journey of *dhyana yog* after *ashtanga yog* is accomplished, the first stage that the *sadhaka* reaches is of *mantra yog*. In the process of *dhyana yog* the *mantra yog* of sixteen limbs is achieved and then he turns to *laya yog*. The fixed stages of the journey are *laya yog, hatha yog* and then *raja yog*. These are not different kinds of *yog* as many people believe today. In the *sadhana* of *dhyana yog* or of any *yog, ashtanga yog* is imperative. It is the core of our *Vedic* culture, or rather of the *sadhana* of life. Even if you are not a *sadhaka* of spirituality, the values of *ashtanga yog* are so important that they have to be cultivated in human life. *Ashtanga yog* is basic for any kind of *yog*. When the *yogi* is heading towards *dhyana yog*, the first stage is *mantra yog* of sixteen limbs. It is followed by *laya yog* of nine limbs, *hatha yog* of six limbs leading to *raja yog* and the point of culmination is *kundalini yog*.

We are going to consider here *laya yog* which is a kind of *yog*. Even if the word 'kind' is used here, please note that it is actually not a kind, but a stage after the *mantra yog* and before *hatha yog*. All these are not kinds but stages in the journey of *yog sadhana*. *Nama yog, nada yog, japa yog, Kundalini yog* are stages of the journey of *yog sadhana*. The word *laya* itself suggests the concept in it. The *laya* of mind or *chitta* is accomplished which keeps the *yogi* away and safe from the three kinds of agonies (*tapatraya*) of human life. An ill person does not feel the ailments when he is asleep, so the *laya yogi* is free from the sorrows. Human beings are subject to physical, mental, intellectual, emotional and so many other kinds of constraints. Man is oblivious of them in his sleep. *Laya* of mind and *chitta* rids the *yogi* of all these human constraints in the same way. We can see the psychology of *laya yog* here.

We can guess about the nature of *laya yog* when we try to understand the physiology and psychology of sleep. Even an ordinary man experiences this *laya*. Moreover, we feel this *laya* or a shade of it, in the waking state at some moments. When we are listening to sweet melodies we become one with those tunes. Other arts also offer us this kind of heavenly experience if we are lost in the appreciation of their beauty. Even the mind of a common man is capable of experiencing this *laya*. His mind or *chitta* sometimes gets *laya*. When we are lost in the enjoyment of the pleasures of senses of sound, touch, beauty, taste or smell, we are in a spellbound state. We forget the outside world when we are reading an engrossing novel that depicts great truths of life. A person may forget everything else when he is watching a great painting or reading beautiful poetry or even while relishing some favourite delicious dish. The enchanting tunes of a violin or sitar or sarod take us beyond or above the mundane world. Even a diseased person is temporarily free from his ailments. Sometimes this makes the patient forget the doctor's instructions and then suffer the consequences. This is a shade of *yogic chitta laya*. That is why they are making a study of the healing effects of music on patients. The tunes of Lord *Krishna's* flute enchanted even the animals. Perhaps the mind of every living being is fit for *laya*. But this is merely to say that every mind is capable of *laya* and we should not overlook the vast difference between *chitta laya* and *laya yog*. They should not be confused with each other.

The Sanskrit word used for the condition of getting *laya* in great happiness is *mantra mugdha*. It is a word in *yogic* terminology. This means enchanted or spellbound. Amusingly, *mantra* means chant or spell. So both the Sanskrit and English languages suggest the same idea of *laya*. Thus *laya yog* manifests the entire psychology of enchantment. Rather we can get to know the physiology, psychology and physical chemistry of enchantment in *laya yog*. *Laya* of *chitta* is a lofty, quiet state of mind which is above normal. It is called supraconsciousness in modern parlance. This is primary knowledge of *laya yog*.

How is this *laya* of *chitta* achieved? *Laya* is achieved because of *mantra* and through *mantra*. The higher psychological state of identification with heavenly music depends upon the appreciation of the tunes. *Mantra* does the same for *laya yog*. *Mantra* is the beginning and core of *laya yog*. Which *mantra* gives this *laya* of *chitta*? The reply is *bija mantra*. There are *bija mantras* of the six *chakras*, of *sadhana* of the deities. *Laya* of *chitta* is achieved through them leading to *laya yog*. *Soham* or *bija mantra* or *hamsa mantra* and *nada* also give *laya* of *chitta*. *Nada* is important in *prana kriya* and *prana sadhana*. The sciences refer to *nadanusandhana*. This *nada* is called *anahata nada*. So *mantra yog* is the foundation of *laya yog* and *ashtanga yog* is the foundation of *mantra yog*. Naturally, *ashtanga yog* contains some components of both *mantra yog* and *laya yog*. So the journey is *laya yog* through *mantra yog* through *ashtanga yog*. There is no by pass for *laya yog*, neither there is a by pass for *hatha yog*.

Some misunderstanding about Hath yog

There are many misconceptions about *hatha yog*, too. They take it to be *yog* of *asanas*, of *pranayama* of *bhastrika*, *shat kriyas* on physical level and so on. They give jerks to the abdomen and call it *uddiyana* or *nauli* and name it as *hatha yog*. So also never forget that *hatha yog* is not an alternative for *ashtanga yog*. The order of *sadhanas* in the science of *yog* is strictly disciplined. There are no short cuts like bypass or open university. *Hatha yog* cannot be achieved without *mantra yog*, because the *kriyas* in *hatha yog* have *mantras* or spells embedded in it. The *bhedana* (piercing) of the six *chakras* or awakening of the *kundalini* in *hatha yog* is not just jolting somebody out of sleep. *Mantra* is the sole way of awakening of *kundalini*. There is no other way of achieving it. The piper makes a snake sway and the tunes of his pipe remove the evil and brutal tendencies in it. It does not hiss or bite even when there are onlookers around. So nothing like *bhastrika, nauli, uddiyana, pranayama* or *shaktichalana* can awaken *kundalini*. Only *mantra* can accomplish it. So the awakening of *kundalini* without *mantra* in *hatha yog* is absolutely meaningless.

Laya yog and Ashtanga yog

Now let us turn to *laya yog*. Even if *laya yog* comes after *ashtanga yog* and *mantra yog*, many of its components are gathered from *ashtanga yog*. The *ashtanga yog sadhaka* who is 'arambhadhikari' also learns many *kriyas*, processes and important points in *ashtanga sadhana* itself. Some stable *asanas* such as *shirshasana, sarvangasana, halasana* make him acquainted with some components of *laya yog* and he is benefited by them. Rather, any *asana* can give the experience of certain kind of *laya* provided it is a *yog asana* and not just a kind of exercise. This *laya* may be different in different *asanas*; for example, the *laya* of *shirshasana* is different from that of *marichasana*. Every *asana* has its own particular *laya* when it is *yog asana*, which is above than a physical *asana*. Different conditions of *laya* are accomplished in the *asanas* of *ashtanga yog* *sadhana*. Particular mention has to be made here of *shavasana*. It is the treasure of *laya yog*. Many a gem of *laya yog* are gathered from the processes, experiences and success in *shavasana*. Components of *laya yog* are collected also from the kinds of *pranayama* used by the *ashtanga yog sadhaka*. *Pratyahara* in *ashtanga yog* contributes immensely to *laya yog*. In short, *laya yog* gets a solid foundation from *pranayama*, *pratyahara* and *shavasana* of *ashtanga yog*.

While thinking of *laya yog*, we have to think of the physiology of it. *Chitta laya* has a particular biochemistry or physiological components in it. It also has neurological, glandular and psychological components of modern sciences in it. It also gets *pranic* components because of *pranayama* or *pranic kriyas*. This part of the five or ten *pranas* such as *prana, apana, vyana, samana, udana, Dhananjaya, Krukara, Devadatta, Naga* and *Kurma* is very important. The *shat chakra kriya* through *asanas, dhyana* and *pranayama* is very important, too. So different parts of *ashtanga yog* give the *sadhana* of *laya yog*. The perspective related to *chitta* also has to be taken into account. *Patanjali* presents a small topic of *chitta prasadana* in the first *pada* of *yog sutras*. It thinks extensively of *laya yog*. Every *sutra* gives some thought about *laya yog* 'प्रच्छर्दनविदारणाभ्यां वा प्राणस्य' 'विशोका वा ज्योतिष्मती' 'वीतरागविषयं वा चित्तं' 'स्वप्ननिद्राज्ञानालंबनं वा यथाभिमतज्ञानात्'. *Laya yog* plays a significant role in all these *sutras* and theories of *chitta pari karma*. The *Ashtanga yog sadhaka* gets acquainted with *chitta* components in it. The *japa, dhyan* and *mantra sadhana* makes the *sadhaka* familiar with *laya yog* components.

We considered many components of *laya yog* here. The

physiological, neurological and glandular ones of them are found in modern sciences but the *pranic* components are not found there. They are found only in the science of *yog*. The components related with six *chakras*, their *bija mantra* and their *sadhana* also are to be found only in the science of *yog*. *Patanjali* has described *chitta pari karma* in the first *pada*. The components related to *chitta* in it can be achieved only in the science of *yog*. Also the components of *mantra*, *dhyana* and *japa* are handled in *ashtanga yog*. All the components described above belong to *pratyahara*. We make movements with joints, muscles, tendons, bones, cartilages and tissues. They are felt keenly in *asanas*. *Pratyahaara* has components related to *japa*, *mantra*, *dhyana*, *prana*, *chakra* and *chitta*. They give solid foundation for *laya yog*. So the foundation of *laya yog* is laid mainly in the *pratyahara* of *ashtanga yog sadhana*. The condition of "स्थिरसुखं आसनम्" in the *asanas* of *yog*, the *siddhi* of *asanas* as *dvandva anabhighata*, *pranayama* and *shavasana* collect components of *pratyahara* or *laya yog*. The components of *pratyahara* are foundation stones of *laya yog*. Rather, *pratyahara* is the *yoni* of *laya yog*. It is necessary to get some knowledge of this *yoni*. So let us think of *pratyahara*.

Our senses have a natural tendency of turning outwards and towards pleasures. The moment we wake up in the morning, our eyes look for what is to be seen, ears are eager to hear something, the skin is waiting for objects to touch and so on. As if the senses ride horses and begin striding after objects. The *Upanishads* have described a meaningful metaphor. The senses are the horses of the chariot of the body whereas the mind is the charioteer and if the charioteer is weak the horses decide where to go. Usually we find that the senses govern the mind and the body. The metaphor comprises a major part of human psychology.

The chariot in the above metaphor in *Katha Upanishad* will go ahead if all the horses proceed in the forward direction but if every horse chooses its own direction, what will happen to the chariot and the charioteer? We face the same plight. The five horses of our five senses dash in their own directions. The afflictions in our life have their source in this plight. That is why it is necessary to control them in spiritual practice or *yog sadhana*. And even if spiritual practice or *yog sadhana* is not our goal, control of the senses is needed for being successful in life. Control of the senses is necessary for succeeding in the worldly endeavours, too. Life becomes wayward without it. The reins of all these five horses must be in our hands. Otherwise they run astray and the purpose is defeated, whether it is spiritual or worldly. *Asanas* help us in this respect. Regulation of the senses is vital in life. So there must be the exercise of culturing of the senses in the spiritual practice or *yog sadhana*; and it is very much there.

Ashtanga yog contains the *sadhana* required for this control or regulation. *Asanas* may be done on physical level but they help taking the reins of the senses in our hands. The discipline of *Ashtanga yog* is effective in the behaviour, conduct, activities, thoughts, philosophy and over all level of life. If *sattva* or merit is achieved with right conduct, knowledge of sciences and penance, the reins of the senses can be in our hands. This regulation is obtained mainly from *pranayama* which is *pranic* regulation. *Japa sadhana, dhyana sadhana* and *shavasana* offer the components of *pratyahara* and other *yogic* components are given by *dhyana, japa, asanas* and *pranayama*.

If we want to control a horse, we must get the specific training of riding. We cannot take the reins or whip in our hands for controlling the horse without this training. Similarly the training for riding the horses of senses for the sake of *pratyahara* is given by *shavasana*. *Pratyahara* is opposed to outward and pleasure-loving tendencies of the senses. In horse riding the horses are to rush ahead but the process is reverse here. The horses of senses have to turn back. This is an amazing phenomenon. *Pratyahaara* means making the senses turn back to *chitta* from outward objects of pleasures. *Laya sadhana* of *chitta* is necessary for this regulation. The senses have to retire from objects of pleasures which can give sensory withdrawal or sensory abstraction. The process of *pratyahara* has *laya sadhana* in it. The relation of the senses, mind and *prana* in the context of senses is presented in a theorem in the science of *yog*. The 80th *shloka* in the 2nd chapter of *Varaha Upanishad* is as follows- इंद्रियाणां मनो नाथ: मनोनाथ: मारुत: मारुतस्य लयो नाथ: तत् नाथं लयं आश्रय ।, Mind is the master of senses, *marut* or *prana* is the master of mind and *laya* is the master of *prana*. So take resort to *laya*. *Laya* controls *prana*, *prana* controls mind and mind controls senses. This can show us the great contribution of the two components of *ashtanga yog* i. e. *pranayama* and *pratyahara*, in *laya yog* Our desires, tendencies of the senses turn to pleasures and indulgence easily and they are prominent enemies of *laya yog*. *Pranayama* and *pratyahara* do culturing of the senses and this can change the whole character of a person. Even a licentious person may undergo total transformation. These desires and tendencies are enemies of *pranayama* and *pratyahara*. *Yogvasishtha* describes the relation between desires, renunciation of desires and *prana* in *shloka* 80 of the 4th chapter in the topic of *upasana*.

वासनासंपरित्यागसमे प्राणनिरोधनं ।

This relation between renunciation of desires and regulation of prana has to be considered in the context of *laya yog* and *pratyahara*, because the desires are hidden behind the senses. *Pranayama* sublimates the senses and the mind. This pranayama is important to move back the horses of senses that are running astray. The importance of *pranayama* in *sadhana* of *laya yog* is immense.

The sciences have established the importance of the relation between *shat chakra* and *prana*. It is stated here that *prana* is related to *pratyahara* and *laya yog*. So the contribution of *shat chakra*, their regulation and *sadhana* is easy to understand. *Ashtanga yog sadhana* joins our mind, breath and *prana* and *pranayama* with *shat chakra*. So *ashtanga yog* creates 'communication'. This *sadhana* provides the background of management of *shat chakra* in *laya yog*. Just now we referred to *Varaha shruti* and *Yogavashishtha smriti* and saw that desires and mind are related to *prana*. So management of *prana* is important in *laya yog*. Management of the five elements in our body also is important. So the *sadhaka* should remember the role of five *pranas*, five elements, and management of five *pranas*, five elements and of *shat chakra*. The advice in *Shandilya Upanishad* is significant in this context. It gives us knowledge of esoteric physiology, because five *pranas* and *shat chakra* are a part of esoteric physiology. Both of them are never found in the gross physiology. This advice in *Shandilya Upanishad* is fundamental and significant.

We have considered in the beginning the various components of *pratyahara* related to *prana*, *chitta* and so on. The *Shandilya Upanishad* says that there are eighteen vital regions in our body. These are spots related to *pratyahara*. The students of *Ayurved* know

362

also the vital parts in the body but they should note that they are altogether different. The number of them, there, are thirty-two and their purpose and objectives are different. They are described in the context of defeating, stunning and disarming the enemy. The vital regions in *pratyahara* here are related to the process of *pratyahara*. This process is to accomplish *laya* of mind in those spots in a definite order and the mind there. This process of *pratyahara* is useful even in *shavasana*. The process is mentioned in the 69th *shloka* of the first chapter of *Shandilya Upanishad*. The spots are the toe, feet, ankles, shin bone, knees, thighs, anus, genital organs, then navei, heart, throat pipe and crown of the head. It is told in the process of *laya yog* that the mind should get *laya* in these spots in this order. So the journey is from toe tip to crown and we considered the stages in it. But remember, the toe is not just toe here; the ankle is not just ankle here; it is a stage in the journey. These are all the stages of *chitta laya* in the journey. The mind gets *laya* here. This is beneficial in *shavasana*.

If we want to understand the beginning of *pratyahara*, we should note that *pratyahara* is an important component of *laya yog*. *Pratyahara* is to turn the senses back. Its beginning shows its relation with *laya yog*. The *yogic* process of *pratyahara* starts well if the *sadhaka* has ample *shama* and *dama* in him. *Shama* is restraint of external senses and *dama* means restraining the mind. The spiritual sciences mention this and applaud it. *Shama-dama sadhana* is very important. The nature of *ashtanga yog* is such that it generates *shama* and *dama* which is the basic component of *pratyahara*. The *laya* of mind in *laya yog* is largely handled in *yogasanas*. *Patanjali* says that *asanas* should reach the level of *ananta samapatti*. The *sadhaka* has to obtain the introvert state and peace of *chitta* in *asanas*. *Yogasanas* are not meant as exercises for the body, muscles and bones. They should be done in such a way that a composed state of peace and balance is achieved and there is no duality on the plane of body and mind. *Laya* of *chitta* is to be obtained at least to some extent. Different *asanas* give different degrees of *shama-dama*. While experiencing them, the *sadhaka* is producing strength and power and he experiences it. *Laya* of *chitta* also is different in different *asanas*. The *laya* of *chitta* in *shirshasana*, *sarvangasana* and in the *asanas* in the position of lying on the back is different. This difference is not due to the change merely in the body posture but changing breathing constallations and those of *prana*. The change occurs in the bio dynamics and bio dynamics of statics. Breathing and *prana* position are different while lying on the back and lying on the stomach. So we experience different kinds of *pratyahara* in the *asanas* because of *pranic kriyas*. So *asana sadhana* gives us management of the five elements and of the six *chakras*. Especially, if we achieve the *kriyaa* and *prayatna shaithilya* of *asanas* up to *ananta samapatti* at least bit by bit, we can increase the amount of these qualities in us. Particularly in *shavasana* the components of *pratyahara* are generated, maintained and raised. The *sadhaka* can experience this even in the beginning of *shavasana*. This *asana* is like a laboratory for the research and development for *pratyahara*.

We achieve *laya* in the context of *ajna chakra* and *vishuddhi chakra* with particular *asanas* and *pranayama*. These plexuses are the resting places of the mind. So the *laya* of mind in particular *chakras* produce the components of *pratyahara* in a great quantity. Particular *mudras* also contribute in this respect. *Viparita karani, shambhavi* and especially *shanmukhi mudra* are immensely effective for *laya* of *chitta*.

Science of *nadi* is a branch of the science of *yog* which contains many important thoughts. The treatise '*Shiva Svarodaya*' throws flood of light on this science of *nadi*. It gives the process and kinds of *shanmukhi vidya*. It says that when the *sadhaka* succeeds in *shanmukhi vidya*, it gives a report of the five elements in his mind and body. This report is like blood reports or pathological reports that we get from a medical check up. The *yogi* can understand from this report which element is ruling him at a particular moment, whether it is the earth or fire or water, etc. He can make changes in it according to his requirements. If he finds that he is controlled by an unwanted element, he can make the necessary changes. This enables him to get the appropriate biochemistry for his body. Suppose, he wants to do *dhyana* and he is under control of the element of wind, this will make him unstable. According to the report given by *shanmukhi mudra* he devises suitable *pranayama* and attains compatibility in the elements for the proposed act or deed, element of ether is necessary for the sake of nobility needed for *dhyana*. He can manage to get the changes. This *dhyana sadhana* is significant in *laya yog*. Breathing through *sushumna nadi* is far useful for *laya yog* than *Ida* or *Pingala nadis*. The *yogi* gets to know from the report which *nadi* is working for his breathing. He can shift to the breathing of *sushumna* or *shunya nadi* and progress in *laya yogs*.

Even though *pratyahara* is a great contributory component of *laya yogs*, there are some other components, too. They are physiological, neurological, endochrynological or glandular, *pranic*, *mantric*, *japic*, *chakric*, *dhyanic* and so on. Let us get acquainted with each of them. The first one is related to physiological. This is physiology of our anger, hatred and attachment. We know these concepts. Anger brings about a total, inward and outward change in the body of man. Anger changes the biochemistry. We relate anger to fire. So it is connected to the element of fire. Our idiom also is based on this, the expressions for anger are flare up, kindle, fume, boil, fire up, etc. So there is physiology of all the emotions like anger, love, lust, depression and so on. Everyone's physiology is different. An ireful person has his physiology and a quiet person also has his own physiology. In short, the condition of *chitta* has its physiology.

Shri Krishnaarpanam astu

✤ ✤ ✤

We were considering the first factor or characteristic of *laya yog* which is physiological. We saw that physiological peace and well being is important for *laya yog*. It must have serenity, nobility, control and balance. As children have hunger and thirst, want toys or an outing and cry because of them. Every child has a different demand but all of them are crying and shouting. Imagine children in the joint families of olden times, not in the nucleus family of today. Imagine how women must have been peeved by the children's crying and shouting in those days. Similarly our body, our organs and mind have hunger, thirst and other desires. All of them are overwhelmed by this hunger and thirst. Every one of these organs has the hunger like a child. As the child cries, the organs also cry and demand. All the organs do not want the same thing at the same time because they want different things at different times. One wants to eat, the other wants rest, some other organ may want to sleep at that time. They make a chaos with these demands. When the children are sleeping, they do not cry for anything. Their demands have stopped at that time. In the same way, if the organs are sleeping, they do not demand and cry, and there is peace. This sleep of organs is hibernation. This calls for *pratyahara* rapidly and then *laya yog* also progresses fast. So *laya yog* needs gratification of all the desires. The whole body, mind, organs and senses should get this gratification of all the desires.

Aasanas, dhyana, pranayama or *sadhana* of *yog* bring a kind of regulation in the body. So these processes of *yog* are very important. They establish physiology of peace and serenity. This is the physiology of cosmos. Even a beginner can experience this to some extent. This *sadhana* of *asanas, dhyana, pranayama* or *japa* can give a balanced state of mind. So this physiology of peace, balance and nobility is significant. The physiology of *pratyahara* and *laya yog* is not just imaginary. The point is that *laya yog* has physical and physiological factors.

We can now turn to the other factor which is a neurological component. People with the knowledge of modern sciences know very well that any action of our body or mind or organs depends on the nervous system. If the eyes see, the nervous system decides how to see, what to see and so on. It is the nervous system that stimulates the body or mind or organs. It goes without saying that the very existence and nature of man has its source in the sympathetic, para-sympathetic nervous system or voluntary nervous system and involuntary nervous system. The common people also know this and its contribution. Now *laya yog, samadhi, dhyana* need a specific contribution of the nervous system. It is more significant for the *chitta laya* of *laya yog*. Rather, it would be correct to say that the nervous system takes the lead role in it. It is not exaggerating if we say that *laya yog* takes place under the guidance of the nervous system.

The nervous system is properly activated in the *sadhana* of *asanas, dhyana, pranayama* or *japa*. Especially brain and its working have an important contribution in the *sadhana* of *asanas, dhyana, pranayama* or *japa*. Also the contribution of *prana* is important. As a piper makes the snake sway with the tune of his pipe, so the *prana* controls the nervous system. The *yogi* controls the nervous system with the naad of *prana* and leads it to the proper point. He is like the ring master in a circus who keeps a tight rein on the beasts with his

368

whip. He curbs the nervous system with *prana* or *parana nada*. He does this for the sake of *dhyana*, undisturbed *dhyana*. He controls the nervous system so that the desires, hunger and thirst should not disturb the *dhyana* and make chaos.

The *yogi* enchants the nervous system with *prana kriya*, *mantra*, *japa* and *dhyana*. They have this power. Once he succeeds in this task, he can control his hunger and thirst, hunger and thirst of body, mind, organs and all kinds of desires. So he can get the contribution of the nervous system to bring about the condition conducive for peace, sublimity, serenity. The science of *nadis* and *pranayama* help this. The glands are used largely for this. Glands have a great contribution to and influence upon our mind, mentality and mental balance. Our kidneys have adrenal glands and they exude adrenaline. The modern sciences tell us that this adrenaline is a boon for our efficiency and energy when it enters the blood. It also influences our mindset. Today steroids work for the sportspersons in the same way. The dope tests show how such medicines bring adrenaline in the blood in a big quantity and create a great fund of energy, strength and vigour.

So the glands and their secretions boost the mental and physical energies. But the same glands have an opposite function in *yog*. They have to pacify the energies and bring peace for *yog tantra*. The *yog kriyas* such as *bandhas* and *mudras* have an access to these glands. *Asanas* in *yog* work upon them. The spot between the eyebrows has pineal pituitary glands. Their control on our mind is vital and they are called master glands. These crown glands are related to *ajna chakra*. Some *yog kriyas* and *asanas* have connection with *ajna chakra* and consequently with these glands. So the *sadhaka* can bring peace and changes in the mentality through these glands by doing those *asanas* and *pranayama*.

The secretions of glands are used to bring balanced mindset. This is the importance of glands. Now if we consider *prana*, it is next to *Omkar* in the *laya* of *chitta* because *Omkar* is the most powerful weapon of *laya* of *chitta*. *Prana* is the chief of all the internal energies. *Prana* is at the centre of human body, mind, organs, senses, will and renunciation and everything. It is fundamental to the existence. *Pranayama* is the working of *prana*. So we can see the importance of the role of *prana*.

Prana and the Chakras

We can consider the role of all the *pranas* they play in the six *chakras* of *muladhara, svadhishthana, manipuraka, anahata, vishuddhi* and *ajna. Udana prana* is in *vishuddhi chakra.* 'हृदये चित्तसंविद्' The name *vishuddhi* itself suggests the purpose and function of it. It can purify the heart, mind and thoughts. Today they use catalytic converters in technology. *Vishuddhi chakra* is like a catalytic converter. *Patanjali sutra* says,

कंठकूपे क्षुत् पिपासा निवृत्ति: ।

The throat pipe quenches and removes all kinds of thirst and hunger. Isn't that a great step towards purification? The *nadis* in the throat pipe enable the *sadhaka* to get it. This is a great contribution of the *vishuddhi chakra. Vishuddhi* is cleansing and purification. It spreads the element of *akasha* or ether in the mind which is nobility and sublimity. These are the significant qualities that bring about *laya* of *chitta. Laya* of *chitta* at the place of *vishuddhi chakra* which is throat pipe, is very effective. *Udana* and *vishuddhi kriyas* are important also in *shavasana*. Rather *shavasana* is a preliminary stage of *laya yog*. This is the importance of *Udana prana*.

We have biological and inborn desires that are difficult for controlling. The *laya* of *chitta* in *muladhara chakra* gives us control of these animal tendencies.

Svadhishthana chakra is the place of human individuality, outfit of 'I'-ness and the related emotions and tendencies. The *laya* of *chitta* in *svadhishthana chakra* destroys our excessive egoistic feelings. *Manipuraka chakra* is the place of the element of fire. We contain many kinds of fire in us. The emotions of lust, anger, greed, jealousy, infatuation are all fires in us when they are intense. We suffer many times because of their intensity. So the *laya* of *chitta* there curbs these fires. Again *Manipuraka chakra* is the place of *vaishvanara* or digestive fire. Digestion of good food there gives us *sattva* and *sattvic* tendencies.

The next *anahata chakra* is the place of *sadhana* of *nada*, concentration on *nada*. This is the place of *anahata nada*. It is *Omkar nada*. This *nada* is heavenly and it gives knowledge and salvation to the *sadhaka*. The *yogi* gets *laya* of *chitta* here which elevates him to the ultimate stage of *laya yog*. The 18th chapter of the *Gita* says,

ईश्वर: सर्वभूतानाम् हृदेशे अर्जुन तिष्ठति । (18 : 61)

The Divinity stays in the heart which is the place of *anahata chakra* and *anahata nada*. To concentrate upon this *nada* of *Omkar* and to be dissolved in it is the salvation. So we can see the importance of *laya* of *chitta* here. We recall a line in an *Upanishad* here.

भिद्यते हृदयग्रंथि: छिद्यन्ते सर्वसंशया:

God-realization cuts as under the web of *karma*, *vasana* or desires, and *kleshas* or afflictions in the heart. Then liberation ensues. The last part of the *shloka* from the *Gita* is as follows,

ईश्वर: सर्वभूतानाम् हृदेशे अर्जुन तिष्ठति ।
भ्रामयन् सर्वभूतानि यंत्रारूढानि मायया ॥ (18 : 61)

371

We are moving in this incessant cycle of *karma*, in the cycle of births and attachments. This is the *maya* or delusion created by God. If we want liberation from this, we have to get *laya* of *chitta* at this place. Even *Patanjali* says,

अंतकाले च मां एव स्मरन् मुक्त्वा कलेवरम् ।
य: प्रयांति स मद्भावं यांति न अस्ति अत्र संशय: ।।
प्रयाणकाले मनसा अचलेन् भक्त्या युक्तो योगबलेन च एव ।।
भ्रुवोर्मध्ये प्राणम् आवेश्य सम्यक् स तं परं पुरुषम् उपैति दिव्यम् ।।
सर्वद्वाराणि संयम्य मनो हृदि निरुध्य च ।
मूर्ध्नि आधाय आत्मन: प्राणम् आस्थितो योगधारणाम् ।
य: प्रयांति त्यजन् देहं स: यांति परमां गतिम् ।।

So the *anahata* place and *kriya,* are important.

The next *chakra* is *ajna* which is mentioned in the 8th chapter of the *Gita*. According to *tantra* also the *bija mantra* of *ajna chakra* is *Omkar*. The shloka in the Gita is'

ॐ इति एकाक्षरं ब्रह्म व्याहरन् माम् अनुस्मरन् । (8 : 13)

"The *yogi* should think of Me at the time of death while uttering *Omkar*. That will lead him to the place of the Divinity. This *dhyana* is to be done after confining the *pranas* at the crown of the head. This may be done by bringing them at the spot between the eyebrows and doing *bandha* there." As the Gita says, the *dhyana* is of *ajna chakra* and at the spot between the eyebrows. The *sadhaka* should remember that it is not for him but it is for the last moment of the life of the *yogi*.

"No doubt the *yogi* who thinks of Me at the last moment of life and abandons the body, reaches Me. His mind is fixed on Me and has the power of *yog* to concentrate at the spot between the eyebrows. He closes all the doors of the body and brings the mind in the heart with *dharana* of *yog* and then gives up the body."

The *shlokas* clearly say that this *dhyana* is for the last moment of life of a *yogi* and not for anyone else. So this is the contribution of the *chakras* in *laya yog*. The next part of *laya yog* and *pratyahara* is *chitta parikarma*.

The *yog sutras* of *Patanjali* have an interesting topic in the first *pada*. We find the core of spiritual psychology in this *chitta parikarma*. It tells of some ways of getting sublimity of *chitta*. It says,

मैत्री करुणा मुदिता उपेक्षाणां सुखदुःख पुण्यापुण्य विषयानां भावनात: चित्त प्रसादनम्

To have friendliness with the happy persons is one way. It is natural to feel jealous about them but jealousy should be overcome. The meritorious persons should be treated with our respect and gladness. So also there should be compassion for the suffering persons. Indifference towards the sinful persons is the right reaction about them. The 33rd *sutra* gives this advice to us. This attitude is a way out in the difficult situations in the *sadhana* of *laya yog*.

The other solution is a particular kind of *pranayama* described in the *sutra* 34. It is described as,

'प्रच्छर्दनविधारणाभ्यां वा प्राणस्य'

The *chitta* gets peace and balance by doing *prana dharana* after *rechaka pranayama*. The 35th *sutra* talks of one more solution-

'विशोका वा ज्योतिष्मती'

The *chitta* should be free from any kind of melancholy and full of light. The 36th *sutra* gives another solution as

"वीतराग विषयं वा चित्तम्"

The *chitta* should think of the persons who have renounced all attachment. They are saints and sages. Thinking about them is a way of beginning to become like them.

The 38th *sutra* advises to take support of the knowledge of how dreams and sleep occur.

स्वप्ननिद्राज्ञानालंबनं वा ।

It also suggests doing *dhyana* on the personal deity. It is a deep subject but let it suffice to note that *chitta parikarma* is an important part of *laya yog*. *Asana*, *pranayama* also make for the factors of *laya yog*. *Sadhana* of *nama*, *japa*, *mantra* and *dhyana* help to make the mind noble. *Mantra* or spell has a power in itself to attract and hold; that is why we use the word 'spellbound'. The word 'bound' also suggests 'bandha'. The *beeja mantra* that is used for the *kriyas* of the six *chakras* is also *mantra*. *Omkar* is *pranava mantra*. This is as important in any *yog* as the soul in the body, so it is significant in *laya yog*, too. The Universe emerges from *Omkar* and gets dissolution or *laya* in *Omkar*. No wonder, *chitta* gets laya in *Omkar*.

Omkar works in *dhyana yog*. The *mantra* of *karma yog* also is *Omkar*. It is expressed as

'हरि: ॐ तत् सत्'

The attitude necessary for *karma yog* is inherent in the words *Hari*, *Om*, *Tat* and *Sat*. The *karma yogi* is working with the spirit of a servant of God. He says,

'ओम् श्री भगवदाज्ञा भगवत् कैंकर्य रूपम्'

Whatever he is doing is done because of the dictate of God. *Omkar* is *pranava*. *Pranava* is the spell which praises God with overwhelming devotion.

'प्रकर्षेण नीयते स्तूयते इति प्रणव:'

Even the *Gitaa* suggests the central place of *Omkar* in the life in the universe. The Lord describes the death of the *yogi*. It is said that the *yogi* reaches the Divinity by thinking of Him with *dharana* and reciting *Omkar* at the last moment of his life.

'ओम् इत्येकाक्षरं ब्रह्म व्याहरन् अनुस्मरन्'

Omkar is essential in any kind of *yog*, and naturally in *laya yog* that we are considering.

Every *chakra* has its *beeja* mantra. The *laya* or *samaadhi* of *laya yog* takes place in the six *chakras*. The *beeja mantra* of *muladhara* is *lammm*, that of *svadhishthana* is *vammm*, that of *manipuraka* is *rammm*. *Anahata chakra* has its *mantra* as *yammm*, *vishuddhi chakra* has *hammm* and *ajna chakra* has *Omkar*. *Sahasrara chakra* has no *beeja* or seed. So, to recap, we should remember that the *samadhi* of *laya yog* takes place at the *chakras* with the means of *beeja mantra* in the respective deities of the *chakras*.

Chakras and their deities

Now let us think about the *chakras* and their deities. *Brahmadeva* is the deity of *muladhara chakra*, *Vishnudeva* of *svadhishthana*, *Rudradeva* of *manipuraka* and also *anahata*, *Panchanana* of *vishuddhi*, *Linga* of *ajna chakra* and *Para Brahma* of the seventh *sahasrara chakra*. These *chakras* are related to five *pranas*, their *beeja mantras* and deities. The *samadhi* of *laya yog* is achieved through these. *Japa sadhana* is understood to get the *laya* of *chitta*. *Japa* of the deity gives the effect like that of hypnotism, because the mind gets *laya* in the personal deity easily. Some *dhyana* oriented *asanas* are useful. Also *shambhavi mudra* or *shanmukhi mudra* are effective. *Shavasana* which is very important in *ashtanga yog sadhana* is almost the mine or laboratory of *laya yog*.

Generally people do *dhyana* on a lotus or an idol of *Krishna* or on *Ganesha* or *Shiva*, but the *dhyana* in *laya yog* is connected to *chakras*. At the primary level of the *sadhana* of the six *chakras* the *sadhaka* does not think of the *beeja mantra* and deities. Only some *kriyas* of *prana*, *asanas*, *bandhas* or *mudras* are used. But in *laya yog*, *laya* is achieved with *dhyana* through the *beeja mantra*.

These *chakras* are lotuses and even *Patanjali* has mentioned that it is important to get *laya* in the heart region.

'हृदये चित्तसंविद्'

Again *laya* cannot be achieved without *ashtanga yog sadhana* of *Patanjali*. The edifice of *laya yog* can be firmly built on the foundation of *ashtanga yog*. All the factors of *laya yog* along with *pranic* technology and *sadhana* are collected, although in the rudimentary form from *ashtanga yog*. It also gets maturity here.

'प्रयत्नशैथिल्यं अनंतसमापत्तिभ्याम्'

This letting go of efforts is a part of *laya yog* and it is practised in *ashtanga yog*. These elements of *laya yog* are tackled with at the level of *asanas* in *ashtanga yog*. *Asanas* are evolved to the extent of *prayatnashaithilya* and *Ananta samapatti* in *Patanjali's* technology. Here the *sadhaka* explores the huge mine of *laya yog* components. The *samapatti* in *Ananta* means *laya* of *chitta* is there.

As told earlier, *shavasana* is the mine of the bio-chemistry of *dhyana*. Even the beginner in *sadhana* can get the experience of peace of *shavasana*. This experience might be 0000000001% of the real effect but it is substantial for the '*arambhadhikari*'. The achievement of *ashtanga yog* leads to *mantra yog* of 16 limbs after which follows *laya yog* of 9 limbs. Since *laya yog* cannot be achieved

देवता : ब्रह्मा

शक्ती : डाकिनि

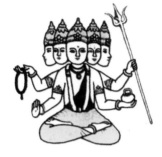

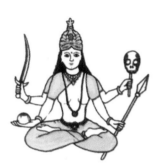

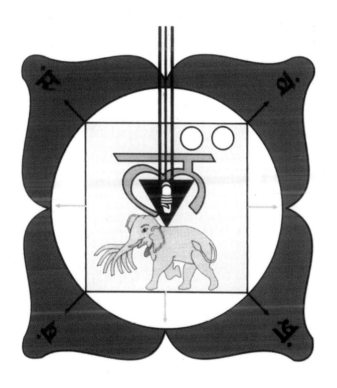

मूलाधार चक्र

देवता : विष्णू 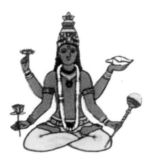 शक्ती : लाकिनि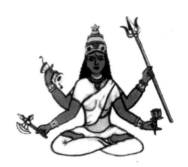

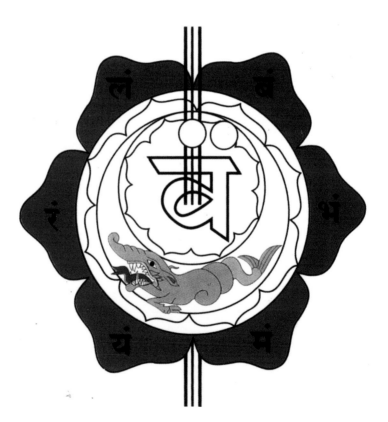

स्वाधिष्ठान चक्र

देवता : विष्णू

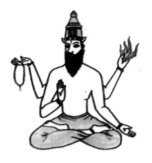

शक्ती : लाकिनि

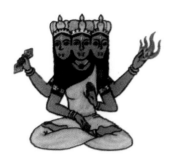

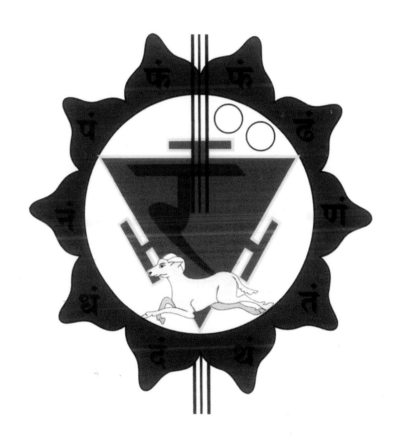

मणिपूर चक्र

देवता : ईश 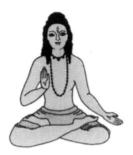 शक्ती : काकिणि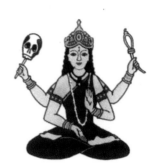

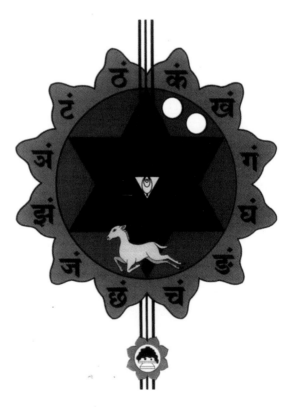

अनाहत चक्र

देवता : सदाशिव   शक्ती : गौरी

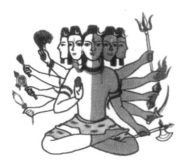

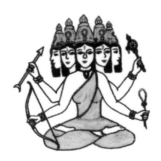

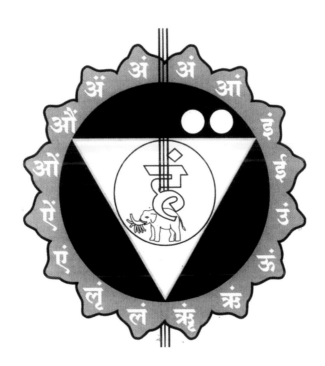

विशुध्दी चक्र

शक्ती : लाकिनि

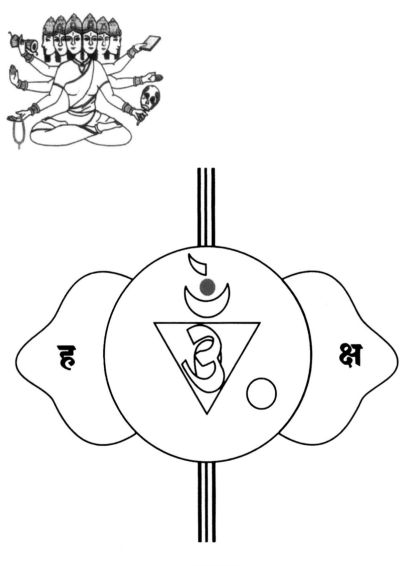

आज्ञा चक्र

without achieving *mantra yog*, it follows that the *kriyas* in *laya yog* are *mantric*. The achievement of *laya yog* leads to *hatha yog*. Today *hatha yog* is taken to be a simple kind of *yog*. They forget that it is the highest *yog* after *ashtanga yog*, *mantra* and *laya yog*. They think that *hatha yog* is a gymnastic feat of *asanas* and *pranayama*. It is not a superhuman demonstration of physical flexibility and steadfastness. The picture of a *hatha yogi* they have before their minds is an irate and merciless man practicing terrible penance and mental torment. Let it suffice to say that *Jnaneshvar* was a *hatha yogi*, his *sadhana* was *hatha yog* and the misunderstanding should be removed. Look at his life story, his character and his serene face. This is *hatha yog* It is not gymnastics of body and mind, please note. We can imagine the qualification of a *hatha yogi* who has achieved *mantra* and *laya yog* that come only after *ashtanga yog*. He has completed such a long and rigorous journey. The ideas prevalent about *hatha yog* today are just foolish. They still think that *raja yog* is of contemplative nature with *dhyana* at the core of it and *hatha yog* needs athletic skill without any mental peace. When we consider the process of *dhyana yog,* we should remember that the inevitable stages of the journey are *ashtanga yog*, *mantra yog*, *laya yog*, *hatha yog* and then *raja yog*.

Now let us think of the limbs of *laya yog*. It has nine limbs. They are *yama*, *niyama*, *sthula kriya*, *sukshma kriya*, *pratyahara*, *dharana*, *dhyana*, *laya kriya* and *samadhi*. This *samadhi* is *maha laya*. So this set does not have *asana* and *pranayama* of *ashanga yog*. *Laya kriya* follows *dhyana*. So the process of *ashtanga yog* is *dharana*, *dhyana* and then immediately *samadhi* but here it is *laya kriya* between *dharana*, *dhyana* and *samadhi*. So these are nine limbs of *laya yog*.

Ashtanga yog has *yama* and *niyama*. *Laya yog* also has them. But since the *laya yogi* is better a *siddha* and is better accomplished

important parts of *sthula kriya*.

The fourth limb is *sukshma kriya*. They are done mainly by *pranayama*. To create appropriate mindset through *pranayama* is *sukshma kriya*, so it is regulation of *prana*. This gives proper grounding for *laya* of *chitta*. The *yog* has to use the science of *svarodaya*. He has to know and use the *svara* of *ida, pingala* and *sushumna* according to the need. This part is very important. The *sadhaka* has already mastered it at the stage of *mantra yog*. According to the science of *svarodaya* the *saadhaka* should know the prominence of energy in his body and whether it is the same as required or expected and he should be able to bring appropriate changes in it. This is energy circulation. The outer atmosphere is made conducive to *yog* in *sthula kriya* and *sukshma kriya* manages it for the inner world with the help of the science of *svarodaya*. Prominence of the appropriate *nadi* and of the appropriate element out of the earth, ether, wind, water and fire is created. *Sthula kriya* makes the necessary changes. *Kumbhaka pranayama* is very important here. Its process is subtle but it is included in *sthula kriya*.

Shri Krishnaarpanam astu

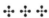

Discourse - 29

Laya Yog - 3

So *sukshma kriya* is done after the *sthula kriya* in *laya yog*. The *pranayama* needed for it is either *kevala kumbhaka* with *bhrumadhya drishti* or eyesight at the middle of the eyebrows or *shunya drishti*. The science of *Shiva Svarodaya* is very important for this. The study of this science tells us which of the five elements of the earth, water, fire, wind and ether is prevailing, which of the *nadis* of *chandra*, *surya* and *shunya nadis* is working, and which *nadi* we need. The *sadhaka* has to get the modification done according to it. He has to modify the *nadis* and *chakras* for compatibility. So he should know this science and make the modification with the help of *sukshma kriya*. He turns to *dhyana* with *Omkar* or does the *sukshma kriya* with the *beeja mantra*. So this is the fourth limb of *laya yog*. The science of *Shiva Svarodaya* is important here. These things are dealt with at the stage of *mantra yog*.

The fifth limb of *laya yog* is *pratyahara* which is a kind of *laya kriya*. *Pratyahara* is important in *ashtanga yog* and also in *laya yog*. It brings back the senses and takes them on the proper path. So it is useful in *laya yog*. The sixth and seventh limbs are *dharana* and *dhyana* respectively. They are based on *Omkar* and the *beeja mantra* of *Soham*. It is repeatedly told that *laya yog* is connected to *beeja mantra*. The *dharana* and *dhyana* are done with the *dhyana* of the *beeja mantra* and its deity. Every *chakra* as well as every deity has its *beeja mantra*. *Gam* is the *beeja mantra* of the deity *Ganesha* and *kleem* belongs to Lord *Krishna* and His *Sudarshana mantra*. Thus the *mantras* are ॐ श्री गं गणपतये नमः and ॐ क्लिम् कृष्णाय गोविन्दाय गोपीजनवल्लभाय पराय परमपुरुषाय परमात्मने.

We get to know this in the science of *mantra*. We have seen that

"राजयोगसमाधि: च उन्मनी मनोन्मनी अमरत्वं लयं तत्त्वं शून्याशून्यं परं पदम् ।

अमनस्कं तथा अद्वैतं निरालम्बं, निरंजनं जीवन्मुक्तिश्च सहजा तूर्या च इति एकवाचका : ।

It clearly says that this supreme state has different nomenclatures such as *raja yog, samadhi, unmani, manonmani, amaratva, tattva, laya, shunyashunya, niralamba, niranjana, jivanamukti, amanaska, advaita, sahaja, turiya*. All this nomenclatures points to the same and one thing only. So there should be no disputes about them. Since all these are one, there is no superiority of one and inferiority of the other. All of them denote one thing only.

A word of caution !

One statement of conclusion has to be made here. *Laya yog* is a post-graduate curriculum and it is of a very high level and it can be done only after completion of *ashtanga yog* and of *mantra yog* of sixteen limbs. So *laya yog* can never be the beginning of *yog sadhana*. *Hatha yog* comes only after *laya yog*. If we find *hatha yog* without these preliminary steps, it is not real *hatha yog*. This dummy *hatha yog* has only gymnastics of body and breathing and exercises of *prana*. There is no *mantra* in it. The *pranayama* and *bhastrika* in it cannot make it *hatha yog*. It is a *yog* at the pinnacle. Just by looking at steps prior to *hatha yog* we can see what it is. It is not for an unprepared, common and ordinary person. We are going to consider it in detail. *Hatha* is not *hatha* in the general usage which means stubbornness. The sciences say that '*ha*' and '*tha*' are two things that make *hatha yog*.

The point is—Accomplishment of *ashtanga yog*,which is made up of *yama, niyama, asana, pranayama, pratyahara, dharana,*

384

dhyana and *samadhi* is the prerequisite. Then the *mantra yog* of sixteen limbs has to be achieved which can bring about the accomplishment of *laya yog* At this point begins the *hatha yog*. This is the whole process of it. When we consider this process, it becomes obvious that *hatha yog*, *mantra yog*, *raja yog*, and *laya yog* are not different. It is important to note that *laya yog* comes after *mantra yog*. The main factors of *laya yog* are from *ashtanga yog*, especially *shavasana*. *Shavasana*, *pranayama* and *pratyahara* of *ashtanga yog* give much contribution for *laya yog*, rather they are the basic components of it. *Japa* or *dhyana* also help it.

Let us conclude the chapter with a theory about *Laya yog*. The sciences say,

इंद्रियाणां मनोनाथ: मनोनाथस्य मारुत: ।
मारुतस्य लयो नाथ: तत् नाथं लयं आश्रय ॥

Mind is the master of senses or organs. Wind or breath or *prana* is the master of mind and *laya* is the master of *prana*. So we see that there is an embedded connection between *laya yog* and *prana*, and the *laya* principle and *laya* process. So we have considered the *laya yog* of nine limbs. In the process of *dhyana yog* what naturally follows *laya yog* is *hatha yog*. So we will take up *hatha yog* now in the next chapter.

Shri Krishnaarpanam astu

has to get the help of some factors of *mantra, mantra yog, tantra* and *laya yog*. In all these processes *prana nadis* and their management are very important. The three *nadis* of *ida, pingala* and *sushumna; Brahma granthi, Vishnu granthi, Rudra granthi; bandha; mudra; kriya;* management of the *chakras* of *muladhara, svadhishthana, manipuraka, anahata, vishuddhi* and *ajna* and *pancha prana* are also at the foundation. The books on *hatha yog* explain *bandha, mudra, kriya* and *chakras*. The management of the five elements of the earth, wind, water, fire and sky/ether have to be achieved. The *sadhana* of the six chakras, *sadhana* of five *pranas* have to be achieved on the level of *dhyana*. *Mirabai* and *Chaitanya Maha Prabhu* had devotion par excellence for *Shri Krishna* and so they could do His *dhyana*. The *dhyana* in *hatha yog* is not like this. Devotion or emotions are not important but management of *pancha prana*, of *pancha* elements, of three *bandhas* and of *granthis* and *mudras* is more important.

The connection of *hatha yog* with *tantra* is significant. Concepts about esoteric physiology in *hatha yog* are according to *tantra*. Its processes and scientific parts are according to *tantra* concepts and *tantra* processes. *Hatha yog sadhana* is impossible without knowledge of *tantra*. This can give us some ideas about *hatha yog*.

The three *bandhas* such as *mulabandha, uddiyana bandha* and *jalandhara bandha* are important in *hatha yog*. They are included in *pranayama*, process of *pranayama, kriya* of *hatha yog*. The *mudra* like *simha mudra, Brahma mudra, shambhavi mudra, yog mudra, kaki mudra, maha mudra, ashvini mudra, amaroli mudra, khechari mudra, shanmukhi mudra, vajroli mudra, sahajoli mudra* also are used in *hath yog*. So *hatha yog* is more of these *bandhas* and *mudras* than exercises of body and breath. The books of *hatha yog* describe them deeply and at length. Many people think that *raja yog* and *hatha yog* are opposite and they have their images as fighting wrestlers. This is ridiculous. In fact they are complementary to each other.

हठं विना राजयोग: राजयोगं विना हठ:
न सिध्यति, ततो युग्मं आनिष्पत्ते: समभ्यसेत् ।। (2: 76)

Treatises on *hatha yog* tell this. So the misunderstanding should be given up. *Raja yog* is made up of *abhyasa- vairagya*. This *abhyasa vairagya* should not be only on the level of our nature and conduct but there has to be contribution of management of *pancha prana*, *nadis*, of esoteric physiology, three *bandhas*, the six plexi, *mudras*, *kriyas* and *pranayama*.

All these must be studied together. *Hatha yog* and *raja yog* are not rivals, so the *sadhana* should be done together until there is accomplishment. It is not wrong to say that when *hatha yog* is accomplished, *raja yog* also is accomplished. They help each other and one cannot exist without the other.

Samkhya philosophy and *samkhya Dharma* conduct is important in *raja yog sadhana* and *hatha yog sadhana* is needed for the ability to follow this conduct. The *hatha yog kriyas* of *prana sadhana* and *nadi sadhana* give this kind of ability and capacity. It can also help through management of the three *gunas* of *sattva*, *raja* and *tama*. This again shows the collaboration between these two *yogs*.

Note one more important point. It is said that *hatha yog* means *asana sadhana* or rather excessive *asana sadhana*. So the ordinary people are eager to learn *siddhasana*, *bhadrasana*, *padmasana*, since they are taken to be important in *hatha yog sadhana*. But the *asana* process in *hatha yog* is totally different. Putting feet on opposite thighs is not *padmasana*. Same is the case with *siddhasana*. They

we get from it? We cannot just imagine that we can get rid of all the physical troubles by doing *padmasana*. So the *padmasana* that is prescribed in *Hatha Yog Pradipika* is not for us even if we have flexible and strong legs. We may not be able to do it just because we have flexible joints of pelvis, knees, ankles and feet. Much more has to be done in it which is done by the *hatha yogi*. Billions of people in the world can do *padmasana*, sit in *padmasana* but how many of them are free from ailments? How many of them are free from ailments on account doing of *padmasana*?

This *padmasana* is not achieved just by putting the feet on opposite thighs. It is not just sitting straight. It is not mere posture and exercise of feet and legs. There is esoteric physiological activity and *tantra* involved in it. We have to bear in mind that the *asanas* explained in *Hatha Yog Pradipika* belong to a very high level. It is a grave mistake to think that *hatha yog* means doing mere *asanas* and that they are just physical postures.

So the explanation in the first chapter of *Hatha Yog Pradipika* makes it clear that we so-called *yog sadhakas* do not actually do the *asanas* of the level of a *hatha yogi*. The second chapter of *Hatha Yog Pradipika* consists of the subject of *pranayama*. At the outset we are made aware that *pranayama* is not exercises of breath. It is much beyond controlling the breath. This *pranayama* reaches management of *nadis*. It has a connection with *prana nadi* and control of the movement of *prana*. It is not just the control of breath going through right and left nostrils. Mainly and importantly, all the *prana nadis* have to be purified and efficient for this *pranayama*. They have to be 'traffic worthy'. If the trafficking is like that on the Indian roads, *prana* cannot be regulated. It is not breath gymnastics. This *pranayama* consists of breathing through *ida nadi*, *pingala nadi* and through *sushumna nadi*. Proficiency in the three *bandhas* such as *mulabandha*, *uddiyana bandha* and *jalandhara bandha* is needed for this *hatha yog pranayama*. Mastery of the trio of *bandhas*, not just doing it on physical level, is needed for *prana* regulation.

Shat Kriyas

Then *shat kriyas* are described. Again, there are many misconceptions about these *shat kriyas*. We think that the *shat kriyas* make *hatha yog*. Actually these *shat kriyas* are not for any layman. They are only for a *hatha yogi*. His caliber is already described at length. He has to be well versed in *ashtanga yog*, *mantra yog*, *laya yog* and then only *hatha yog* emerges which is like a post-graduate course of *sadhana*. Today veteran teachers are teaching these *shat kriyas* to raw beginners. This is not more foolish and ridiculous than admitting a primary class student in a medical college class. It is unfortunate that ordinary people are saying that they are doing *neti*, *basti* and so on. Some people claim that they use them as medical treatment or therapy. It is a sheer fad. They are remedial but are so purely for the *hatha yogi*. It has to be categorically stated again that these *kriyas* may be studied academically but they are to be performed only by the *hatha yogi*, the *hatha yogi* whose *nadis* are purified and who is a *yogi* out and out, in conduct, thought, habits and mind.

This can be elucidated with an example. We have a garbage can in our house. We throw garbage in it and close it. After some time we empty it. Suppose, we put a vibrator in it. What will happen? The garbage will spread in the whole house. So the vibrator must not be working in the garbage can. These *kriyas* are like a vibrator in the body. Then imagine its effects in the body if it is not pure. The impurities in the personality will be spreading and churning in the

393

existence. Bathing, etc. can remove only the impurities of the body. This is a partial and incomplete purification. Complete purification can be done if only the thinking, food habits and conduct become pure. So the ordinary people should not venture to do *kapalbhati*, *nauli* and so on as a therapy.

After the second chapter of *pranayama* and *kriyas* the third chapter deals with *mudras*. They are important in the awakening of *kundalini*. As *kundalini* is mystical, the *kriyas* are used. We cannot do these *mudras*. They are various *mudras* such as *simha mudra*, *Brahma mudra*, *shambhavi mudra*, *yog mudra*, *kaki mudra*, *maha mudra*, *ashvini mudra*, *amaroli mudra*, *khechari mudra*, *shanmukhi mudra*, *vajroli mudra*, *sahajoli mudra*, *viparita karani mudra*. The *tantra* of all these *mudras* is kept in coded language which is beyond our ken. None but a *hatha yogi* has the capacity to follow this language.

Remember one more point. *Mudras* are used to awaken *kundalini* which is the culminating point of *sadhana*. So this is the final stage of *sadhana* of a *hath yogi*. Isn't it preposterous to go for them in the pre-primary stage of our so-called *sadhana* when there is no purification of our personality? Whatever we do by following even a veteran teacher is something merely physical. This is like a child studying History in the first standard. He does not claim to be a historian at that stage. So these *mudras* for *kundalini* awakening were handled by supreme *yogis* like *Matsyendranath*, *Nivruttinath*, *Gorakshanath, Jnaneshvar*. Think of their status and appreciate the fact that all these factors are solely for them. The bow of God *Shiva* can be lifted only by *Rama* and nobody else should think of more than respecting *kundalini* from a distance.

Today they have another misconception that there is no spirituality in *hatha yog*. This misunderstanding is based on the wrong impression that *hatha yog* means physical feats, exercises of breath, holding breath for two-three minutes, sitting under water and so on. But read the biography and literature of *Jnaneshvar* and remember that *Jnaneshvar* was an accomplished *hatha yogi*. If we want to know *hatha yog* we can look at *Jnaneshvar*. His nature is that of a *hatha yogi*. If this is the acme of *hatha yog* the misunderstanding about *hatha yog* will melt away in a moment. The sixth chapter of the *Jnaneshvari* expounds on *hatha yog* and *kundalini yog*. Read it and the inflated ideas about *hatha yog* like a wrestlers' *yog* will be removed.

The fourth chapter of *Hatha Yog Pradipika* explains *samadhi* and its different kinds. All the processes of these *samadhis* are based on *mudra*, *prana* and *nadi*. This is its peculiarity. Their structuring has the foundation of use of *mudra* and science of *prana* and *nadi*. The *samadhi* in *Patanjali yog sutras* and that in *Hatha Yog Pradipika* are vastly different. The *samadhi* in *Patanjali's samprajnata samadhi* chapter or in the third chapter about various *samadhi* giving *siddhis* is different. The *samadhi* in *ashtanga yog* is of the beginning stage and that of *hatha yog* is very much advanced. It is of a high level because a *hatha yogi* is not a *sadhaka*, but he is a *siddha*.

The *samadhi* in *hatha yog* is mainly based on *mudras* and *prana*. Our body contains the five elements and *hatha yog* describes five kinds of *samadhi* based on these elements of the earth, water, fire, wind and ether. *Hatha Yog Pradipika* also tells about *nada samadhi* which has *anahata nada* as its locus. There are the *bindu samadhi* and *granthi samadhi*. We have *Vishnu granthi*, *Rudra granthi*, *Brahma granthi* in us which are used on a higher level of *yog* and *hatha yog*. The *granthis* or knots are cut as under in *granthi bhedana samadhi*.

So the *samsadhis* in *hatha yog* belong to a high level. Now let us think of the *samadhis* of a *hatha yogi*.

The first is *prana samadhi*. This *prana samadhi* follows the process of bringing the *prana* in the *Brahma randhra*, the hole in the crown of the head. The *hatha yogi* applies this *samadhi* at the time of death or departure from the world. We must note that this is not a kind of *samadhi sadhana* of every day. He does not use it frequently but only once and that, too, in the end. This *samadhi* is to be applied at the end of the last birth among the many births of the birth cycle. This moment gives *Nirvana* to the *yogi* and he gets salvation after that. This is *Kaivalya* and the *yogi* does not get birth again. In this *prana samadhi* he brings all *pranas* in the *Brahma randhra* or *sahasrara chakra* which is at the crown of the head. In this important process the *yogi* reaches salvation through *Archiradi* or *Devayana pantha*. The science of eschatology gives this information.

This *prana samsadhi* is described in the eighth chapter of the *Gita*. Lord *Krishna* says, "O *Arjuna*, the scholars of the *Vedas* call the highest abode as *Omkar*. What does the *yogi* who desires and deserves to reach that place do?

The *shloka* 12 of chapter 8 tells,

सर्वद्वाराणि संयम्य मनो हृदि निरुध्य च ।
मूर्ध्न्याधाय आत्मन: प्राणं आस्थित: योगधारणाम् ।।

He controls all the senses and takes them away from the objects of the senses, draws the mind to the heart, steadies there and takes *prana* in the crown of the head. Then he is stable in the *yog dharana*, utters the *mantra* of *Omkar* and leaves the body while thinking of the meaning of *Omkar Brahma*. He reaches the place of salvation. So according to the *Gita* this *dhyana* is for the end of life. The Lord says,

अंतकाले च मां एवं स्मरन् मुक्त्वा कलेवरम् ।

य: प्रयाति स मद् भावं याति न अस्ति अत्र संशय: ।।

One who leaves the body while thinking of Me becomes one with Me. What is the process of it? It is described in the *shloka* 10,

प्रयाणकाले मनसा अचलेन, भक्त्या युक्त: योगबलेन च एव ।

भ्रुवार्मध्ये प्राणं आवेश्य सम्यक् स तत् पदं पुरुष: उपैति दिव्यम् ।।

At the time of death he brings his mind between the eyebrows properly. He is thinking of Me with concentration, strength of *yog* and devotion. He reaches the highest and holiest spiritual place.

So this is *prana samadhi* with the utterance of *Omkar*. Many simpletons venture to imitate this and say that this advice is in the *Gita*. They sit with their sight fixed at the middle of the eyebrows but actually what they do is invite diseases. It is said very rightly by Alexander Pope, "Fools rush in where angels fear to tread".

This is the first kind of *prana samadhi*. The other kind is called *bhu samadhi* or *murchha samadhi*. This is achieved with *mantra* or medicinal herbs because it gives *tantra*. This has a kind of hypnotism. Of course, some discretionary power to use it must be there, otherwise it is annihilating for this *samadhi*.

The third kind is *dhyana yog samadhi*. This is found in the *shlokas* 7 and 8 of the *Gheranda Samhita*. This *samadhi* is achieved in *shambhavi mudra*. It is already told that *hatha yog samadhi* is based on *mudra*. *Dhyana yog samadhi* is helped by the *shambhavi mudra*.

Then the kind of *nada yog samadhi* is described which depends upon *khechari mudra*. The *shloka* 9 of 7th chapter of *Gheranda Samhita* explains this. Another *samadhi* is *rasananda samadhi* which depends upon *bhramari kumbhaka*. We find it in the *shloka*s 10 and 11 of 7th chapter of *Gheranda Samhita*.

Bhaktisiddha samadhi depends upon the *dhyana* of the personal deity and we find it in the *shlokas* 14 and 15 of 7th chapter of *Gheranda Samhita*. *Raja yog siddha samadhi* is described in the *shloka* 16 of 7th chapter of *Gheranda Samhita* which depends upon *ajna chakra kumbhaka*.

Thus we have briefly considered *prana samadhi, murchha samadhi, dhyana yog samadhi, nada yog samadhi, rasananda samadhi, bhaktisiddha samadhi, raja yog siddha samadhi*. We have understood that they are far different from *ashtanga yog samadhi* and their processes and they depend upon *mudras* and *prana kriyas*.

Shri Krishnaarpanam astu

Discourse - 31

Hatha Yog to Kundalini Yog

We were considering the kinds of *samadhi* in *hatha yog*. *Prana samadhi* is the *samadhi* at the time of departure. This is called *bhu samadhi* or *murchhakalina samadhi*. It has a kind of *mohini tantra* or casting spell. It is achieved through *yantra, tantra* or *mantra*.Then there is *dhyana samadhi* and it depends upon *shambhavi mudra* and its application. *Nada yog samadhi* depends upon *khechari mudra*. *Rasanand samadhi* depends on *bhramari kumbhaka, raja yog siddha samadhi* on *ajna chakriya kumbhaka* which is described in the 7th chapter of *Gheranda Samhita*, and *laya siddha samadhi* on *yoni mudra*. *Bhakti siddha samadhi* can be achieved by the *dhyana* of *Ishta* or personal deity. So these are some kinds of *samadhi* in the *hatha yog* system.

The *Shandilya Upanishad* describes *samadhi* based on the five elements of the earth, water, wind, fire and ether. These five elements have their respective deities and there are *samadhis* based on the *sadhana* and *beeja mantra* of these deities. So the *Shandilya Upanishad* suggests that there can be the kinds of *samadhi* as *bhu samadhi, jaliya samadhi, vayaviya samadhi, tejiya samadhi*, and *akasha samadhi. trishikhi Brahma Upanishad, jabala darshana Upanishad* and *Vashishtha samhita* also describe these *samadhis*. Those interested should see the original books. These books describe these *samadhi* of the five elements. So the *samadhi* processes in *hatha yog* are different from those of *ashtanga yog*. Now we have to think of the six *kriyas*. *Dhauti* is a *kriya* or a *karma* among the six *karmas*. *Dhauti* has three kinds-*jala dhauti, vastra dhauti* and *sutra dhauti*.

Basti is a *kriya*. *Jala neti* and *sutra neti* are two kinds of *neti*. *Tratak, nauli* and *kapalabhati* together with the preceding *kriyas* form the six *kriyas*. All these are *sadhanas* of *hatha yog*. These *kriyas* belong to the post-graduate level in *yog*. It has to be repeatedly instructed that they are not for the beginners among the *sadhakas*. It is unfortunate that today they are being offered to ordinary people at random. The important point is that the *hatha yogi* is not doing *yog* or *asanas* merely on the physical level. His has an advanced status. This may be called the third storey built on the foundation of *ashtanga yog*. The first floor is *mantra yog* the second one is *laya yog*, and the third is *hatha yog*. The science of *nadi*, of *prana nadi*, *bandha, mudra, kriya* are important here and they are more important than physical *asanas*. Another misconception is that the *hatha yogi* is one who does miracles and he possesses superhuman powers. There are strange foolish ideas that he can walk on water, bury himself under the ground, stay without breathing or stop his heart. Remember, *hath yogis* are not stunt men. The stunt men can do such feats that ordinary men cannot do. The *Hatha Yogi* has no such powers but has a retiring mindset and extreme renunciation. Look at *Jnaneshvar*, for example. If we see his mind set, life and inclinations and consider his humanism, genius and compassion we can get the picture of a *hatha yogi*. So we have spent much time on what a *hatha yogi* is not while trying to understand what *hatha yogi* is. But that was inevitable in this age with prevalence of idiotic ideas about *yog* and *hatha yog*, in particular. Now we can turn to *raja yog*.

Raja yog

One popular meaning of *raja yog* is the *raja* i. e. king of the kinds of *yog*. This word is used also in astrology and there it means the *yog* that comes in the form of a king. We have seen in the process of *dhyana yog* that *raja yog* has the highest place as it is reached after *ashtanga yog*, *mantra yog* and *laya yog*. *Raja yog* has the highest place in the *hatha yog* sect. There is a *raja yog* also in the science of the *yog* of *Patanjali*. There are three levels of advice in the science of the *yog* of *Patanjali*. The *yog sutras* of *Patanjali* give advice to the *sadhakas* and *siddhas* of three levels of *adhamadhikari*, *madhyamadhikari* and *uttamadhikari*. It will be proper to call the *yog* of the *uttamadhikari* as *raja yog*. The *yog* advised in the *samadhi pada* of the *yog sutras* of *Patanjali* is of *uttamadhikari*. It is said,

अभ्यासवैराग्याभ्यां तन्निरोध:

The control of fluctuations is achieved by efforts to steady the mind and renunciation. Afterwards it is told that the *samprajnata* and *asamprajnata samadhi* belong to the *uttamadhikari* and then the *yog* of the highest category, of the supreme *bhakta* or of *Ishvara pranidhana* is related there. So the *yog* in the *samadhi pada* of *yog sutras* of *Patanjali*,is the supreme *raja yog* which is achieved by *Ishvarapranidhana* and that, too, is based on *ashtanga yog*. The hierarchy is *ashtanga yog*, then *kriya yog*, *abhyasa- vairagya yog* and then *samprajnata* and *asamprajnata*. *Ashtanga yog* is for the *arambhadhikari*, *kriya yog* for the *madhyamadhikari* and *samprajnata* and *asamprajnata* or *abhyasa -vairagya yog* for the *uttamadhikari* and that can be called the supreme *raja yog*. There are three kinds of *yog sadhana* in the *yog sutras* of *Patanjali*. In the 27th *sutra* and further in the 2nd *pada* we find *ashtanga yog* of the *arambhadhikari* as *yama, niyama, asana, pranayama, pratyahara, dharana, dhyana*, and *samadhi*. The *kriya yog* as

'तप स्वाध्याय ईश्वरप्रणिधानानि क्रियायोग'

Is found in the first *sutra* and further in the beginning of the 2nd *pada*.The *yog* of the *uttamadhikari* is told as

वितर्कविचारानंदास्मितारूपानुगमात् संप्रज्ञात: ।
विरामप्रत्ययाभ्यासपूर्व: संस्कारशेष: अन्य:

Samprajnata and *asamprajnata yog* are described in
this way

This can be called *raja yog* because it belongs to the *yogi* of the
highest authority and caliber. Its limbs are *abhyasa* and *vairagya*.
These two also must be of the supreme level. The *abhyasa* must be
the highest as an effort for stability of mind and *vairagya* must be
supreme and such as belongs to a *sanyasi* with utmost renunciation.
It is the *yog* of a *yogi* who possesses this kind of *vairagya* or the
devotion of a *Tukaram*. Perhaps we can call him a *raja yogi*. He has
done *yog sadhana* for many births to reach that level. It is said in the
Gita

'अनेकजन्मसंसिद्धौ ततो याति परां गतिम्'

This *yogi* is an accomplished *yogi*. Here we find the essence of
dhyana, *karma* and *bhakti yog* together, so it is *raja yog*. The *yog* of
a supreme *siddha* can be *raja yog*.

How does the *yog* of the *uttamadhikari* begin? It starts with
pranayama. When he sits for *pranayama*, he finishes the primary
sthula kriya quickly and reaches the *sukshma kriyas* which is achieved
within no time. Because of this *pranayama* he does *pratyahara*
immediately. In this condition he naturally gets *Omkar* and this *Omkar*
gives him *samadhi*. The *yogi's chitta* is absolutely pure and noble at
this time and so *Omkar* resounds naturally in his mind. It turns into
anahata nada; *dhyana*, *dharana*, *samadhi* attached to *Omkar* and
he gets *samadhi*. This is the way of his *sadhana*.

His *samadhi* has two levels. One is *samprajnata* or *vitarkavichara*,
ananda asmita anugata. All the *sthula* (gross), subtle and supremely

subtle elements are revealed to him in this *samadhi*. The next is *asamprajnata samadhi* which is the *nirodha* of all the fluctuations of the mind. His journey towards *Kaivalya* is very fast. In the first *pada* of the *yog sutras* some ways for the ennobling of his *chitta* are suggested. They are called *chitta parikarma*. He makes his *chitta* nobler and *yogic* with this *chitta parikarma*. The *samadhi* takes place in such a *chitta*. The *vairagya* of this *raja yogi* has the level of *vashikara sanjna vairagya* and *parama vairagya*. There are four kinds of *vairagya* as *yatamana vairagya*, *vyatireka vairagya*, *ekendriya vairagya* and the highest is *vashikara*. This *yogi* achieves the highest level of these where he gets divine revelation in *samadhi*. He gets the blessings of *dhyana yog* and also flawless knowledge. He gets the fruit of *jnana yog* easily and then *parama vairagya* which leads to the highest state of *bhakti*. He is heading towards *Kaivalya*.

So the *raja yog* is a supreme *yog*. Nowadays people are equating *raja yog* with so many things as if it is only a subject of meditation, or contemplation of the *Upanishads* or any contemplation with closed eyes or *dhyana*. In fact, it is not a cup of an ordinary man. It is not like a sitting posture so that mere *dhyana* in an *asana* can give *raja yog*! Never forget that it can be achieved only after *sadhana* of many births and it has great *abhyasa* and *vairagya*. After *sadhana* of these two the two limbs become one and then it is *Ishvarapranidhana*. If we want this kind of *raja yog*, it is found in the first *pada* of *sutras* of *Patanjali*. We searched for it in the *yog shastra* of *Patanjali* in order to give justice to the commentary of *Swami Vivekananda*. But the nomenclature of *raja yog* is used in a different sense in the tradition. In short, what is the concept of *raja yog*? If we want to build *raja yog* in *ashtanga yog*, we have to collect the foundational factors of *mantra yog*, *laya yog*, *hatha yog*, *raja yog*, *japa yog*, *nama yog*, *nada yog*, *jnana yog*, *karma yog*, *dhyana yog* and *bhakti yog*. *Ashtanga yog* is built on these factors. When this *ashtanga yog* is in an advanced state, it becomes kriya yog. If *kriya yog* is successful, it becomes *raja yog*. So it is an ultimate step of *vairagya* and *abhyasa*. There is a mistaken idea that *raja yog* can be without *asanas*. Remember, *raja yog* stands upon the foundation of *ashtanga yog*. *Hatha yog* is already there in its constitution. They think that *raja yog* and *hatha yog* belong to two opposite kinds of people. This is a stark misconception. The process of *hatha yog* contains *raja yog* and vice versa. *Hatha Yog Pradipika* has a statement-

हठं विना राजयोग: राजयोगं विना हठ: ।

न सिध्यति

तस्मात् प्रवर्तते योगी हठे सद्गुरुमार्गत: ।

There is no *raja yog* without *hatha yog* and no *hatha yog* without *raja yog*. The sciences of *yog* state this clearly. The main point is that the *yog sadhaka* has to be accomplished in the *tantra* of both *raja yog* and *hatha yog*. Even the 6th chapter of the *Gita* and the first *pada* of *Patanjali's yog sutras* say that the *yog* of the *uttamadhikari* is *raaj yog*. The constitution of *raja yog* shows that it has the five *prana kriya*, management of five *pranas*, management of five elements, management of *nadis* and process of purification of *nadis* in *hatha yog* are essential in it. Also the management of six plexii and management of the *kriya* of the six plexii in *hatha yog* are needed. Even skill of *japa yog* is necessary. *Pranava japa* has to be done with *japa yog*. The skill of *tantra* of *mantra japa* and *Omkar* also are prerequisites for this.

The *raja yogi* has to get *chitta laya* in this *pranava* so he has to be skilful in *laya yog*. *Jnana yog* also is needed and must be achieved because the meaning of *pranava* is found in the principles of *jnana yog*. So also *bhakti yog* has to be achieved because *bhakti* with great devotion is necessary for *Ishvarapranidhana*. As *Vyasa* says the first *pada* of the *Patanjali yogasutras* is *bhakti pranidhana*, so it is *Ishvara pranidhana*. Therefore, it is *bhakti yog* and *dhyana yog*. The *tantras* of *dhyana yog* are useful here. So the success in *jnana yog*, *mantra yog*, *karma yog*, *dhyana yog*, *japa yog*, *bhakti yog*, *laya yog* and *hatha yog* has to be there. Then only *raja yog* can be achieved. *Raja yog* is supreme and it is not without *asanas* and *pranayama*.

If we want to see the traditional meaning of *raja yog* we cannot get it completely, and with its *tantra*, in the *Patanjali yog sutras*, and not even in the sixth chapter of the *Gita*. We have to turn to *Upanishads*. It is mentioned in *Yog Shikha Upanishad*, *Yog Tattva Upanishad*, *Hatha Yog Pradipika*, *Gheranda Samhita* and *Shiva Samhita*. Let us see what these *Upanishads* and *hath yog* books say about *raja yog*.

It has to be noted at the outset that *Yog Shikha Upanishad*, *Yog Tattva Upanishad*, *Hatha Yog Pradipika*, *Gheranda Samhita* and *Shiva Samhita* suggest that *raja yog* means the completion, fruition and acme of *hatha yog*. *Mandala Brahma Upanishad* says that if *hatha yog* has thought about six *chakras*, *raja yog* has thought about nine *chakras*. We know six *chakras* and *raja yog* discovers more *chakras* and their use/application. It mentions *talu chakra*, *bhu chakra* and *akasha chakra*. There is a *shloka* in the 4th chapter of *Mandala Brahma Upanishad*.

"नवचक्रं षडाधारं त्रिलस्वं व्योमपंचकं सम्यक् एतन्न जानाति स योगी नामतः भवेत्"

One who knows the nine *chakras*, six *adharas* and five kinds of *akasha* is a *raja yogi*. This *akasha chakra* is for three kinds of introversion and intercession. They are internal, external and intermediate. Now the question is-why is it called *raja yog*? First of all, this has no connection with king or kingship. This is not the king of *yogs*. *Shlokas* 136 and 137 of the first chapter of *Yog Shikha Upanishad* contain mystical description of this *yog*. The word '*raja*' in *raja yog* comes from the verb '*raja*'. *Raja* is an ovum cell. We know *raja* and semen from biology. Reproduction takes place from the union of *raja* and semen. So the word *raja yog* is formed because of the relation with '*raja*'.

"योनिमध्ये महाक्षेत्रे जपाबन्धूकसंनिभम् ।
रजो वसति जंतूनां देवीतत्त्वं समावृतम् ।।
रजसो रेतसो योगात् राजयोग इति स्मृत: ।
अणिमादिपदं प्राप्य राजते राजयोगत: ।

The meaning is as follows. *Raja* of the beings stays in the great area of the vagina. It is like the flower of *japabandhuka* and is a protected principle representing *Shakti* or goddess. The union of *rajas* and *retas*/semen becomes *raja yog*. This is union of *Shiva* and *Shakti*. The *yogi* can get *siddhis* like *anima* with this *raja yog*. This is the meaning of *raja yog*. Ordinarily males have semen and females have *raja* but a *yogi* has both. The union of these two in the *yogi* takes place in the *sahasrara chakra*. This is union of *Shiva* and *Shakti*. Some people think that it is called *raja yog* because it is *raja* or king. If this is the *raja* of *yog*, can there be a beggar of *yog*? So there is nothing like *raja* or beggar *yog*. All the *yogs* are *raja yog* in a way. *Raja yog* happens when *raja* and semen of the *yogi* are taken upwards after crossing the six plexii and their union is achieved. This definition of *raja yog* is found in *Yog Shikha Upanishad*. The inquisitive *sadhaka* should consult the *Upanishad* for himself. *Yog Tattva Upanishad* describes *raja yog* in the *shlokas* 129 and 130.

They are

ततो भवेत् राजयोगो न अंतरा भवति ध्रुवम् ।
यदा तु राजयोगेन निष्पन्ना योगिभि: क्रिया: ।।

The next *shloka* is

"तदा विवेकवैराग्यं जायते योगिनो ध्रुवं विष्णुर्नाम महायोगी
महाभूतो महातपा: तत्त्वमार्गे यथा दीपो दृश्यते पुरुषोत्तम: '

It says that *raja yog* is accomplished after all the *kriyas, bandhas, mudras*, especially *vajroli mudra* and *amaroli mudra*, from *hatha yog* are achieved. Usually semen flows downwards but in the *yogi* it goes upwards for which *vajroli mudra* and *amaroli mudra* are prescribed in *hatha yog*. The *yogi* has to possess this skill. *Raja yog* takes place by discretion, renunciation and *Purushottama darshana* along with the union of *rajas* and *retas*/semen. In the 16th *shloka* of 7th chapter of *Gheranda Samhita* is clearly connected with *hatha yog*.

'मनोमूर्च्छां समासाद्य मन आत्मनि योजयेत्
परमात्मा समायोगात् समाधिं समवान्पुमान्'

The *samadhi* of *hatha yog* that gives *manomurchha* is *raja yog*. Thus *raja yog* is not opposite to *hatha yog* but the culmination of *hatha yog*. This point has to be understood. The second *shloka* of the first chapter of *HathaYog Pradipika* clearly says that *hatha yog* culminates in *raja yog* and they are not different. The 15th *shloka* of fifth chapter of *Shiva Samhita* tells that there are four kinds of *yog*. It describes the process in which *mantra yog* is followed by *hatha yog*, then by *laya yog* and then comes *raja yog*.

Shiva Samhita has a short chapter on *raja yog* in the fifth chapter itself after *shloka* 196. The process of *raja yog* is described there as culminating from *hatha yog*. *Shloka* 203 says that the union of *kundalini* and the soul is *raja yog*. *Shloka* 229 clearly says

हठं विना राजयोगो, राजयोगं विना हठ: न सिध्यति
तस्मात् प्रवर्तते योगी हठे सद्गुरुमार्गत: ।

There is no *raja yog* without *hatha yog* and vice versa. The tradition says that all the *sadhana* is connected to *chakra, bandha* and *mudra*. If we want to grasp the meaning of *raja yog* in the tradition we have to turn to *Mandala Brahma Upanishad, Yog Shikha Upanishad, Yog Tattva Upanishad, Hatha Yog Pradipika, Gheranda Samhita* and *Shiva Samhita*. They explain the meaning of *raja yog* and according to them *raja yog* is union of *Shiva* and *Shakti*. Depending on the tradition we can venture to say that the *yog* described by *Patanjali* in the first *pada* also is not *raja yog*. The *yog* described by *Swami Vivekananda* as *raja yog* is not *raja yog*.

Patanjala yog sutras do not have union of *Shiva* and *Shakti* and the raising of *kundalini*. Raising of *kundalini* belongs to *hatha yog*. So it is partially meaningless when it was said that *raja yog* is *Patanjala yog* because the main aspect of *raja yog* is union of *Shiva* and *Shakti*. Even the *Jnaneshvari* says that the *yogi* makes the the union of his own *raja* and *semen* in the *sahasrara chakra* in *kundalini yog*. So the *Patanjala yog* may be of *adhamadhikari, madhyamadhikari* or *uttamadhikari*, but it is not at all *raja yog*. *Raja yog* belongs to the tradition of *tantra*. It is in the process of *mantra yog, hatha yog, laya yog, raja yog*. It comes in the context of *bandha, mudra, kriya, pranayama, nadi* and *chakra*. *Raja yog* or its tradition uses *tantra* in the context of raising of *kundalini shakti* but *Patanjala yog* is based on the knowledge of *samkhya* and *Vedanta*. It also has *bhakti* and *Ishvarapranidhana* in it.

'समाधिसिद्धि: ईश्वर प्रणिधानात्'

Ishvarapranidhana gives *samadhi* and *siddhi*. It has *pranava* *sadhana*. *Patanjala yog* develops through *sadhana* of *bhakti* and knowledge. This *samadhi yog* or *yog* in *samadhi pada* is not *raja yog*. This science has developed in *tantra, mantra, yantra* or our *agama*. The supreme stage in the tradition of *mantra yog, hatha yog, laya yog* is *raja yog* which we have considered is *Raj yog* here. The higher step of *raja yog* is *rajadhiraja yog* or *kundalini yog*.

Kundalini yog

Now we are going to think about *kundalini yog*. This is a supreme *yog*. It is esteemed as *rajadhiraja* in the process of *mantra yog, hatha yog, laya yog*. We will think of it in detail in the next chapter. *Yog vidya* speaks about the six *chakras* - *muladhara chakra, svadhishthana, manipuraka, anahata, vishuddhi* and *ajna*; and the seventh *sahasrara*. There is the science of *nadis*. Also the three *bandhas* such as *mulabandha, uddiyana bandha* and *jalandhara bandha*; *ida, pingala, sushumna* and the ten *mahanadis* and *kriyas* are integral parts of *yog sadhana*. They have originated in *tantra* of *hatha yog*. The hierarchy of *mantra yog, laya yog, hatha yog, raja yog* in *sadhana* is supported by *tantra*. All these *sadhanas* and *yogs* are concluded at one place and that place is called *rajadhiraja yog* or *kundalini yog*. Whatever concepts are there in all these types of *yog* are given by *tantra*. The following long list of concepts can give us an idea of the enormous contribution of *tantra*.

The four kinds of *dhauti* as *jaladhauti, vastradhauti, sutradhauti, dandadhauti*; the kinds of *basti*; *jalaneti, sutraneti, tratak, nauli, kapalabhati, uddiyana, simha mudra, brahma mudra, shambhavi mudra, yog mudra, kaki mudra, maha mudra, ashwini mudra, amaroli mudra, khechari mudra, shanmukhi mudra, vajroli mudra, sahajoli mudra*; the three *bandhas* such as *mulabandha, uddiyana bandha* and *jalandhara bandha*, *bija mantras* of the six plexii, the ten *mahanadis* like *ida*, *pingala*, the *svara* concepts of *prana* like *surya svara*, *chandra svara*, *shunya svara* and their *sadhana*; *kala sadhana* like *bindu sadhana*, *tejovalaya sadhana*, and *prakasha sadhana*; *varna sadhana* i. e. *sadhana* of the letters from *a* to *ksha* and their *sanket*; every *mantra* has its *mata* and so the *matruka sadhana*; thought of *mantra*, *Kulakulachakra* for *mantra anushthana*, *shashi chakra*, *arakata chakra*, *nakshatra chakra*, *akadama chakra* for *mantra anushthana*; the positive and negative poles of energy in the body; *mandala japa*, *mala*, *varna*, *mantra* , concept of *bija mantra*, concept of *asanas* like skin of tiger or that of deer or the *asana* made of *kusha* grass; thought of *purashcharana*; *mantra purashcharana*; *anga nyasa*, *kara nyasa*, *matruka nyasa*, *pitha nyasa*. All these concepts are gifted by *tantra*.

All these thoughts have come from the source of *tantra* and they are scattered in various treatises of *yog*. For example, *tantraloka*, *Shivasamhita* in *Shaivagama*, *jnanarnava tantra*, *dhyanasankalini*, *kashmiri Shaivagama*, *Bhairavi tantra*, *Sharadatilak*, *Tripurasundari Rahasya*, treatises of *hatha yog*, *siddhasiddhanta paddhati*. The thoughts were scattered in these books. So it is difficult to search in all these books in order to study *kundalini yog* through the way of *mantra yog* , *laya yog*, *hatha yog*, *raja yog*. It is like searching in a dense forest. But this complicated task is simplified by *Jnaneshvar* and so the job of the *yog sadhakas* has become easy. We can get this *yog* in the sixth chapter of *Jnaneshvari* and we have been spared the trouble of browsing in all these books. The type of this study has not only become easy and simple but also pleasant because of the grace of the kind Master, *Jnaneshvar* whose style is so blissful.

The *samadhi* in *kundalini yog* and that in *ashtanga yog* of *Patanjali* are different. *Samadhi* in *ashtanga yog* of *Patanjali* takes place by *Ishvarapranidhana* i.e. by *pranava dhyana* and devotion. *Samadhi* of *kundalini yog* happens when the dormant *kundalini* is taken upwards after crossing the six plexii through *sushumna,* and union of *Shiva* and *Shakti* is achieved. The journey of *kundalini yog* takes place after achieving success in *ashtanga yog* followed by *sadhanas* of *mantra yog, laya yog, hatha yog* and *raja yog.* These are factors of *hatha yog.* The steps in the long list above have to be followed. The useful factors in the eight limbs of *ashtanga yog* and *mudra, kriya* etc are freely taken in *kundalini yog.* Even though it is said that the *samadhi* in *kundalini yog* and that in *ashtanga yog* of *Patanjali* are different; *ashtanga yog sadhana* uses useful factors from *kundalini yog* without inhibitions.

In *kundalini yog* each of the six *chakras* has *bija mantra.* The *bija mantra* opens the locks of *chakras* related to the five elements of the earth, wind, water, fire and ether. The *mantras* are used like keys and the journey towards *sahasrara chakra* is completed. The *sadhaka* goes ahead by doing *dhyana* of the respective *bija mantra* of each *chakra* and conquering it with the help of *tantra.* The *bija mantra* Omkar is for *ajna chakra* in *hatha yog* or *tantra* but in all the *samadhis* of *Patanjali*'s *ashtanga yog,* Omkar is the *mantra.* In *kundalini yog* and *hatha yog* Omkar is the denoter of Divinity, as it is said in the *Gita.* Devotion is necessary. In *kundalini,* Omkar is to stimulate *ajna chakra* or to uplift *kundalini* and it is used with caution for *tantra* and *mantra.* In short, Omkar in *kundalini yog* is for acquiring certain powers and in *Patanjali yog* for creating devotion.

Nowadays there are many so-called *yogis* who are distributing *kundalini yog* among the common people and supposed *sadhakas,* like hot cakes. So many masters are available to teach them to move and twist the upper part of the body like a haunted person and then they call it *Shakti chalana*. Many of them ask to move the neck fast and call it *Brahma mudra*. Many are there who start the engines of *bhastrika* and *kapalabhati* and say that they are raising *kundalini*. They ask you to concentrate on the central point between eyebrows and brag that they will show you the union of *Shiva* and *Shakti*. This will give you nothing but headache and incurable diseases of nerves. This so-called spiritual propaganda and their promoters is found in any corner of the town. It is important to note that we must not go for such *gurus* and such display of fake *yog*.

Where does this *kundalini yog* start? First the *samadhi* of *sadhana* of *ashtanga yog* has to be accomplished through *yama, niyama, asana, pranayama, pratyahara, dharana, dhyana*. Then *mantra yog* of sixteen parts has to be achieved. These sixteen parts are *bhakti*, purification, *asana, panchangasevana*, five aspects of worshipping deities, *achar, dharana, divyadeshasevana, pranakriya, mudra, tarpana, havana, bali* or sacrifice, offerings to deities, *yag* or a form of worship, recitation of the hymns like *hridaya stavana* or *kavacha*, the Gita or *Sahasranam, japa, dhyana* and *Samadhi*. Then *Hath yog* of six limbs has to be followed. *Asana, pranayama, pratyahara, dharana, dhyana, samadhi* and then the six *kriyas* of *dhauti, basti, neti, tratak, nauli, kapalabhati* have to be achieved along with all the *mudras* like *simhamudra, shambhavi mudra, khechari mudra* that are mentioned above. The *pranayama* of *chandra, shunya* and *surya nadis* have to be achieved. The five *dhyanas* of the five elements of the earth, wind, water, fire and ether have to be achieved. The *sadhana* of the six *chakras, sadhana* of five *prana* have to be achieved on the level of *dhyana*. After accomplishing *mantra yog* of sixteen limbs the *laya yog* of nine limbs has to be achieved. Then comes *hatha yog* of six limbs,. The *yama* and *niyama* in it have to be followed. These *yamas* and *niyama* are not those of *Ashtanga yog*. They are on the level of conduct or thinking. The way Jnaneshwar, Ramdas, Tukaram followed *yama* and *niyamas* are of a different kind. It is the conduct of a *siddha purusha*. *Laya yog* has to be achieved through *sthula kriyas*, *sukshma kriya*, *pratyahara*, *dharana*, *laya kriya*, *samadhi*. Then follows *raja yog*.

Kundalini yog is accomplished only through *hatha yog*. There is no other way for it. This is accomplished after the five *yogas* of *ashtanga*, *mantra*, *laya*, *hatha* and *raja yog* are achieved. There is no short cut for *kundalini yog*.

Shri Krishnaarpanam astu

✦ ✦ ✦

Discourse - 32

Kundalini Yog

It is a reality that *vedic sadhana* and penance have made a natural and profound contribution of *tantra* in it. Right from yore, the *tantra* of *agama* has entered the *vedic* religion, *vedic sadhana*, *vedic* penance and *vedic* science. The contribution of *tantra* in disclosing the secrets of mysticism that was added to the *vedic* knowledge is certainly seminal. It is valuable. The *vedic sadhana,* values, emotions and feelings while worshipping the personal Deity, the devotion is definitely important but *tantra*, *yantra*, and *mantra* are no less important. These *tantra*, *yantra* and *mantra* were not only assimilated in the *vedic sadhana* but became one with it. This is a fact. Rituals are important in *yajna*, worship and *mantra* and they are amply used in it. They are strictly stipulated. This is *tantra*. *Tantra* has stipulated the rituals of worship. The contribution of *tantra* of *agama* is great. *Shaiva agama*, *Vaishnava agama*, *Shakta agama* have constructed these rituals. The construction of *Vaishnava* temples, its sculpture and designs are scientific. This science has come from *agama*. So also *Shaiva* temples have *Shaiva agama* behind them. Temples of *Shakti* have *Shakta agama*. *Tantras* are always there behind all worship and prayers. They are found in the respective *agamas*. The rituals of worship of *Laxmi, Shakti, Durga* and the rules of the temples of *Shakti* and other deities are framed by *agamas*. *Tantra* has created its own significant place in the *yog vidya* that has come from the *vedic* origin. The excellent revelation of the blending of *yog vidya* and *tantra agama* is *kundalini yog.*

Yog vidya has the study of six plexii or *chakras*. They are *muladhara, svadhishthana, manipuraka, anahata, vishuddhi* and *ajna* and the seventh is *sahasrara chakra*. *Yog sadhana* also has the knowledge of the three *nadis* of *ida, pingala* and *sushumna,* ten *maha nadis,* three *bandhas* such as *mulabandha, uddiyana bandha* and *jalandhara bandha,* various *mudras* and many kinds of *yog kriyas* as its integral parts. These *kriyas* are given by *tantra* only. The hierarchy of *mantra yog, laya yog, hatha yog, raja yog* in *sadhana* is supported by *tantra.* All these *sadhanas* and *yogs* are concluded at one place and that place is called *rajadhiraja yog* or *kundalini yog.* Whatever concepts are there in all these types of *yog* are given by *tantra.*

The following long list of concepts can give us an idea of the enormous contribution of *tantra.* The four kinds of *dhauti* as *jaladhauti, vastradhauti, sutradhauti, dandadhauti;* the kinds of *basti; jalaneti, sutraneti, tratak, nauli, kapalabhati, uddiyana, simha mudra, brahma mudra, shaambhavi mudra, yog mudra, kaki mudra, maha mudra, ashwini mudra, amaroli mudra, khechari mudra, shanmukhi mudra, vajroli mudra, sahajoli mudra;* the three *bandhas* such as *mulabandha, uddiyana bandha* and *jalandhara bandha, bija mantras* of the six plexi, the ten *mahanadis* like *ida, pingala,* the *svara* concepts of *prana* like *surya svara, chandra svara, shunya svara* and their *sadhana; kala sadhana* like *bindu sadhana, tejovalaya sadhana,* and *prakasha sadhana; varna sadhana* i.e. *sadhana* of the letters from *a* to *ksha* and their *sanket;* every *mantra* has its *mata* and so the *matruka sadhana;* thought of *mantra, kulakulachakra* for *mantra anushthana, shashi chakra, akadaha chakra, nakshatra chakra, akadama chakra* for *mantra anushthana;* the positive and negative poles of energy in the body; *mandala japa, mala, varna, mantra,* concept of *bija mantra,* concept of seats like skin of tiger or that of deer or the *asana* made of *kusha* grass; concept of *purashcharana; mantra purashcharana; anga nyasa, matruka nyasa, pitha nyasa.*

415

All these concepts are gifted by *tantra*.

All these concepts have come from the source of *tantra* and they are scattered in various treatises of *yog*. For example, *tantraloka*, *Shivasamhitaa* in *Shaivagama*, *Jnanarnava tantra*, *jnanasankalini*, *kashmiri Shaivagama*, *Bhairavi tantra*, *Sharadatilaka*, *Tripurasundari rahasya*, books of *hath yog*, *Siddha Siddhanta Paddhati*. The thoughts were scattered in these books. So it is difficult to search in all these books in order to study *kundalini yog* through the way of *mantra yog*, *laya yog*, *hatha yog*, *raja yog*. It is like searching in a dense forest. But this complicated task is simplified by *Jnaneshvar* and so the job of the *yog sadhakas* has become easy. We can get this *yog* in the sixth chapter of *Jnaneshvari* and we have been spared the trouble of browsing in all these books. The type of this study has not only become easy and simple but also pleasant because of the grace of the kind Master, *Jnaneshvar* whose style is blissful.

Jnaneshvari tells the entire *sadhana*, concepts, science and techniques of *kundalini yog*. There is vast difference between *samadhi* of *kundalini yog* and *samadhi* of *ashtanga yog* of *Patanjali*. The *samadhi* of *Patanjali* is accomplished with *Ishvarapranidhana* or *Omkar* and devotion. The *samadhi* in *kundalini yog* is accomplished by raising the dormant *kundalini* in *muladhara* and then pulling it through *sushumna* to the *brahmarandhra* or the hole at the crown of the head which is union of *Shiva* and *Shakti*. The journey of *kundalini yog* takes place after *ashtanga yog* is accomplished and then the *sadhana* of *mantra yog*, *laya yog*, *hatha yog*, *raja yog* is completed in this same order. A well planned *sadhana* of all the things that are described in the long list above has to be completed in this journey. While practising *hatha yog* many things have to be achieved through the consolidated *sadhana*. *Yama*, *niyama*, *asana*, *pranayama*, *pratyahara, dharana, dhyana, samadhi* are the limbs of *ashtanga yog* of *Patanjali* and the *sadhaka* chooses the useful and complementary things among them. *Sadhana* of the five *pranas*, selected *mudras*, three *bandhas* and *japa sadhana* for the sake of *dhyana* are accepted for elevating level of *yog*. In *kundalini yog* each of the six *chakras* has a *bija mantra*. The *bija mantra* opens the locks of *chakras* related to the five elements of the earth, wind, water, fire and ether. The *mantras* are used like keys and the journey towards *sahasrara chakra* is completed. The *mantra* of *muladhara*, *chakra* is *lammm*, that of *svadhishthana* is *vammm*, that of *manipuraka* is *rammm*, that of *anahata* is *yammm*, that of *vishuddhi* is *huummm* and that of *ajna* is *Omkar*. The *sadhaka* goes ahead by doing *dhyana* of the respective *bija mantra* of each *chakra* and conquering it with the help of *tantra*. The *bija mantra Omkar* is for *ajna chakra* in *hatha yog* or *tantra* but in all the *samadhis* of *Patanjali's ashtanga yog* such as *samprajnata* and *asamprajnata Omkar* is the *mantra*. In *Patanjali's sutras Omkar* is the denoter of Divinity. The *Gita* says,

ॐ इति एकाक्षरं ब्रह्म व्याहरन् मां अनुस्मरन् ।

So *Omkar* is for Divinity. The utterance should have devotion. *Omkara* is the *bija mantra* in *kundalini yog* to open the lock of *ajna chakra*, to stimulate the *kundalini* and then to take it up through *ajna chakra*. It is used taking care of the discipline of *mantra* and *tantra*.

Beware !

Nowadays there are many so-called *yogis* who are distributing *kundalini yog* among common people and supposed *sadhakas* like hot cakes. So many masters are available to teach them to move and twist the upper part of the body like a haunted person and then they call it *Shakti chalana*. Many of them ask to move the neck fast

417

and call it *Brahma mudra*. Many are there who start the engines of *bhastrika* and *kapala bhati* and say that they are raising *kundalini*. They ask you to concentrate on the central point between eyebrows and brag that they will show you the union of *Shiva* and *Shakti*. This will give you nothing but headache and diseases of nerves that shall not be cured by medicines. This so-called spiritual propaganda and the promoters are found in any corner of the town. It is important to note that we must not go for such gurus and such display of fake *yog.*

Where does this *kundalini yog* start? First the *samadhi* of *sadhana* of *ashtanga yog* has to be accomplished through *yama, niyama, asana, pranayama, pratyahara, dharana, dhyana*. Then *mantra yog* of sixteen limbs has to be achieved. These sixteen limbs are *bhakti*, purification, *asana, panchangasevana, achara, dharana, divyadeshasevana, pranakriya, mudra, tarpana, havana, bali* or sacrifice, *yaga, japa, dhyana* and *samadhi*. Then *hatha yog* of six limbs has to be followed. *Asana, pranayama, pratyahara, dharana, dhyana, samadhi* and then the six *kriyas* of *dhauti, basti, neti, tratak, nauli, kapalabhati* have to be achieved along with all the *mudras* like *simhamudra, shambhavi mudra, khechari mudra* that are mentioned above. The *svara* concepts of *chandra, shunya* and *surya* and the *pranayama* of all the *nadis* have to be achieved. The five *dhyanas* of the five elements of the earth, wind, water, fire and ether have to be achieved. The *sadhana* of the six *chakras, sadhana* of five *prana* have to be achieved on the level of *dhyana*. After accomplishing *mantra yog* of sixteen limbs, the *laya yog* of nine limbs has to be achieved and then there is *hatha yog* of six limbs. The *yama* and *niyama* in it have to be followed. These *yamas* and *niyamas* are not those of *ashtanga yog*. They are on the level of conduct or thinking.

The way *Jnaneshvar, Ramdas, Tukaram* followed *yama* and *niyama* is of a different calibre. It is the conduct of a *siddha purusha.*

Laya yog has to be achieved through *sthula kriya, sukshma kriya, pratyahara, dharana, laya kriya, samadhi*. Then follows *raja yog*. The *yogi* has to get the union of his *virya* with *rajas* within himself. *Raja yog* means the union of the *virya* that exists in the form of *ojas* and *tejas* with his own *rajas* in the *yogi*. The union of *pum bija* or semen with *stri bija* or ovum in oneself by internal intercourse is the union of *Shiva* and *Shakti*. It is *raja yog* or the climax of *raja yog*. The *Shakti* in *muladhara* gets united with *Shiva* in the *Brahma randhra*. This is *kundalini yog*. This *kundalini yog* is accomplished only through *hath yog*. There is no other way for it. This is accomplished after the five *yogs* of *ashtanga, mantra, laya, hatha* and *raja* are achieved.

There is no short cut for *kundalini yog*. Some great master puts his index finger at the spot between the eyebrows of his disciple and within a tremendous flash of a split second *yog* is accomplished. We read and hear of such miracles. We hear that a master touched the *ajna chakra* of his disciple with his index finger and made the upsurge of his *Shakti* for giving *Diksha* or initiation. But the guru and the disciple have to be of that caliber for such a miracle to happen There are only very few examples of this kind such as *Ramakrishna* and *Vivekananda, Muktabai* and *Visoba Khechar, Nivruttinath* and *Jnaneshvar, Visoba Khechar* and *Namdev. Nivruttinath* could have created many *Jnaneshvars* by touching the *ajna chakra* of his disciples with his index finger and *Jnaneshvar* would have produced many *yogis*. But this does not happen. We ordinary people should only hear this *yog* with pure minds. We should read about it and try to understand it. That is enough. We should not go for any higher expectations than this. At the most we can start the *sadhana* with

419

ashtanga yog. It may not be completed within twenty-five or thirty years. The *Jnaneshvari* says,

तो गीतेमागे षष्ठीचा । प्रसंगी असो आयणीचा ।
जैसा क्षीरार्णवी अमृताचा । निवाडु जाहला ।।

After many births a *sadhaka* can accomplish *yog* and the fulfilment.

We should remember this and continue the necessary *sadhana*. We must not aspire for the *kundalini yog* and be content with knowing about it. It is not everybody's cup of tea. Knowledge of it should satisfy us.

Previously we had to search for *kundalini yog* in awful, dense, complicated, terse and mysterious treatises. It was like wandering in a vast forest. But the condition changed before seven hundred and fifty years.

Kundalini Yog in Jnaneshvari

Today we have *kundalini yog* in the beautiful book of *Jnaneshvari*. *Jnaneshvar* has motherly affection for his readers and he has related the subject with the same concern and affection in the sixth chapter. So the subject is transferred from the mysterious, vast forest to a pleasant orchard of the book. We have to turn to *Jnaneshvari* to know this *yog*. This sixth chapter is a discourse of this *yog*. *Jnaneshvara* himself says that the aspiring *sadhakas* should try to understand this *yog* first. In the tenth verse he tells us that it is adventurous to go for this *yog*.

आता योग चळाचा निमथा । जरी टाकावा अभि पार्थी ।

420

तरी सोपाना या कर्मपथा । चुका झणी ।।
येण यमनियमाचे तळवटे । रिंगे आसनाचिये पाऊलवाटे ।
येई प्राण्यामाचेनि आडकंठे वरौता गा ।।
मग प्रत्याहाराचा आघाडा । जो बुद्धिचिया ही पाया निसरडा ।
जेथ हठिये सांगती होडा । कळेल ग ।।

"In the churning process of the sea of milk ambrosia came up. In the same way the sixth chapter gives us the excellent knowledge and advice. We should not try to interfere in it or to have the audacity to start *sadhana* of it. He instructs that our *sadhana* should begin with *ashtanga yog* only. *Kundalini yog* is the peak of the mountain of *hatha yog* and we should only have a look at it. We must follow *ashtanga yog* according to the proper order of the steps of it. Even we must not audaciously skip the steps. We must take the way of *karma* with appropriate steps of *achar*/conduct, thoughts, food, study of the *vidyas* and company of saints. He says that we should not venture to climb the top by skipping the stairs. He says in the verse 186,

मग तेथ आपण । एकाग्र अंतःकरण ।
करूनी सद्गुरु स्मरण । अनुभविजे ।।

Jnaneshwar tells the sadhaka to concentrate on the thoughts of Guru.

The *sadhaka* should not skip the path of *karma*. On this way he first meets the bottom of *yama* and *niyama*. Then there is the small path of *asanas*. Then there is the ridge of *pranayama* on the mount of *yog*. *Pratyahara* is a half cut ridge of which it is dangerous. Even intellectuals can slip from this and reel down. Even *hatha yogis* had

421

to give up their vows here and they did give them up.

O *Arjuna*, only renunciation can prove to be prevention from slipping down. The *sadhaka* can proceed safely only if he is equipped with strict renunciation. He goes on riding the horse of *Pranapana* on the spacious road of *dharana* towards reaching the peak of *dhyana*. This is described nicely in the verse 54-58. *Kundalini yog* is accomplished through *ashtanga yog*, *mantra*, *laya*, *hath* and *rajayog*. It is achieved through sitting *asanas* that are useful for and conducive to *dhyana*. Remember that it is related to *dhyana*. *Jnaneshvar* says that the *sadhaka* sits in the *asana* and begins with thinking of his master. Of course, the *yogi* of *kundalini* has to be an accomplished *yogi* who has achieved *samadhi*. He is not a mere *sadhaka*, and never a *sadhaka* like us. He has already climbed the steps of *ashtanga yog*, *mantra*, *laya*, *hatha* and *raja yog*. Such an accomplished *yogi* with *siddhi* of *samadhi* starts *dhyana* after praying to his master. What should he do after taking *asana*? The blessings of the *Guru* are extremely important.

He experiences bliss when he remembers his *guru*. What happens when the greatest disciple like *Jnaneshvar* remembers the great *guru Nivruttinath*?

जेथ स्मरतेनि आदरे । सबाह्य सात्त्विके भरे ।
जंव काठिण्य विरे । अहंभावाचे ।

What could be the pride of such a saint as *Jnaneshvar*? But when a blessed disciple thinks of his *guru* all the eight divine tendencies upsurge and pride vanishes. Of course, it is not our pride. If a mountain falls on our pride, it will shatter but our pride will remain intact. The next lines contain touching poetry. They say that all the desires dissolve when pride vanishes. The longing for pleasures of senses is removed. This longing is not like that of ordinary people. It belongs to the level of a disciple like *Jnaneshvar*. But when the mind becomes calm and quiet, the turmoil of doubts is over. The *yogi's* body takes care of itself. The fluctuations of the mind are quiet.? *Pranapana* are stable. *Samadhi* stage is not far away now.

आगळे अभ्यासू सरे । बैसत ठेवो ।

So as soon as the *yogi* sits in the *asana* posture his efforts to calm the mind and his *sadhana* are fulfilled. The description in the verse 191 shows that the *yogi* becomes calm & stable just by sitting in the *asana*. We ordinary people struggle and flounder in the *asana* for hours and hours but *yog* is far away from us. Our mind is just tossing and turning restlessly. But the power of the *kundalini yogi* is immense.

What is his *asana*? *Jnaneshvar* describes it fully. It looks like a physical *asana* but is not merely physical. What type is the *asana*? It is only one. One foot is kept on the other in such a way that both the soles stay fixed under the *muladhara chakra*. The right heel is pressed between the space of genital organ and anus. So the left foot is fixed properly on the right foot. There is four finger distance between anus and penis. It should be placed exactly in the centre of the space mentioned above i. e. four finger space. With the pressure on the heel the spine should be ascended. *Jnaneshvar* calls this *mulbandhasiddhavajrasana*. When this *aasana* is fixed on the *muladhara chakra* the downward road is closed. The *yogi* goes up from inside.

The verse from 193 to two hundred have this description. The palms should be placed one over the other with the left at the bottom, right at the top and the palms should be curled to the shape of a *drona*, a vessel. So the two shoulders are broadened and the head is firmly set between them. The closed upper eyelids come down and those down go further downwards. The eyesight is slit opened. The inward sight is inside and if it comes out it turns only to the tip of the nose. When the eyesight turns inward, the mind is without any desires and fluctuations. The cylindrical throat pipe is narrowed. The chin is put into the notch and it makes *jalandhara bandha*. The *jaalandhara bandha* of *kundalini yogi* does not take place just by putting the chin in the notch but it is a *pranic*, inward action. The navel supports it. The abdomen goes inside. The heart is exhilarated like a lotus.

O *Arjuna*, at that time the *bandha* that occurs on the *svaadhishthaana chakra* down the navel is *uddiyana bandha*. Verses 201 to 210 give this description. *Jnaneshvar* says that when the three *bandhas* as *mula*, *uddiyana* and *jalandhara bandha* take place in the *kundalini yogi*, they seem to be physical but it removes the fluctuating nature of the mind. Such a *yogi* is sleepless. This does not mean that he has insomnia but his sleep is over. His hunger also is over. His *apana* comes up and forcefully rushes to the *manipuraka chakra*. Then the hollow of the abdomen is churned and all the dirt accumulated from the childhood is thrown out. This *vayu* has no way to turn inward and so enters the excretory channels. It finishes the cough and bile. It crosses the sea of seven *dhatus*. It shatters the hills of fat. It brings out the bone marrow.

Remember, this can happen only in case of a *yogi*. Do not try to imagine what will happen if we were to face this. This turmoil of *manipuraka* disentangles the *nadis* and relaxes the limbs. *Jnaneshvar* says that this scares even the *yogi* but he should not give up his courage and sincerity. Sometimes this gives rise to some ailments or even removes them.

Here we have to explain an important point. The treatment suggested in *hatha yog* is for this *yogi*, and never for us. The six *kriyaas* of *neti*, *dhauti* and so on are remedies of ailments but that too for the *yogi* and not for the ordinary people. This should never be forgotten. The turbulence and the heat of *vajrasana* awakens dormant *kundalini* and quickly rushes to the navel. Like a hungry snake, it eats up the *vayu* under the heart. It also eats the flesh near the heart and around. *Jnaneshvar* says that it finishes up all the fat and flesh in the body. The skin now sticks to the bones. It helps itself with bone marrow and life in the nerves. The growth of the hair is stunted. Of course, all this happens with a *yogi*. Its thirst dries the sea of seven *dhatus* in one sip. It creates severe heat in the body. Verses from 210 to 235 describe all this.

Then in the embrace of *prana* and *apana* the six plexii remain just like skeletons, because it finishes the whole element of earth as bones, skin, hair and flesh. The water element in the form of urine, mucus, blood, sweat and semen also are exhausted. When these two elements are finished, it is full. How would the *yogi* look then as there are no elements of earth and water and not their signs? When *kundalini* is full, it becomes tender. It comes to *sushumna* and vomits the firy poisonous matter inside. Verses from 235 to 240 narrate this process. How does the *yogi* live then? The reply is that he lives on the ambrosia exuded from the mouth of *kundalini*. This gives life to his *prana*. Even if fire comes out in the form of poison it cools the body inwardly and outwardly. The *yogi's* feeble body becomes strong again. This new strength is extraordinary. The physiology here is metaphysical. The modern science or medical experts will not be able to imagine it. The natural tendencies of the body are not now valid for his body. His nerves stop flowing. This is a wonderful phenomenon. This *yogi* has to be a *hatha yogi* and in *samadhi* and not in action. His *ida* and *pingala* become one and their knots are disentangled. The three *bandhas* are over. The next description is mystical and engaging.

Jnaneshvar presents a poetic description then. He says that there is a lake of ambrosia of the moon in the head. This is reality. This is reality of the esoteric physiology. This lake gets a jog and tilts. The ambrosia falls in the mouth of *kundalini*. It is full to the brim and then it spreads in the whole body. So, even the *pranavayu* is soaked at its place. The elements of earth and water no longer stay in his body. In a way he is without his body. He gets new nails and new teeth. This is described in the verse 263. In 260, *Jnaneshvar* relates that the *yogi* gets childhood. Today we hear of the concept of Time Machine. This machine can take a person in the past. Similarly the *yogi* goes in the past. *Jnaneshvar* has described this act of going in the past seven hundred and fifty years ago. The *yogi's* palms become red like a red lotus. The body gets golden complexion. The verse 268 tells us that the *yogi's* body becomes light like the air. Then *kundalini* comes to the *chakra* at the heart. The turmoil of *manipuraka* is over. Now starts *ajapajapa*. The *anahata* sound resounds incessantly. It is the sound of *Soham*. He tells in 278 that this *anahata* sound continues until *pranapana* are there. In the 300th verse he says that

तेवेळी कुंडलिनी हे भाष जाये । मग मारुती ऐसे नाव होये ।

Kundalini becomes *Maruti* when *Soham* begins. Then it crosses *Jalandara*. It goes beyond *vishuddhi chakra* and enters *ajna chakra* which has *Omkar* form. Then it goes to the area of head, keeps the foot on the *Omkar* and crosses speech of *pashyanti* to enter *para* speech. The half *matraa* of mind in *Omkar* is left behind. It reaches

426

the head as a river meets the sea. So *kundalini* starts from *muladhara*, becomes *Maruti* at *anahata*, crosses *Omkar* of *ajna chakra* and is stable in the *brahma randhra* of *sahasrara* in the head to repose in the embrace of the emotion of *Soham*. So the curtain of the five elements goes away. *Shiva* and *Shakti* are united. The *atma* is united with *Paramatma*. This is *kundalini yog*. This is *siddha yog*. This is a brief and moving description of the union in the cerebral space.

Why is this *yogi* a *siddha yogi*? The reason is that he has accomplished *raja*, *hatha*, *laya*, *mantra* and *ashtanga yog* before turning to this *yog*. After achieving the *samadhis* of these *yogs* he has achieved this supreme *samadhi*. So this *yog* is for the *Jnaneshvar* of *Jnaneshvaras*. An ordinary man should not try to think of achieving this *yog*. He should begin with *sham-dama sadhana* and *ashtanga yog sadhana* first.

According to *Patanjali*, a *yogi* can go to the supreme achievement through *ashtanga yog sadhana*. This journey is different from that of *kundalini yog*. *Ashtanga yog* turns into *kriya yog*. From that arise *samprajnata yog*, *asamprajnata yog*, *Dharma megha*, continuous shower of *viveka khyati*, *klesha karma nivrutti*, then the cessation of *guna vyapara* of *prakriti* out of this *nivrutti*, then *pratiprasava* and ultimately *Kaivalya*. Then there is the climax of the spiritual life which is supreme in the hierarchy of spiritual achievements. But this entire journey takes place with the support of *Omkar*. The climax of *samadhis* of all categories is achieved through *Omkar* which is at par with the Almighty. The foundational *mantra* of all the *samadhis* is *Omkar*. The highest accomplishment is achieved through this *mantra* only.

There are similarities and differences between *Patanjali* and *kundalini yog*. In a way they are different and even they are not different also. Scholars have shown the differences at many places. Both of them end in *Kaivalya*. As both of them offer supreme accomplishment on the spiritual path, they are similar from that point of view. We have considered *kundalini yog* as it is explained in the *Jnaneshvari*. We have understood the fact that there is *ashtanga yog* at its foundation. So this discussion of *kundalini* is concluded here.

Shri Krishnaarpanam astu

✠ ✠ ✠

Discourse - 33

Nada Yog - 1

Now we are going to think of *nada yog*. There are many kinds of *yog* such as *mantra yog*, *laya yog*, *hatha yog*. Another *yog* emerges in this process. It is *nada yog*. We remember here one *shloka* from the *Smritis*. "समस्वराश्च गाथाश्च सर्वा: नाद समुद्भवा:" *Nada* pervades the whole universe. If we close our ears, we hear the noise, chaos and turmoil. The heartbeats are going on. The *Upanishads* say that the *vaishvanara* fire inside us is making some irritating noise of hunger. There is chaos in the hollow of the stomach. The nerves are sending messages from the brain to the organs and from the organs to the brain with a speed of more than two hundred miles. The Upanishads say that there is a trafficking of tremendous speed in our vessels. Our body contains noise of a market place or of a road in a metropolitan city which is full of vehicles. The metropolis of our body bears the enormous traffic of the network of nerves as long as six thousand miles and that of vessels that are as long as sixty thousand miles. Imagine fifty little children put in a room, what will be the chaos inside? One is asking for food, another crying for water, still another shouting for something else. The innumerable cells in our body are making a similar chaos or turmoil inside.

But suppose, a *yogi* or *muni* closes his ears; what will he hear? He will listen to the inward music which is *Omkar*, which is the recitation of the name of his deity. He has an altogether different experience. In this ocean of false *maya* and chaotic world, he hears the sound of bells. *Varaha Upanishad* says that the devotee hears the name of his deity in his heart. *Kabir* or *Hanuman* hears the name of *Shri Rama*. Some *yogi* will hear *Omkar* or *Soham*. This is *nada yog*.

Nada yog is a branch of *laya yog* and we can get the knowledge about it in the books about *laya yog*. Rather we find the *samadhi* of a *laya yogi* or *mahalaya* in *nada yog*. The process of concentration on *nada* in *nada yog* is found in *laya yog* itself. *Laya yog* is discovered in *nada yog*. *Nada yog* is discovered in *laya yog*. This is a queer relationship between them. Concentration on *nada* is of vital importance in the science of *yog*. It is the centre of *yog*. This is true of any kind of *yog*. So *nada yog* is extremely important in *yog sadhana*. The dissolution of mind in *laya yog* is achieved in *nada* only. That *nada* is *omkar* or *soham*. So also the *Bija mantras* of the plexii give *laya* because they have *nada*, they are in the form of *nada* only.

The science of *yog* and *mantra yog* tell us that *mantra* makes the mind dissolve. The mind dissolves in the *mantra* as salt dissolves in water. *Nada yog* can be called the accomplishment of *mantra yog* or completion of *laya yog*. The *mantra* in *mantra yog* is always given by the *guru*. This is called *sampradaya mantra*, *mantra* of the particular sect. The pupil gets it if he is accepted by the *guru* as his regular disciple. This is extremely sacred and it has to be kept secret. It is not to be disclosed in any condition. When the *yogi* reaches *dhyana* through *mantra*, all his organs, mind, body resound with the vibrations of the *mantra*. They are dissolved. *Shri Hanuman* was the true devotee of *Shri Rama*. His heart beats were not like ours. If a stethoscope is used, one could hear the recitation of the name of *Rama* there. His heart beat with the name of *Rama*. We can see the final stage of *nada yog* here. We know sonography, ultrasound in the modern medical science. What would be the infrasound of *Prahlada*, the great devotee of *Vishnu*? It would have been the *mantra* of *Om Namo Bhagavate Vasudevaya*. *Swami Ramdas* recited the name of *Rama* for thirteen crore times. So his body was vibrating with the name of *Rama* only. The great saint *Tukaram* had the vibrations of the *mantra Rama Krishna Hari* all the while in every cell of his body. The effect of *naada* is of this kind, of this extent.

So-ham

In the *yog* tradition of the spiritual sciences *ajapajapa* is a *mantra*. It is *soham*. It is also called *hamsa mantra* or *hamsa sadhana*. This is the infrasound of the heart. This is not cardiac heart but mystic heart. In this mystic heart the *mantra* of *Soham* is resounding ceaselessly. Only in *kumbhaka* the '*So*' vanishes, '*ham*' goes and the *Omkar* remains. This is explained in the science of *nada yog*. This is the seminal *mantra* of *nada yog*. The sound of inhalation is ssss and that of exhalation is *ham*; so the sound of inhalation and exhalation together make the effect of *Soham*. Our spiritual sciences explain the theory of *Soham* in this way.

There is an interval of a split second between inhalation and exhalation. Exhalation, subtle interval and inhalation is the process of our breathing. The mysticism of *yogshastra* tells us that *Soham* is created out of this process. *Omkar* remains in *kevala kumbhaka*. *Yogashastra* explains the relation of it with *prana*. *Nada yog* is accomplished by *mantra* and there are many well known *mantras* in our spiritual *yog sadhana*. Some of them are ॐ नम: शिवाय, ॐ नमो नारायणाय, ॐ नमो भगवते वासुदेवाय। They are basic ingredients of *nada yog*. The *mantra* may be *vedic* or of a deity, it has *Omkar* before it. Every *mantra* has its hypostatization in *Omkar*. It has a metaphysical meaning. The whole universe may have smell, form, taste, touch but basically it has *Omkar*. It is created out of the sound of *Omkar* and this world with matter and life is going to end in the sound of *Omkar* only. *Nada* is there in the beginning, middle and end of this universe. The variety in the phenomena of this world is

431

unfathomable but it has its origin in *Omkar* and it is homogeneous from this point of view. This homogeneity is there in all the expressions, stages and phases of this universe. This *nada* is there in the *naadis* of the body. It is very significant in the context of *yog sadhana*. So the *nadis* should be sensitive and resonant for these inward vibrations. The cords of an instrument lose their resonance and vibration if it is out of use. Similarly the *naadis* do not remain sensitive for the nada if they are not pure. *Naada* is pulsating in the whole body through the *nadis*. They must be pure in order to be resonant to this *nada*. So purification of *nadis* is important in *yog sadhana*.

So also *pranayama* with *mantra* is important because it makes the *nadis* resonant to *nada*. The science of *yog* tells us that the three matras of *Omkar* are *a*, *u* and *m* and they are for *puraka*, *rechaka* and *kumbhaka*. The *Omkar mantra sadhana* is fundamental for *nada yog*. It creates resonance in *nadis*, nerves and cells. Like some sound ringing in a palace, the *akara*, *ukara* and *makara* should ring in the *nadis*, nerves and cells. They have to be sensitive enough for that. *Darshan Upanishad* gives some information about *samantraka nadishodhana pranayama* which is useful in this respect. It says, inhale through *ida* - left nostril. Do *kumbhaka*. At the same time take *apana* upwards. Do this with *akara*. It has sixteen *matras*. After the *puraka* of sixteen *matras kumbhaka* of *ukara* has sixty-four *matras*. Then there is *rechaka* of *makar* which has thirty-two *matras*. This is *nadishodhan pranayama* of *ida* and *pingala nadis*. Each of these *matras* must be accompanied with the pronunciation of *Omkar*. The *Upanishad* suggests that it should be pronounced on mental level and not with *vaikhari*. *Vaikhari* is described as the fourth kind of speech in the Indian tradition of mysticism. *Matras* are given for *rechaka, puraka* and then *kumbhaka* of *pingala*; and then for *rechaka*, *puraka* and *kumbhaka* of *ida*. *Matras* of *Omkar* also are divided in that. In this way *nadishaodhana paranayama* goes on the respective and particular *nada*. This is very important in *nada yog*.

The third chapter of *Yog Shikha Upanishad* has a statement-*Nasti.* नास्ति नादात्परो मंत्र: । No *mantra* is greater than *nada*. There is one more *kandika/shloka* in it. *Aksharam----*. This is called *Shabdabrahma* in the *Vedanta*. This *nada* is at *muladhara*. *Nada* is the strength of *muladhara*. *Muladhar* is the place of creation, *brahma* and power. *Nada* itself always gives voice to *mantra*. That is why it is said in the beginning

नादरूपो स्मृतो ब्रह्मा नादरूपो जनार्दन: ।
नादरूपा पराशक्ति: तस्मात् नादात्मकं जगत् ।।

Nada yog describes four kinds of speech--*Para, Pashyanti, Madhyama* and *Vaikhari*. Speech comes out through these four levels. The third chapter of *Yogshikha Upanishad* describes these four kinds of speech. The student of *yog* should see it for himself. This is the description of *Shabdabrahma*. *Muladhara* is the origin of *Shakti*. It is also called *bindu*. *Bindu* is a technical word in the science of *yog*, which is named as *Aksharabrahma, Paramabrahma*. *Paramabrahma* is achieved from *bindu*. *Para* speech is *bindu*, *Pashyanti* is *anahata nada*, *madhyama* is the speech of the mind and *vaikhari* is the actual audible speech with our speech organs with the letters from a to z. It has audible sound. When we go to the origin of speech, we go to *bindu*. The journey from *bindu* to *vaikhari* is the journey through the four stages of speech. The eighth shloka says,---समस्वराश्च गाथाश्च सर्वा: नादसमुद्भवा: ।

Shri Krishnaarpanam astu

Discourse - 34

Nada Yog - 2

We were discussing the four kinds of speech, *Para, Pashyanti, Madhyama* and *Vaikhari*. *Para* is called *bindu* in the science of *yog*. Our ancient spiritual sciences describe the stages of *nada*. *Bindu* or *para* creates *pashyanti* which is silent or voiceless voice. This gives rise to mental speech or *madhyama*, then follows *vaikhari* which is the audible speech of letters from *a* to *ksha / jna* According to our metaphysics these are the stages of speech. This journey from *bindu* to *vaikhari* is described in the following line- ''समस्वराश्च गाथाश्च सर्वा: नादसमुद्भवा:'' The *Yog Shikha Upanishad* has depicted this journey of sound or *Shabdabrahma* upto the seven notes in Indian music. *Soham* or *ajapajapa* in this *Nada yog* is very important. It is also called *Hamsa Vidya*. *Hamsa Upanishad* relates *naada yog*, *hamsa vidya* and *Soham sadhana*. It tells that the *sadhana* of *hamsa vidya* blesses the *yogi* with nine kinds of *nada*. He experiences these nine *nadas* that are *Chinha, Chinha Chinha, Ghanta nada, Shankha nada, Tri nada, Tala nada, Venu nada, Bheri nada* and *Mrudanga nada*. We often read and hear about this *Soham sadhana* and *hamsa sadhana*. One important point to be noted here is the *yogi* experiences *nada* and they are nine.

Hatha Yog Pradipika tells that the confluence of *prana* and *apana* takes the form of *nada* and *bindu*. A *hatha yogi* experiences this. *Maitrayani Upanishad* also gives some explanation of *nada yog*. The 22nd shloka of the 5th Chapter of this *Upanishad* says that when the *nada yogi* closes his ears, what sound does he hear? We have seen in the beginning of this chapter of *nada yog* that we hear noise if we close our ears. Our body is a chemical complex. It has many kinds of sounds and loud noise. But when the *nada yogi* with his tranquil mind closes his ears, he has an altogether different experience. He hears *Omkar* or *hamsa mantra*. One more source is available for the curious persons. It is the *Nada Bindu Upanishad* about *nada*. The three *matras* of *Omkar* are explained here with a beautiful metaphor. It is *vairaja pranava*. *Vairaja* is the god of birds. How is the god of birds? *'A'kara*, the first *matra* of *Omkar*, is his right wing. *'U'kara* is the left wing. *'Ma'kara* is his tail and the half *matra* is his head. The three *gunas* of *sattva*, *raja* and *tama* are his feet. His body is Truth, right eye is *Dharma* and left eye is opposite of *Dharma*. His body represents the seven *lokas* or worlds. His feet have the *Bhu*, knees have *Bhuvah*, waist has *Suvah*, back has *Svah*, his naval has *Maha*, heart has *Jana*, throat has *Tapa* and *Satya loka* rests between his eye brows. Thus is the *vairaja pranava* as depicted in the *Nada Bindu Upanishad*. The *'a'kara* of *pranava* is related to the element of fire, *'U'kara* is the element of air and *'Ma'kara* is refulgent crescent of the sun called '*Bijatya*' and the half *matra* is *Varuna* and *Turiya*. This *Upanishad* describes twelve kinds or forms of *Omkar*.

These twelve forms are as follows. *Goshini*, *Vidyut*, *Patangini*, *Vayuvegini*, *Namadheya*, *Aindree*, *Vaishnavi*, *Shankari*, *Mahati*, *Dhruti*, *Nari* and *Brahmi*. Of course, only a *nada yogi* can understand these concepts. We can only see the names. His experience of *Omkar* is different; his experience of life is far different because he belongs to a higher level of life. For us *Omkar* is only one, whereas he perceives twelve forms of *Omkar*. The science of *yog* explains this. The 41st *shloka* says that the mind becomes one with *nada*. This is the nature of mind. As salt or sugar dissolves in water, so does mind dissolve in *nada*. We can experience this with respect to music on our mundane level, too. We have to note one important point that if the mind or *chitta* has to dissolve, it can dissolve in *nada*. The control of mind and its fluctuations are related with *nada*. We must not forget this significant point in *yog shastra*. We take control of mind as silence and peace, a soundless condition. But *chitta* dissolves in *nada* and the control of mind is *nada*. The 41st *shloka* says "नादमेवानुसंदधानादे चित्तम् विलीयते" This is a very meaningful and pertinent statement for the *yogi*.

It is important to consult *Brahmavidya Upanishad* also in this context because it refers to *nada vidya* which is nothing but *hamsa vidya*. It gives the meaning of *hamsa* as 'Prana Apana Samanata' from which *nada* and *hamsa* emerge. This *Upanishad* describes *rechaka*, *puraka* and *kumbhaka pranayama* in the way that has *nada* and *hamsa*; so it brings 'Prana Apana Samanata.' This *samanata* or equality cannot be brought by counts or measurements. This can be achieved by *rechaka*, *puraka* and *kumbhaka pranayama*. In the efforts or *sadhana* of *naada* devotion for *guru* is very important. The 30th *shloka* of *Brahmavidya Upanishad* mentions that without devotion *samanata* is impossible to achieve. This is not a matter of calculation and you cannot bring *samanata* by taking, say, 50 gram *apana* and 50 gram *prana*. This is ridiculous. The student of *yog* must remember that for devotion to *guru*, the mindset of this devotion is indispensable. Only that can bring this *samanata*.

The second chapter of *Yog Shikha Upanishad* presents two very significant *shlokas*. Listen to these *shlokas* 20 and 21 carefully.

न अस्ति नादात् परो मन्त्रो न देव: स्वात्मन: पर: ।

नानुसंधे: परा पूजा न हि तृप्ते: परं सुखम् ।।

गोपनीयम् प्रयत्नेन सर्वधा सिद्धिम् इच्छता

Nada is the greatest spell and it is God only. It is the most blessed mode of worship. There is no greater happiness than you receive in this. Your concentration on *nada* gives you the proper mindset of worship. That is the worship of a *sadhaka* with *sattva guna*. *Nada* can give the greatest bliss. This *nada* and *mantra* can give *siddhi* and it should be kept secret. This is an instruction in this *Upanishad*.

Sadhana of Nada Yog

Now let us think about the *sadhana* of *naada yog*. Purification of *nadis* is the pivotal and the most important requisite for the *sadhana* of *nada yog*. Without purification of *naadis* neither they nor the mind or *chitta* can become sensitive and susceptible for *nada*. Purification of *nadis* is fundamental and seminal in the *sadhana* of *nada yog*. There is *nadi shodhana pranayama* in *yogshastra*. There are mantras for *nadi shodhana*. As some *mantras* can put a cobra under spell and make him sway, so can they get the *nadis* under spell. *Mantras* are not only for the ears or for *siddhis* but they can purify the *nadis*. Therefore, *samantraka nadi shodhana pranayama* is very important. It brings resonance in the *nadis* along with making them sensitive. Again *dhyana* of *pranava* is vital for *nada yog* and mainly in *nadi shodhana pranayama*. If the *sadhaka* can concentrate on *nada* he is exempted from many conditions. But otherwise the *sadhaka* has to do purification of *nadis, nadi shodhana pranayama, pranayama* with *pranava* and other things that are needed in *hatha yog*. The *sadhaka* has to be accomplished in so many things for *mantra yog, laya yog, dhyana yog, kundalini* or *raja yog* and this penance is very rigorous and rigid. But remember that a sincere devotee is not required to go into the hardships. If his heart is overflowing with true devotion, it makes up for everything else. He does not have to go for the process of *nadi shodhana* or *chakra bhedana* or *pancha prana* management. The *sadhaka* has to do management of three *gunas*, three *nadis* of *ida*, *pingla* and *sushumna*, five elements, three glands, three *doshas* and so on for any kind of *yog*. But the true devotee can bypass all these steps with the great strength of his devotion. His *sadhana* of *nama* or recitation of God's name accomplishes everything for him. *Nama sadhana* makes his efforts complete. The importance of *nama sadhana* is described in all the mythologies and it is lauded in the *Kali Yuga* especially. *Nama sadhana* consists of all the subtleties of *nada sadhana*. Devotion is everything here. So *bhakti yogis* say that if *nada yogis* incorporate devotion or *bhakti* or *nama sadhana* in their *yog* much of the hardship can be spared.

The hardships are well known. The *sadhaka* has to follow *ashtanga yog*, the rigorous *sadhana*, *mantra yog* of sixteen parts, *laya yog* of nine parts, *hatha yog* of six parts, various *kriyas* and *mudras* and he has to go through all the similar acid tests. These *sadhanas* need many and many births. Devotion can be equal to all these efforts. In a mythological story, Lord *Krishna* was being weighed and they were putting enormous wealth at the other end of the scale. No amount of wealth could be equal to Lord *Krishna*. When *Rukmini* put a leaf of *tulasi* with devotion at that end, it became equal to Lord *Krishna*. So devotion has immeasurable value. We can see that music enhances the emotion of devotion or rather both enhance each other. So *nada* is important in *bhakti yog*. *Nada* or music keeps *bhakti* away from any kind of dryness or coldness. This should also remove one general misunderstanding of the people. They think that *yog sadhana* is dry and sapless. *Nada yog* can show that there is music in it, there are emotions in it. It has *laya*. Consider all the meanings of *laya* in Sanskrit. *Laya* means rhythm, *laya* means being one with the other and *laya* means surrender. We can see how *nada yog* has the aspects of music and also of *nama yog*. *Nama* has *nada* in it and both of them have the power to bring *laya* or *vilaya* in the *chitta*. The name of the beloved or lover can bring a kind of *laya* to the *chitta*. Naturally the name of God with great devotion of the *bhakta* can easily bring *laya* in the *chitta*. *Nada yog* and *nama yog* are very close to each other.

All this is easy for understanding for those who know the power of music. They know the experience of *nada* and they are aware how it leads to a stage almost similar to *samadhi*. They can understand the concept of *nada brahma*, the truth of it and hence *nada yog*. Ancient Indians believed that, though music is heard but unseen, it can bring changes in the seen and unseen world. The flute of Lord *Krishna* had a tremendous effect not only on the people but also on the animals. Hundreds of folktales can tell us about this belief. *Sur* in Marathi has two meanings-musical notes, and gods. Certainly musical notes are like gods and the notes in *Omkar* are divine. The *ragas* in Indian music are related to emotions. Every *raga* has the expression of some particular emotion through the notes. Great musical maestros are capable of creating a heavenly atmosphere and giving even an experience of a kind of *samadhi* to the listeners. This is the power of music. So we commonly use the word *nada samadhi*. The root of this *nada samadhi* and its science is in *nada yog*. One cannot go to heaven without great deeds of merit but the ladder of the seven musical notes can lead one to heavenly bliss. *Nada yog* is behind all this music. And the origin of *nada*, *nada yog*, tunes, words, utterances is *Omkar*.

Vyasa says in *Brihan Narada Purana*,

ॐ ऽऽऽऽ

हरेर्नाम, हरेर्नाम, हरेर्नाम हि केवलम्,
कलौ नास्ति एव, नास्ति एव, नास्ति एव
गति: अन्यथा ।

In the present age *nama* of *Hari* is the only way of great sadhana. Lord *Krishna* says in the *Gita*, यज्ञानां जपयज्ञ: अस्मि *Nama japa* is the greatest *yajna*. *Nama sadhana* and *japa sadhana* are like saviours for mankind for all times, especially in this present age which is called *Kali yug* or age of *Kali*. The Hindu tradition believes in the concept of four *yugas-Satya*, *Dvapara*, *Treta* and *Kali*. *Kali* is taken to be the present *yug* and as being the vicious and decadent *yug*. This *sadhana* can help man in all his afflictions. Not only *Vyasa* but also sages and saints of yore have told the importance of *nama sadhana*. Recitation of God's name is pivotal in spiritualism. The philosophy of every saint has a place for *Nama sadhana*. In the *anushasana parva* of the *Mahabharat, Yudhishthira* asks his grandfather, *Bhishma* about the solution of different problems and afflictions in human life. *Bhishma* advises *nama sadhana* like *Vishnu Sahasra Nama* at that time. Every *vaidic* longs for spiritual development and then he always remembers from *Vishnu Sahasra Nama* that he can progress only with the help of *nama sadhana*. Man can avoid all evils with the help of recitation of God's name. Recitation of God's name gives knowledge to *Brahmanas*, victory to *Kshatriyas*, wealth to *Vaishyas* and happiness to *Shudras*. People of the four *varnas* achieve their goals through this *sadhana*. Man receives fame, health and brightness through the recitation of God's name. As it is said,

अचलां श्रियं आप्नोति श्रेय: प्राप्नोति अनुत्तमम्

440

Indian tradition values *nama sadhana* very much but even all the religions have advised recitation of God's name for their followers.

Mythologies are filled with famous examples of persons who became happy with *nama sadhana*. *Ajamila* achieved salvation only by recitation of the name-*Narayana*. *Nama sadhana* is *japa sadhana*. They are almost synonymous. *Japa* is recitation but there is a science of it. What is *japa*? Is it just uttering a name or a word? Recitation of just any name cannot be *japa*. Lovers of mammon recite the word money; but it cannot be called *japa*. Then what is the meaning of *japa*? "जकारो जन्मविच्छेद: पकारो पापनाशक: तस्य जप इति जन्मपापविनाशक:" *Japa* has two letters-*ja* and *pa*. *Ja* stands for *janmavicchedaka* or removal of the cycle of births. *Pa* stands for *papanashaka* or reducing *papa* i.e. sins. So the words for the *japa* must be such as will bring reduction of births and sins. *Agni Purana* gives this definition of *japa*. *Jabala Darshana* and some other *Upanishads* also have discussed classification of *japas* and their significance.

The classification of *japa* is a vast subject for studying because *japa* is done with different purposes and in different ways. The ways are various because purposes are different. *Japa* is done for removing sins, for exonerating oneself, for worshipping a deity. So it is done for *Dharma*, for *karma* or for *upasana*. It is done for knowledge or for achieving merit. It is done for exoneration of some known or unknown sin. It is done for peace of mind or for health. There are *mantras* for recovering from ailments and so *japa* of those *mantras* is done.

There is a classification of the ways of doing *japa*. It is of two kinds-vocal and mental. Vocal *japa* is of two kinds-*uchchayee* and *upanshu*. *Uchchayee* is done loudly and *upanshu* is done without any sound. So the vocal *japa* is explicit and implicit. The mental *japa* has two kinds-contemplative and meditative. The classification suggests the methods of doing the japa but the science of *yog* says that these are not just the differences but grades. There is a hierarchy. The meditative one is the highest kind, then follow contemplative, *ujjayi* and then *upanshu*. *Kurma purana* says that silence or muteness is necessary for making the *japa* powerful. This may seem contradictory or paradoxical but this is muteness for religious or yogik purpose. The *sadhaka* should sit straight and still for *japa*. He should choose a holy place for *japa* and himself should be physically and mentally clean and pure. There are also rules about the sitting positions for *japa*. In a silent *japa* the *saadhaka* should not show his teeth.

Bhagavata purana has *Bhagavata Mahatmya* in its beginning. The 73rd *shloka* of its fifth chapter says that the *japa* should be supported by knowledge. The *sadhaka* should know what he is reciting and its meaning. His mind should be one with the deity. He should concentrate on it. *Vishnu purana* also offers an important piece of advice. This *purana* values emotions very much but the advice is very practical. It suggests that the *japa* should be without any pride. The *sadhaka* should not make a show of his religiosity or spiritual mindset or purity. The most remarkable part of the advice is that we should not give up or neglect our duties for it. We have duties towards our family, our society. They must not be sacrificed for the sake of *japa*. The critics of old culture should particularly note this practical and sane kind of advice given in the olden days.

There is a science and methodology of *japa*. So the *sadhakas* of *japa* should not forget that observance of *yama* and *niyama* are imperative in *japa sadhana* in the spiritual field. It cannot be neglected in *yog sadhana*. Otherwise the *japa* becomes futile and proves to be

442

hypocrisy. The science of *japa* is clear about it. Faithful observance of *yama*, *niyama* and the discipline make the *japa* successful and powerful, too. The discipline of *japa* consists of the thought of *asana*. *Mantra shastra* advises which *asana* is fit for which *japa*. *Asana* in Sanskrit means the position of sitting and also the seat used for sitting. Both of them are important. The kind of *japa* decides whether the *sadhaka* should sit in *veerasana* or *svastikasana* or some other *asana*. The kind of *japa* also decides whether the *sadhaka* should use the seat made of cotton or a particular type of grass or the skin of deer or tiger. The kind of *japa* depends on the deity for whom the *japa* is being done. This decides the direction the *sadhaka* should face. He may be required to face the east or north for the *japa* of particular deities. *Japa shastra* is related to *mantra shastra* and both of them have to be considered for *japa*. The directions in *mantra shastra* are important for the ways of doing *japa*. In short, *japa* should be done as a part of penance faor God and the *mantra* and techniques in *mantra shastra* are essential in it.

Nama sadhana

Nama sadhana does not need all these rituals and rules. What counts in it is the sincerity, devotion and longing of the *bhakta* for God. The devotion decides the rules. When sincerity is there, some rules are naturally followed. The *bhakta* naturally takes care of cleanliness and purity. *Nama yog* is not strict about the rules like *japa yog*. Devotion is supreme in *nama yog*. A saint poet has described the importance of devotion in a *purana* which is very moving.

भावेन लभ्यते सर्वम् भावेन देवदर्शनम् ।
भावेन परमं ज्ञानम्, तस्मात् भावावलंबनम् ॥

443

भावात् परतरं न अस्ति, त्रैलोक्ये सिध्दं ।
भावो हि परमं ज्ञानं ब्रह्मज्ञानं अनुत्तमम् ।।
भावात् परतरं न अस्ति येन अनुग्रहो भवेत् ।
भावात् अनुग्रहप्राप्ति: अनुग्रहात् महान् सुखी ।।
भावेन लभ्यते सर्वं भावाधीनं इदं जगत् ।
भावं विना महाकाल: न सिद्धि: जायते क्वचित् ।।
भावात् परतरं नास्ति भावाधीनं इदं जगत् ।
भावेन लभ्यते योग: तस्मात् भावं समाश्रयेत् ।।

He says that devotion can do and give anything for the devotee.
It can give knowledge, happiness and blessings of God. It can give
siddhi. The world subsists only because devotion is there. Devotion
is necessary even for *yog*. *Patanjali* has said in an aphorism,
'तत् जप: तदर्थभावनम् ।' that japa should be done with the
understanding of it. So devotion is important and it is more important
in *nama yog*. It is the heart and core of it. *Japa* will be mechanical
without it. *Yama, niyama, titiksha, uparati*, etc. are desirable in *nama
yog*, so also *pranayama* and other elements of *ashtanga yog*. But
they are taken care of by devotion. As water does cleaning, fire or
wind does cleaning, so God's name, nam does cleaning of the heart.
Nama of God has all kinds of powers. It is called the holiest and the
most auspicious in the *Gita* and in *Vishnu Divya Sahasranama*. Just
remembering and reciting the *nama* of *Narayana* can bring purity in
the heart.

This purity is required for all kinds of worship and penance and
sadhana, whether it is *japa sadhana* or *mantra sadhana* or *yog
sadhana*. It is needed for any kind of *yajna*. *Nama* creates and gives
this purity. *Nama* alone cannot do this but the devotion which is behind
nama brings this about. Just uttering the name of God cannot do

this. Saint *Kabir* has nicely laughed at the recitation which is devoid of devotion. He says that the person is telling the beads and his mind is wandering in all the ten directions. Such *japa* is utterly useless. On the other hand, if *nama* is recited with devotion, then the *sadhaka* may be in any condition, the same is redeemed. In the *Mahabharata, Draupadi* was brought in the court of the *Kauravas* in a helpless condition. She recited Lord *Krishna*'s name with devotion and the condition was redeemed; purity was created. She was helped by God. This is the greatness of *nama* and devotion.

Nama has a great power to change and transform life. Sage *Valmiki* is an historical example of this. He was *Valya* or *Ratnakara*, a dacoit looting travellers on the road. He even killed many people for money. When he met *Narada* he was advised by the blessed Muni. He did penance, became a sage and poet and then composed the great epic, the *Ramayana. Valya* became a sage and bard. This is the alchemy of *nama*. Many saints like *Surdas, Namdev, Kabir, Jnaneshvar, Ramdas, Mirabai* followed and advocated this *nama sadhana*. They made their lives meaningful and also redeemed the society around. *Japa* is the important medium of *nama sadhana*. We have seen that *japa* is done for various purposes and in different ways. The variety of purposes creates variety of methods and rituals. *Japa* is a part of penance, and there come different rules and discipline of *japa* in that respect. *Japa* becomes a part of the worship we offer to deities and gods. It is an integral part of idol worship and rituals of worship. It is an element of some *karma. Japa* is for retribution and exoneration, too. It is done out of remorse for known or unknown sins. So it is for removal of sins but it is done also for attaining merit. *Japa* helps discipline and control and also sublimation of mind. It can be *mantra sadhana, yog sadhana* and *tantra sadhana*.

It is a mental and emotional worship. It can be an exercise for the mind and for the speech. It is for mental peace and satisfaction. It is *dhyana* and *yog*. So *japa* is of several types. The *yog sadhaka* and *japa sadhaka* have to do all these kinds of *japa*. He is benefited by it. He has to do *japa* for all the purposes described above; for mental peace, penance, *mantra sadhana*, *yog sadhana* and *tantra sadhana*, retribution and exoneration, sublimation of mind, removal of known or unknown sins. This will tell us what all *japa* can do for us. *Japa* can help a common man, a *sadhaka* of *yog* and a *bhakta*. *Japa* has vast dimensions. It is a panacea. It gives purity, bliss, *siddhi*, merit, love and blessings of God, power and strength. It helps also on physical level. The example is *Omkar*. It has three *matras*, *a*, *u* and *m*. Long '*a*' gives exercise to stomach by compressing it. '*U*' compresses chest and '*m*' 'mind' compresses brain and gives them exercise. Words and *mantras*, rather the whole series of letters give exercise to the body by its utterance. *Mantras* are remedies for physical and mental afflictions. *Mantras* are a part of knowledge, part of worship, part of *dhyana* and *karma*, too. There is no *yog* without *japa*. *Japa* is there in *jnana yog*, *karma yog*, *hatha yog*, *raja yog*, *dhyana yog*, *laya yog*, *bhakti yog*, *kundalini yog*, *nada yog* and each and every kind of *yog*. In every *yog* it is there in its own way. So *japa* is for achievements in the world, in the spiritual field and in the other worldly pursuits. So Lord *Krishna* has said in the *Gita*, यज्ञानां जपयज्ञ: अस्मि I (10.25) *Japa* is a great type of *yajna*. This is not just a metaphor or hyperbole. It is reality. So *japa* must be studied as an independent subject. The gifts and benefits of japa have to be studied separately. With the *japa* of *Gayatri* a person can progress from physical and mental health to self-discipline, and to emotional and intellectual heights and he can become a great genius. History provides evidences of this. A genius like *Sayanacharya* reached the great height with this *mantra*. The range of *japa* goes from this world to the other world. So the subject is boundless.

So we have considered here all the kinds of *yog* that are mentioned in our tradition. *Jnana*, *karma*, *bhakti* and *dhyana* are the main types and we also discussed the kinds of these four *yogas*. They are *mantra yog, laya yog, hatha yog, dhyana yog, bhakti yog, kundalini yog, nada yog, japa* and so on. Thus we have thought about all the kinds of *yog* that come in the ken of *Yog Vidya*.

Shri Krishnaarpanam astu

Glossary

Matruka : Matruka are literal sound forms which compose the mantras. Therefore, they are constituting literal sound forms which have to be consecrated and worshipped before Mantra and Tantra Sadhana.

Vyahritis : Vyahritis are words that denote the worlds in the universe from the earth to those above. Bhuh is the earth, the terrestrial plane. The rest are celestial planes.

Adhidaivik : Aadhibhoutik, Adhidavik and Adhyatmik are theree planes of creation. Aadhibhoutik is elementally constituted, Adhidavik is celestially constituted and Adhyatmik is spritually constituted.

Adhiyajna : Adhiyajna is divinity which is imminent in every particle of matter and imminent in all metaphysical, spiritual principle. This concepts is exclusively found in the Gita.

Achamana : Achamana is a sip of water taken with consecration in religious and spiritual rituals.